METHODS IN MOLECULAR BIOLOGY™

Series Editor
John M. Walker
School of Life Sciences
University of Hertfordshire
Hatfield, Hertfordshire, AL10 9AB, UK

For other titles published in this series, go to
www.springer.com/series/7651

Immunotherapy of Cancer

Methods and Protocols

Edited by

Patricia Yotnda

Center for Cell and Gene Therapy, Baylor College of Medicine,
Houston, TX, USA

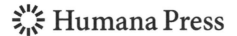 Humana Press

Editor
Patricia Yotnda
Center for Cell and Gene Therapy
Baylor College of Medicine
Baylor Plaza One
77030 Houston Texas
USA
pyotnda@bcm.tmc.edu

ISSN 1064-3745   e-ISSN 1940-6029
ISBN 978-1-60761-785-3   e-ISBN 978-1-60761-786-0
DOI 10.1007/978-1-60761-786-0
Springer New York Dordrecht Heidelberg London

Library of Congress Control Number: 2010931996

Humana Press is part of Springer Science+Business Media (www.springer.com)

Preface

Immunotherapy for the treatment of cancer has been a long-standing, continuously evolving strategy. The emergence of new therapeutic molecules, increased knowledge of gene regulation and protein interactions, and the development of novel technologies have maintained this therapeutic approach at the forefront of cancer treatment. The numerous results and observations obtained from clinical trials have allowed a greater understanding of the in vivo mechanisms and pathways involved in the anti-tumoral response; and therefore, have also provided for the improvement of cancer immunotherapy.

The idea of using immunotherapy to eradicate cancer emerged in the 19th century when Dr. William Coley discovered the effect of bacteria on tumor regression. A few years later, Drs. Richet and Héricourt injected patients with "antitumor-serum" generated in animals to provide them with antibodies directed against tumor associated proteins, a technique called passive immunotherapy. Early on, the BCG vaccine was also used to stimulate the immune system (active immunotherapy) and eradicate cancer. More recently, cancer immunotherapy has included the use of immune cells infused during bone marrow transplant (adoptive immunotherapy), antibodies, and cytokines. It has since been associated with a combination of various other approaches, e.g. cell and gene therapy. Stem cell-based therapies, tissue engineering, and targeting have also contributed to the latest successes in pre-clinical immunotherapy studies.

A large array of techniques is required for the implementation of these continuously developing immunotherapeutic approaches. It is therefore very important that scientists have access to the latest protocols of various techniques. This *Immunotherapy of Cancer* volume of the *Methods in Molecular Biology* book series describes detailed procedures for trainees and experts in the area of basic, clinical science who wish to undertake their own new immunotherapy studies. In addition to the protocols, general overviews provide useful updates in each area, as well as summaries of recent pre-clinical and clinical trials.

Patricia Yotnda

Contents

Contributors

DARYA ALIZADEH • *Division of Neurosurgery, City of Hope Medical Center, Duarte, CA*

BEHNAM BADIE • *Division of Neurosurgery, City of Hope Medical Center, Duarte, CA*

MICHAEL A. BARRY • *Mayo Clinic, Rochester, MN*

LINDA J. HOWLAND • *Cancer Immunology Program, Peter MacCallum Cancer Centre, East Melbourne, Australia*

MALCOLM K. BRENNER • *Baylor College of Medicine, Methodist Hospital and Texas Children's Hospital, Houston, TX*

MICHAEL J. BRONIKOWSKI • *Jet Propulsion Laboratory, California Institute of Technology, Pasadena, CA*

DARIO CAMPANA • *Laboratory Research, Department of Oncology, St. Jude Children's Research Hospital, Memphis, TN, USA*

SUNIL CHADA • *Intrexon, Blacksburg, VA*

XOCHITL CORTEZ-GONZALEZ • *The Laboratory of Immunology, Department of Medicine and Moores Cancer Center, University of California, San Diego, La Jolla , CA*

PHILLIP K. DARCY • *Cancer Immunology Program, Peter MacCallum Cancer Centre, East Melbourne, Australia; Department of Pathology, University of Melbourne, Melbourne, Australia*

BIAGIO DE ANGELIS • *Center for Cell and Gene Therapy, Baylor College of Medicine, The Methodist Hospital and Texas Children's Hospital, Houston, TX*

ANTONIO DI STASI • *Center for Cell and Gene Therapy, Baylor College of Medicine, The Methodist Hospital and Texas Children's Hospital, Houston, TX*

GIANPIETRO DOTTI • *Departments of Medicine and Immunology, Baylor College of Medicine, The Methodist Hospital and Texas Children's Hospital, Houston, TX*

ARTHUR E. FRANKEL • *Cancer Research Institute, Scott and White Memorial Hospital, Temple, TX*

NICOLE M. HAYNES • *Cancer Immunology Program, Peter MacCallum Cancer Centre, East Melbourne, Australia*

DANIEL HIRSCHHORN-CYMERMAN • *Memorial Sloan-Kettering Cancer Center and Weill Medical College of Cornell University, New York, NY*

SEAN E. HOFHERR • *Mayo Clinic, Rochester, MN*

MICHAEL HUST • *Department of Biotechnology, Institute of Biochemistry and Biotechnology, Technische Universität Braunschweig, Braunschweig, Germany*

CONSTANTINE G. IOANNIDES • *Department of Experimental Therapeutics, The University of Texas of M.D. Anderson Cancer Center, Houston, TX*

BABAK KATEB • *Brain Mapping Foundation and International Brain Mapping & Intraoperative Surgical Planning Society (IBMISPS), West Hollywood, CA*

RAJIV KHANNA • *Tumour Immunology Laboratory, Division of Infectious Diseases and Immunology, Australian Centre for Vaccine Development, Queensland Institute of Medical Research, Brisbane, Australia*

EUN-MI KIM • *Department of Internal Medicine, Division of Immunology, Roy J. and Lucille A. Carver College of Medicine, University of Iowa, Iowa City, IA*

NATALIA LAPTEVA • *Baylor College of Medicine, Houston, TX*

DEAN A. LEE • *Division of Pediatrics, Cell Therapy Section, University of Texas M.D. Anderson Cancer Center, Houston, TX*

YU-JEN LEE • *Cancer Research Institute, Scott and White Memorial Hospital, Temple, TX*

HONGTAO LI • *Department of Molecular Medicine, Mayo Clinic, Rochester, MN*

HARISH M. MANOHARA • *Jet Propulsion Laboratory, California Institute of Technology, Pasadena, CA*

DAVID M. NEVILLE • *Angimmune, LLC, Bethesda, MD, USA*

FATMA V. OKUR • *Baylor College of Medicine, Methodist Hospital and Texas Children's Hospital, Houston, TX*

GUANGYONG PENG • *Division of Immunobiology and Department of Internal Medicine, Saint Louis University, Saint Louis, MO*

MIGUEL-ANGEL PERALES • *Memorial Sloan-Kettering Cancer Center and Weill Medical College of Cornell University, New York, NY*

CONCETTA QUINTARELLI • *Center for Cell and Gene Therapy, Baylor College of Medicine, The Methodist Hospital and Texas Children's Hospital, Houston, TX*

RAJAGOPAL RAMESH • *Department of Thoracic and Cardiovascular Surgery, The University of Texas of M.D. Anderson Cancer Center, Houston, TX*

JACK A. ROTH • *Department of Thoracic and Cardiovascular Surgery, The University of Texas of M.D. Anderson Cancer Center, Houston, TX*

BARBARA SAVOLDO • *Center for Cell and Gene Therapy, Department of Pediatrics, Baylor College of Medicine, The Methodist Hospital and Texas Children's Hospital, Houston, TX*

THOMAS SCHIRRMANN • *Department of Biotechnology, Institute of Biochemistry and Biotechnology, Technische Universität Braunschweig, Braunschweig, Germany*

COREY SMITH • *Tumour Immunology Laboratory, Division of Infectious Diseases and Immunology, Australian Centre for Vaccine Development, Queensland Institute of Medical Research, Brisbane, Australia*

ANNA MAY SWANSON • *Baylor College of Medicine, Methodist Hospital and Texas Children's Hospital, Houston, TX*

NANCY SMYTH TEMPLETON • *Gradalis Inc., 2545 Golden Bear Drive, Suite 110, Carrollton, TX, 75006*

MICHAEL R. VERNERIS • *Hematology/Oncology Section and Division of Blood and Marrow Transplant, University of Minnesota, Minneapolis, MN*

ERIC A. WEAVER • *Mayo Clinic, Rochester, MN*

JUNG HEE WOO • *Cancer Research Institute, Scott and White Memorial Hospital, Temple, TX*

DANLI WU • *Baylor College of Medicine, Methodist Hospital and Texas Children's Hospital, Houston, TX*

VICKY YAMAMOTO • *Keck School of Medicine, University of Southern California, Los Angeles, CA*

PATRICIA YOTNDA • *Baylor College of Medicine, Methodist Hospital and Texas Children's Hospital, Houston, TX*

MAURIZIO ZANETTI • *The Laboratory of Immunology, Department of Medicine and Moores Cancer Center, University of California, San Diego, La Jolla, CA*

NICHOLAS ZAVAZAVA • *Department of Internal Medicine, Division of Immunology, Roy J. and Lucille A. Carver College of Medicine, Veterans Affairs Medical Center, Immunology Graduate Program, University of Iowa, Iowa City, IA*
LEYING ZHANG • *Division of Neurosurgery, City of Hope Medical Center, Duarte, CA*
XIAOLIU ZHANG • *Biology and Biochemistry, University of Houston, Houston, TX, USA*

Chapter 1

Hypoxic Tumors and Their Effect on Immune Cells and Cancer Therapy

Patricia Yotnda, Danli Wu, and Anna May Swanson

Abstract

The abnormal decrease or the lack of oxygen supply to cells and tissues is called hypoxia. This condition is commonly seen in various diseases such as rheumatoid arthritis and atherosclerosis, also in solid cancers. Pre-clinical and clinical studies have shown that hypoxic cancers are extremely aggressive, resistant to standard therapies (chemotherapy and radiotherapy), and thus very difficult to eradicate. Hypoxia affects both the tumor and the immune cells via various pathways. This review summarizes the most common effects of hypoxia on immune cells that play a key role in the anti-tumor response, the limitation of current therapies, and the potential solutions that were developed for hypoxic malignancies.

Key words: Hypoxia, aggressive cancers, radio- and chemoresistance, metastasis, immuno-suppression.

1. Introduction

A large number of human solid tumors profoundly lack oxygen, exhibiting hypoxic and anoxic tumor areas; this condition called hypoxia is due to an imbalance between delivery of oxygen and nutrients via the blood circulation and consumption by cancer cells. To survive in this hostile environment, cancer cells upregulate key genes that are involved in the survival and proliferation pathways. Hypoxic cancers are generally aggressive and metastatic and thus correlated with a poor prognosis. Furthermore, these hypoxic tumors are of major concern because they are resistant to traditional radiotherapy, phototherapy, and chemotherapy, and also to conventional cancer immunotherapy. Thus it is important

P. Yotnda (ed.), *Immunotherapy of Cancer*, Methods in Molecular Biology 651,
DOI 10.1007/978-1-60761-786-0_1, © Springer Science+Business Media, LLC 2010

to expand our understanding of hypoxic tumors and their interaction with the immune response in order to adjust and propose alternative cancer immunotherapy strategies. In this review we have summarized important concepts that need to be taken into account to develop efficient cancer immunotherapies for these hypoxic tumors.

2. Hypoxic Tumors

Hypoxia is an abnormal decrease of oxygen levels in tissue. In healthy tissues, the level of oxygen varies depending on the organ but is well adapted to the needs of the corresponding cells. In pathological tissues, however, the oxygen tension is low compared to the corresponding healthy tissue, and this decrease can lead to anoxia, a total deprivation of oxygen. Compelling evidence has been presented demonstrating reduced tissue oxygenation in both malignant and non-malignant conditions like chronic inflammation (chronic inflammatory bowel disease, ischemia/reperfusion injury, and rheumatoid arthritis), heart disease, stroke, diabetic retinopathy, cystic fibrosis, chronic bronchitis, psoriasis, vascular diseases, wounds, infections, and kidney disease.

In solid tumors, the incidence of hypoxia is high and has long been correlated with aggressive and metastatic tumor phenotypes. An increasing list of cancers with hypoxic regions has been reported over the last decade and includes endometrial carcinoma, ovarian, melanoma, lymphoma, breast, bladder, brain, head and neck, renal, colon, gastric, pancreatic, prostate, and non-small cell lung cancers (1–10). These hypoxic tumors are resistant to conventional radiotherapy, chemotherapy, and cell therapy (1–5). For the purpose of diagnosis, various methods of detection have been used to localize and evaluate the extent of tumor hypoxic regions. Such methods include immunohistochemistry on biopsy sections using antibodies specific for endogenous proteins expressed or overexpressed in low oxygen tension such as hypoxia inducible factor (HIF), carbonic anhydrase IX (CAIX), glucose transporter-1 (GLUT-1), lysyl oxidase (LOX), and lactate dehydrogenase (LDH). Exogenous probes, often nitroimidazole-based hypoxia markers (i.e., pimonidazole and EF5) injected into the host or directly injected intratumoraly (before surgical removal of the tumor tissue) and detected by immunohistochemistry are also used for analysis of hypoxic tumors. These detection techniques are limited by the necessity of invasively harvesting tissue samples. Methods of measurement using PO_2 electrodes allow a non-invasive detection and quantification of hypoxia. However, this technique is limited to easily accessible tumors. Techniques based on detection of proteins released during hypoxia (i.e., circulating human vascular endothelium growth factor (VEGF) and osteopontin) have also been developed and used to quantify hypoxia both in animal tumor models and in human tumors, but the lack of information on the localization and extent of the hypoxic zone results in incomplete diagnosis. Other techniques include the classical blood-oxygen-level-dependent (BOLD) MRI and more recently electron paramagnetic resonance imaging (7). Finally, non-invasive imaging techniques like positron emission tomography (PET)/CT-scan using radio-labeled nitroimidazole compounds like ^{18}F-Fluoromisonidazole (8, 10) that specifically bind hypoxic cells have also been tested and are now widely implemented in clinics to reveal hypoxic tumors. For all these techniques, the spatiotemporal variations of hypoxic areas in tumors should been taken in account for the analysis, diagnosis, and therapeutic strategy proposed for each tumor.

3. Causes of Hypoxia

In tumor masses, hypoxia can arise via a number of mechanisms. Fast growing hypoxic tumors have poor vessel bio-distribution (vascular architecture) and/or low vessel number (vascular density). Furthermore, the tumor vasculature also has increased vascular defects. Indeed, inadequate neo-vasculature with irregularities such as abnormal vessel wall, blind ends, arterio-venous anastomosis, distortions, twists, and elongation of vessels can compromise the supply of oxygen to tissue. Abnormal smooth muscle or enervation, and an incomplete endothelial lining or basement membrane have also been observed in hypoxic tumors (11) and contribute to defective tissue oxygenation. The tumor vessels can also be damaged by activated neutrophils, stimulated via hypoxia-mediated release of inflammatory cytokine, increasing vessel permeability.

Highly proliferating cancer cells that outgrow the neovascularization also participate in the formation of hypoxic areas in the tumors. The augmented proliferation directly increases the distance of diffusion for oxygen and nutrients, thus creating hypoxic regions in the enlarged tumors. This high proliferation rate of cancer cells is associated with a high consumption of oxygen and nutrients, also causing hypoxia. Tumor growth itself can also lead to compression of the blood vessels by the tumor mass and high interstitial pressure, again impeding oxygen delivery. Finally, anemia resulting from the disease or the treatment regimen, or the treatment itself can be a contributing factor (9). Any combination or all of these mechanisms can result in a hypoxic tumor.

4. Problems in Hypoxic Tumors

It is now accepted that the tumor and its microenvironment exert an influence on the progression of the disease via various mechanisms and also play a role in the response to cancer therapy. Because of their poor response to treatment, hypoxic cancers and their microenvironment are an important area of investigation; a better understanding of these hypoxic cancer cells (proteomic and genomic changes, interaction with the immune system, etc.) would allow tailoring of efficient therapies and better outcomes.

4.1. Tumor Environment of Hypoxic Tumors

Low oxygen tension directly affects tumor environment parameters such as pH, level of lactic acid, level of growth factors and nutrients (amino acids and glucose), metabolism, and the extracellular matrix (ECM) structure and cell composition (6). Changes in these parameters due to the lack of oxygen have a wide range of side effects on immune cells and alter the efficacy of the antitumor response.

In an environment deprived of oxygen, tumor cells switch from oxidative respiration to glycolysis, and as a result they produce large amounts of lactic acid. To survive, tumor cells export the toxic lactic acid into the extracellular microenvironment. In hypoxia, membrane located transporters, exchangers, and pumps are upregulated (12), facilitating the removal of this acid from the intracellular space to the extracellular space, but thereby decreasing the extracellular pH (12). Hypoxia also creates this acidification via the upregulation of carbonic anhydrases (13) and the production of CO_2 (14). There is evidence that acidic pH promotes an invasive phenotype in certain cancers (15, 16) and that severe tissue acidosis impairs the immune response. Moreover, due to the high glucose consumption by hypoxic tumor cells, the availability of glucose is low in these tumors. Glucose is delivered via blood vessels and thus its concentration in the tumor masses decreases with the disappearance of functional blood vessels, which also contributes to the overall reduction in glucose availability. In response to these events and as a survival mechanism, hypoxic tumors tend to switch to autophagy (17). This adaptive metabolic response limits the production of endogenous reactive oxygen species (ROS) and thus prevents cell death (18–20).

Accumulation of waste products such as ROS and nitrate (NO), as well as necrosis products, also changes the hypoxic tumor microenvironment and affects immune cell function. NO has been shown to promote tumor cell growth and to select for p53 tumor mutants. Several studies including ours (unpublished data) have shown that ROS is detrimental to the survival and adequate function of immune cells.

The ECM and associated stroma regulate the diffusion of oxygen and nutrients, but also secrete regulatory molecules (e.g., angiotensin II); its density impacts the infiltration of tumors by immune cells. Hypoxia modulates the ECM compartment via HIF-mediated production of lysyl oxidase (which catalyzes collagen) and matrix metalloprotease (MMP) and allows tumor metastasis. Stromal cell derived factor-1 (SDF-1) is increased in hypoxic tumors and recruits bone marrow stem cells for the formation of new blood vessels (21, 22), thus further favoring the malignancy by allowing metastasis. Moreover, the secretion of SDF-1 leads to the attraction of mesenchymal stem cells, which are known to be immunosuppressive (23). In this manner the ECM impairs various immune cells, thus reducing their antitumor efficacy and supporting tumor proliferation.

Hypoxia has also been reported to induce hemoconcentration, leading to higher blood viscosity, the aggregation of blood cells including immune cells within the vessels, and reduced blood flow (24), resulting in acute hypoxia. This increased hemoconcentration also reduces the delivery of chemotherapeutic drugs, or antibodies, and prevents immune cells from infiltrating tumor masses by trapping them in the vessels. As mentioned previously, high interstitial pressure is also characteristic of hypoxic tumors and has a detrimental effect on the viability and function of immune cells, and thus on their capability to react to tumor-antigen targets. Together, these events induced by hypoxia in tumor masses and the tumor microenvironment have important implications for the immune response and thus on cancer immunotherapy.

4.2. Hypoxic Cancer Cells

Cancer cells have developed methods by which they can survive periods of low oxygen availability. Central to this process is hypoxia-inducible factor 1 (HIF-1), a key factor in cellular adaptation to hypoxic conditions, including cell survival, angiogenesis, and the switch from aerobic to anaerobic metabolism. Overexpression of HIF-1 in human cancers has been shown to correlate with poor prognosis and increased tumor aggression. In mouse models examining immune function, HIF-1 has different roles in the various immune cells (e.g., protection of myeloid cells from apoptosis but promotion of apoptosis in thymocytes) (25). The HIF complex is a heterodimer, composed of HIF-1α and HIF-1β subunits. While the β subunit is unaffected by oxygen levels, the α subunit is stabilized in hypoxia and targeted for rapid proteosomal degradation in normoxia. As a potent transcription factor, HIF-1 activates numerous target genes via binding to hypoxia response elements (HRE) present in their promoter region. Through this gene regulation, HIF mediates the expression of several key proteins like VEGF, erythropoietin (EPO), CAIX, GLUT-1, and a cluster of glycolytic enzymes (i.e., phosphoglycerate kinase 1, lactate dehydrogenase A). These proteins are involved in different pathways (angiogenesis, erythropoiesis, pH regulation, glucose uptake, etc.) that compensate for altered metabolic needs and enable the survival and proliferation of hypoxic tumors by various mechanisms. A new role for HIF as tumor suppressor has recently been reported by Scortegagna et al. with their finding that HIF prevents epithelial-mesenchymal transformation (26).

Angiogenesis is important to support the proliferation of tumor cells; it allows the supply of oxygen and nutrients necessary for continued growth. VEGF is a key growth factor for new vessel formation, as it promotes the proliferation, migration, elongation, network formation, and branching of endothelial cells (27–29). Tumor growth factor-beta (TFG-β) is also upregulated during hypoxia to resist glucose starvation (30), and it is released by tumor cells or hypoxia-associated T regulatory (Treg) cells; HIF-1 and TGF-β act in synergy to upregulate VEGF production (31).

Hypoxic tumors are highly metastatic; to metastasize, cancer cells must detach from the tumor mass and spread via blood circulation and lymphatic system (32). Such metastatic potential is regulated by HIF-1-mediated repression or induction of several genes. One example is the adhesion protein E-cadherin, which acts by dimerizing with other E-cadherin molecules on nearby cells, contributing to maintain a normal tissues structure (33). HIF-1 downregulates E-cadherin and consequently frees the tumor cells to migrate, facilitating local invasion and metastasis. In addition, it has been reported that the detachment of hypoxic tumor cells is also mediated by decreased adhesion to vitronectin and downregulated expression of integrins (34). HIF-1 also induces the expression of MMPs and LOX that disrupt the structure of the ECM. The expression of these proteins in hypoxic tumors can have a prognostic value. Also important for metastasis are chemokine receptors, which allow attachment of the migrating tumor cells at a new site. One such is CXCR4, the expression and function of which is enhanced by HIF-1 on malignant cells. CXCR4 expression is correlated with poor prognosis in many cancers and has been shown to be important in cell migration and metastasis. Other genes like autocrine motility factor, keratins, receptor tyrosine kinase c-Met (35), and, as mentioned before, SDF-1 are also regulated by HIF-1 and actively participate in the metastasis of cancer cells. Finally, as mentioned above, acidosis generated by hypoxic tumors also promotes metastasis.

The natural cellular response to sustained hypoxia is apoptosis. Thus, the pressure of a hypoxic tumor environment can act in selecting cells with alterations of apoptosis pathways, particularly cells that acquire p53 mutations and deletions (36–38), thus allowing their survival. These residual surviving hypoxic cells often evolve into a more aggressive phenotype (36). The overexpression or activation of p53 blocks the accumulation of HIF-1α. Similarly, p53 mutation significantly reduces the apoptosis rate in hypoxic tumor cells showing that the tumor suppressor protein p53 is a powerful negative regulator of HIF-1 (36). Likewise, cancer cells also cheat hypoxia-induced death by overexpressing the anti-apoptotic protein Bcl-X_L (39). Molecules involved in DNA repair are inhibited by hypoxia, with concomitant increase genome instability leading to higher rates of mutation in hypoxic cells and to their survival (40, 41). Finally, the role of HIF-1 in the increase of telomerase activation via overexpression of human telomerase reverse transcriptase (hTERT), and the resulting prolonged life span of hypoxic tumor cells was recently reported by Bell et al. (42), showing that different survival pathways are "turned on" by HIF-1. Therefore, therapies for hypoxic cancers should preferentially target HIF, or multiple mechanisms supporting cancer progression, rather than any one individual survival pathway.

Hypoxic tumors are highly immunosuppressive; they modulate the immune response directly or indirectly by recruiting other cells. They directly affect immune cells via the expression or upregulation of several molecules known to be immunosuppressive, the most important being TGF-β, which strongly impairs tumor-specific T cells. Another example is HLA-g, a nonclassical major histocompatibility complex (MHC) molecule. In non-pathological conditions its expression is restricted to immune privileged sites such as the trophoblast and the eyes, and its main function is to prevent immune attack of these privileged tissues by ablating T and natural killer (NK) cell functions. However, numerous studies have shown that secreted or membrane-bound HLA-g molecules are expressed in a large number of tumor types as well as overexpressed in hypoxic tumor areas, leading to a drastic decrease of the antitumor response. Similarly, expression and secretion of soluble of MHC class I chain-related molecules (MICs) is upregulated by many hypoxic cancers (via NO), favoring their immune escape by MIC-induced downregulation of NKG2D receptors, which suppress NK-cell activation (43). Hypoxic tumors also indirectly suppress immune cells by promoting the infiltration of TGF-β-producing myeloid suppressor cells (MSC) (44) and T-reg cells. Once present in the tumor, T-reg cells also inhibit a variety of immune cells by contact-dependent mechanisms (31). Hypoxic tumors are known to recruit a high numbers of macrophages and granulocytes, leading to the hyperproduction of reactive oxygen species (ROS) with consequent NF-kB inhibition, and the production of pro-inflammatory cytokines such as interleukin (IL)-10 and TGF-β. Finally, these tumors induce the activation and survival of neutrophils that damage the vessel and worsen the disease. Thus, via immunosuppression, HIF expression, and genomic changes, hypoxic cancer cells can survive and progress toward aggressive and metastatic malignancy. Overall, the immunosuppressive milieu fostered by the tumor and enhanced by hypoxia results in the inability of the immune system to control tumor growth and the resistance of tumors to cell therapy.

4.3. The Effect of Hypoxia on Immune Cells

To eradicate hypoxic cancers immune cells need to infiltrate the tumor mass, to survive, be fully functional, and persist. It has been reported by several groups including ours that the hypoxic tumor exerts its influence on key actors of the antitumor response by a range of mechanisms, all of which contribute to a suppression or attenuation of the anti-tumor response. To propose an effective immunotherapy it is crucial to understand the interactions between the hypoxic tumor, its microenvironment, and immune cells.

4.3.1. Macrophages

Tumors mediate an influx of infiltrating macrophages, which once resident in the tumor are identified as tumor-associated macrophages (TAM). In rapidly growing tumors, a high number of TAM correlates with the aggressiveness of the malignancy. Hypoxia upregulates the expression of integrins α_M and β_2 and MMP (45) in macrophages, facilitating their migration from the vasculature into hypoxic tissue. Hypoxia also inhibits expression of the chemokine receptors CCR2 (46) and CCR5 (47), to keep them in the tumor mass (48). This entrapment is further reinforced by hypoxia-mediated upregulation of their mitogen-activated protein kinase phosphatase (MKP-1) leading to indirect inhibition of the expression of chemokine receptors (48). In the oxygen-deprived microenvironment, TAMs secrete inflammatory cytokines (e.g., IL-1), which chemoattract immune effector cells. However, macrophages in hypoxia have been shown to have a reduced phagocytic capacity (49), likely due to the requirement for oxygen conversion into ROS within the phagocytic vesicle for cytotoxic activity. Still, more investigation is required since contradictory finding have been reported (50).

HIF-1 decreases the effectiveness of TAM to present tumor antigens (51, 52), and thus indirectly prevents the activation of T cells. Hypoxia reduces the expression of CD80 on monocytes and macrophages (51) leading to an altered induction of immune response. Finally, TAM NO production is reduced by tumor-mediated acidosis (53). These hypoxic TAMs switch from immune cells (54) to pro-tumor cells (55, 56) and like tumor cells they adapt to low oxygen tension (57) by becoming resistant to apoptosis (58). Among the other genes upregulated in macrophages during reduced oxygen is inhibitor DNA binding-2 (Id2), which is involved in the survival and differentiation of many cells. In addition, IL-4, IL-10, and TGF-β1 secreted by hypoxic tumor cells prompt macrophages to release factors that promote tumor proliferation (fibroblast growth factor 2 (FGF2), platelet-derived growth factor (PDGF), acidic/basic FGFs (a/bFGFs) (59), and epidermal growth factor (EGF) (60–62)) and metastasis (macrophage inhibitory factor (MIF) (63), tissue factor (TF) (64)). These hypoxic TAMs are polarized toward the M2 phenotype and release prostaglandin E, IL-10 and TGF-β, factors which suppress T-cell activation (65). In conjunction with this inhibition of the antitumor response, they express VEGF (66, 67) and MMP (57), which stimulate angiogenesis and extracellular matrix restructuration, thus further promoting tumor progression and metastasis (65, 68, 69). TAMs also produce interferon gamma (IFN-γ) in reduced oxygen tension (52) such as in hypoxic tumors; however, IFN-γ molecules are very labile in an acidic milieu and thus have limited activity. Altogether, TAMs promote tumor progression and deflection of a robust antitumor response.

4.3.2. Neutrophils

Hypoxic environments like inflammation and tumors recruit large numbers of neutrophils (70). In tumors devoid of oxygen, the upregulation of chemokines (IL-1 and IL-8) and polypeptides exerts a strong chemotactic and activation activity on neutrophils (71, 72). Hypoxic monocytes and macrophages also upregulate chemokines with the potential to attract neutrophils (73). Once in the hypoxic environment, neutrophil susceptibility to apoptosis is reduced, via HIF-1-mediated modulation of the NF-κB pathway (74, 75). Hypoxia also regulates neutrophil adhesion via reactive oxygen species (76), LFA-1 (77) and IL-1, and increases their survival (78). In vivo, neutrophils have been found in large numbers in hypoxia areas (79). Hypoxia exerts a deleterious effect on neutrophil function by limiting their killing activity (80, 81) and migration (82). Low pH in pathological microenvironments activates neutrophils (83) and modulates their oxidative burst (81). Indeed as it appears that HIF-1 protein stabilization and degradation in tumor cells is regulated by ROS (hydrogen peroxidase alters HIF-1 expression) (84), thus reduction of ROS released in the tumor microenvironment would promote tumor development. Of note, the effect of ROS on hypoxic cells depends of the form and the cellular location of the free radicals produced. Activated neutrophils can participate in extracellular acidification (85), and thus probably also affect T- viability and function. Eltzschig et al. reported that adenosine induced during low oxygen tension acts as an anti-inflammatory signal to attenuate extreme neutrophil accumulation (86, 87). These results were recently confirmed by studies showing the role of HIF-induced netrin-1 (Ntn1) expression in this phenomenon (88, 89). Finally, neutrophil-mediated injury (90) also leads to blood vessel damage and thus prevents T and NK cells infiltration. Still, the full extent of the consequences of hypoxia on neutrophils remains to be fully appreciated.

4.3.3. Dendritic Cells

Dendritic cells (DC) play a central and important role in the immune response as they are powerful antigen-presenting cells (APC). They have the capacity to process and present antigen to T cells. DC-mediated activation and regulation of the T-cell response is dependent upon their differentiation and maturation status. Indeed, their inadequate or incomplete maturation leads to a change in cytokine secretion and in decreased expression of co-stimulatory molecules, resulting in the defective activation of T cells, or worse in the induction of T-cell anergy/tolerence and T-reg. In colorectal cancers, DC have been positively correlated with T-reg and disease progression (91), probably due to the presence in these tumors of high amount of VEGF and IL-10 that have been described to inhibit DC maturation (92–94). Hypoxia decreases the capacity of mice DC to uptake antigen (both in presence or absence of LPS stimulation) and increases IL-6 production following LPS activation (95). Surprisingly, the induction of T-cell proliferation in a MLR assay was higher following stimulation with LPS-treated DC in hypoxia (95). This study underlined the oxygen independent role of HIF in LPS-treated DC. Elia et al. demonstrated that in hypoxia, immature human DC have a reduced antigen uptake and an altered chemokine secretion pattern that shows an increase in molecules that promote inflammation via the recruitment of neutrophils (via NAP-3 (CXCL1), CXCL8) rather than lymphocytes (96). Indeed, they reported in hypoxic immature DC a downregulation of CCL18 and MCP-1 (CCL2) chemokines that are known to be T-cell attractants (97–99) and an upregulation of IP-10 (CXCL10) that increases adhesion of T cells to the vessel wall (100). Their study also revealed that despite these changes, hypoxia has no unfavorable effect on the maturation of DC and that their ability to induce proliferation of allogeneic and antigen-specific T cells was preserved. Other studies reported that hypoxia inhibits DC migration via a decrease of MMP (101–103). Mancino et al. found detrimental effects of hypoxia on human DC differentiation (from monocytes) and maturation, as identified by the decreased expression of CD40, CD80, CD83, and CD86 co-stimulation molecules, and an impaired stimulation of T cells (as measured by decreased proliferation of allogeneic T cells and interferon gamma (INF-γ) production) (104).

The effect of hypoxia-associated microenvironmental changes on DC, such as acidosis and increased level of adenosine, have also been investigated. Gottfried et al. reported that lactic acid affects

DC phenotype and decreases IL-12 secretion (105). Adenosine is a product of ATP degradation, and its production is increased during hypoxia. Adenosine was shown to affect DC function (106) by inhibiting IL-12 production in mature DC and to act as a chemotaxin for immature DC (107). Furthermore, adenosine was also shown to inhibit vesicular MHC class I cross-presentation by resting DC, but had no effect on immature and CpG-activated DC (108). There have been an increasing number of publications on DC and hypoxia in recent years; however, the impact of hypoxia on DC is still controversial. Indeed, some studies have found the effects of hypoxia to be detrimental on DC (73, 96, 104, 105), whereas others have found no impairment of the maturation and function of DC and reported that DC matured in hypoxia upregulate genes associated with cell movement and migration (109), or show positive effects of acidosis on antigen uptake and presentation by DC (110). It is crucial when comparing studies of the impact of hypoxia on DC to take into account the duration of exposure to hypoxia, as well as the kinetics of DC maturation following stimulation pre- or post-hypoxia. From a clinical point of view, it is important to consider the fact that tumor-associated DC could be exposed to hypoxia for long periods of time and that their maturation could occur either before or after entering hypoxic areas.

4.3.4. T and Natural Killer (NK) Cells

While there has been undeniable data stressing the importance of cellular immune response in the control of cancer proliferation, it is clear that T-cell growth and survival is profoundly impaired at low oxygen tension (111–113) and, thus, that hypoxic tumors escape T-cell attacks. Hypoxia has the potential to adversely affect the consequences of T-cell receptor (TCR) activation by antigen (25, 114–116) leading to the inhibition of naïve T-cell differentiation into cytotoxic T lymphocytes (CTL). Hypoxia mediates a decrease of Kv1.3 protein levels (depolarizing the T cell) (115) and a decrease in Ca^{2+} signaling (117), both of which are involved in T-cell activation (118), thus preventing T-cell activation, and hence T-cell proliferation. Caldwell et al. have reported that the cytokine pattern is also altered in hypoxic T cells (116). Indeed, hypoxia decreases IL-2 production (119–121), which is required for full T-cell activation. T cells that survive hypoxia have an altered the Th1:Th2 cytokine secretion pattern, inducing release of Th2 cytokines such as IL-1, IL-6, and IL-8, and a decreased in the Th1 cytokines IL-2 and INF-γ, which are required for an efficient cytotoxic T-cell response. Hypoxia was also found to increase the level of pro-apoptotic proteins (BNIP3 and BAX) and decrease the level of anti-apoptotic proteins (BCL-xL) (122, and Yotnda unpublished data) in T cells. In a recent report, Kiang et al. indicated that inhibiting inducible nitric-oxide synthase (iNOS) rescues T cells from hypoxia-induced apoptosis (123) revealing the role of NO in T-cell death. Loeffler et al. found in an in vivo EMT6 tumor mouse model that the number of T cells infiltrating hypoxic tumor areas is equal to T-cell numbers in normoxic areas (79). However, in a xenograft mice model of hypoxic lymphoma, we found that T cells are able to well infiltrate the normoxic tumors but detected only minimum infiltration in the hypoxic areas of these tumors (121). IP-10, a chemoattractant for T cells, is produced during hypoxia (124) and is in part responsible for T-cell homing to the tumor sites. However, the compromised survival of the infiltrating T cells after several hours or days in hypoxia or anoxia would explain the absence of T cells in tumors lacking oxygen. Of note, the lytic activity of T cells, which develops in hypoxia, is amplified (116); similarly, their protection from activation-induced cell death (AICD) is enhanced in low oxygen tension (116, 121). Makino et al. suggested that HIF-1 is responsible for the survival of antigen receptor-driven T cells (111). However, using HIF-1α-I.1-deficient mice, Lukashev et al. showed that both HIF-1α and an activation-inducible short isoform I.1 of HIF downregulated T-cell function (125).

Lactic acid released in hypoxic tumors inhibits the chemoattraction of leucocytes. Fisher et al. demonstrated that tumor cell-derived lactic acid affects the proliferation and killing activity of human T cells (126). Low pH was also reported to decrease T-cell proliferation in response to IL-2 (127) and NK activity (128). Finally, the LAK activity of lymphocytes is inhibited by an acidic pH (129–131). In addition to hypoxic effects of tumors, T cells are also particularly susceptible to the detrimental effects of repeated hypoxia and reoxygenation, such as ischemia reperfusion injury.

Reactive oxygen species (ROS) are produced by most tumors and are detrimental to T-cell viability and function (132, 133). ROS such as superoxide anions, hydrogen peroxide (H_2O_2), hydroxyl radicals and hypochlorous acid are involved in a wide panel of reactions including DNA damage and are produced by various mechanisms. After antigen stimulation and expansion, only a limited number of cells will survive and become memory T cells. The majority of these activated T cells will die by apoptosis (both through the FAS and Bim pathways) to maintain a constant T cells number (homeostasis). This death is related to an increased level of ROS (7, 134) (both superoxide and hydrogen peroxide) generated by T-cell receptor stimulation (135, 136). T cells are also susceptible to ROS produced by surrounding cells. Hypoxia generates ROS as a result of anaerobic metabolism. Reperfusion after ischemia also causes ROS production in various tissues due to a decrease of their intracellular level of pyruvate. In a tumor microenvironment, ROS are produced by the malignant cells themselves (132, 137), while in the context of inflammation it is produced by granulocytes. In tumors, ROS regulates

HIF expression (84). Macrophage-mediated protective response against pathogens involves the production of ROS, which affect the functions and survival of the surrounding T cells (138, 139). Macrophages can also mediate ROS production indirectly via secretion of tumor necrosis factor (TNF)-α (140). Several studies have demonstrated that heat shock generates ROS, impairing T cells and downregulating the TCR-CD3 complex as well as production of IL-2 (141–143). ROS abolishes IFN-α stimulation in CD8, NK/T and NK cells (138), thereby reducing the cellular immune response. Among all the ROS, H_2O_2 is the most stable (longest half-life) and the most damaging to T cells. In the presence of H_2O_2, the function of memory T cells is drastically diminished (144); they lose their ability to secrete IL-2, TNF-α and IFN-γ following activation with phorbol myristate acetate/ionomycin. These T cells die within 6–8 h after exposure to extracellular H_2O_2. Among the memory T-cell populations, effector cells are the most susceptible. Altogether, ROS produced by hypoxic tissues cancer suppress immune effector cells.

Adenosine is produced during the degradation of purine and is present in inflamed and malignant tissues. Sitkovsky et al. have extensively investigated the immunosuppressive effect of extracellular adenosine on T cells during hypoxia (25). Their studies showed that adenosine levels increase in hypoxia, and lymphocytes (T and NK) expressed the A2AR or A2BR adenosine receptors; moreover, the increase in adenosine correlates with the impairment of T-cell activation and function (145–149) as well as with the decrease of lytic activity (150) and cytokine production (150–152) in NK cells.

Regulatory T-cell induction, proliferation, and survival are promoted by tumor cells that secret IL-10 and TGF-β, as well as by defective dendritic cells. T-reg cells are further supported by hypoxia-mediated adenosine production (153). Hypoxia upregulates FoxP3 (154), which is important for T-reg cells, as well as ecto-apyrase (CD39) and ecto-5'-nucleotidase (CD73), which promote extracellular adenosine production (155) and thus further increase adenosine levels in the tumor microenvironment.

Finally, prostaglandin (PGE) a product of the cyclooxygenases (COX-1 and-2) is released during inflammation and hypoxia and correlated with poor outcome (156). Like adenosine, PGE also plays an important role in immunosuppression (157), and impacts NK function (158).

4.3.5. B Cells

Fewer studies have explored the effect of hypoxia on B cells. However, it is known that hypoxia does not affect the production of antibody. Furthermore, HIF-1α deficiency has been linked to altered differentiation of B1 cells, impaired maturation of B2 cells, as well as to autoimmunity (159, 160). Piovan et al. recently reported that hypoxia regulates CXCR4 expression on B cells

(161), and this molecule is expressed on many B-lymphomas; notably, we have found that B-lymphomas have hypoxic areas. Similarly to what has been reported for other cells, HIF-1α is involved in the survival of B cells and in their progression into the S phase of the cell cycle (162).

5. Therapies Targeting Hypoxic Cancers

5.1. Limitations of Standard Therapies

Hypoxic cancers are aggressive and metastatic and consequently detrimental to the disease outcome. Hypoxic areas of tumors are often resistant to chemo- and radiotherapy, since locally deficient drug biodistribution and altered cellular metabolism reduces the efficacy of these agents (163, 164). Additionally, residual surviving hypoxic cells may evolve into a more aggressive phenotype (36), and as hypoxia also has the potential to adversely affect the cellular immunotherapy of tumors (165) it is a major concern for cancer therapy.

Radiation kills tumor cells via the production of free radicals derived from oxygen, subsequently inducing DNA fragmentation. Hypoxia confers resistance to radiation therapy due to the lack of oxygen, and to a decrease in DNA repair systems, lowering the efficacy of radiation. Chemotherapy on the other hand uses a wide range of mechanisms of action leading to a broad range of effects. Hypoxic tumor resistance of to chemotherapy is mainly due to the fact that several of the most widely used drugs require oxygen to produce toxic free radicals that will kill the tumor cells. Furthermore, the reduced proliferation rate of hypoxic tumors affects the efficacy of drugs that target highly proliferative tumor cells, such as antiproliferative drugs or drugs that take advantage of events occurring during proliferation. The abnormal vasculature of hypoxic tumors also prevents the efficient distribution of drugs thereby affecting their efficacy. Downregulation of pro-apoptotic molecules Bid and Bax by hypoxia in tumor cells (166) also reduces tumor susceptibility to chemotherapy. Finally, proteomic and genomic changes also diminish the effect of anticancer drugs, i.e., hypoxia selects p53 mutated cells that are no longer sensitive to several chemotherapies. Likewise, hypoxia upregulates proteins such as the glycoprotein multidrug resistance (MDR1) that confer resistance to therapeutic drugs (167). Acidosis was also reported to confer protection against drugs such as topotecan, vincristine, teniposide, as well as cisplatin cytotoxicity (168). Cell therapy alone or combined with other therapies has been successful for many cancers, as killing via T or NK cells was proven an efficient therapy for certain malignancies. However, as described previously, hypoxic tumors suppress T and NK cells, decrease antigen presentation by DC, and inhibit the killing activity of macrophages, leading to a poor cellular antitumor response. In view of these factors, it is evident that an assessment of the hypoxic tumor (localization, accessibility, extent (large or small area), grade (chronic or acute), and evolution) is critical before deciding on a therapeutic strategy.

5.2. Potential Solutions for Therapy of Hypoxic Cancers

Given the current problems faced when treating hypoxic tumors, it is crucial to rethink and improve non-surgical therapies for these malignancies. Over the years many therapies have been proposed to eradicate tumors deprived of oxygen.

Chemotherapy adapted to treat hypoxic tumors has made tremendous progress with the development of bioreductive drugs, which are non-toxic in vivo and only become cytotoxic after one electron reduction in hypoxia. A number of these drugs have been evaluated for their safety and efficacy. The most commonly used is tirapazamine (TPZ), which has a low non-specific toxicity (169) and PR-104 (170). Recent clinical reports using the bioreductive anthraquinone banoxantrone prodrug (AQ4N) showed preferential activation of the drug only in hypoxic tissues (170, 171). Antioxidants are also upregulated in hypoxic cancers and activate drugs like Mitomycin C, vitamin E, and folate, resulting in tumor cell death; these drugs have been evaluated for their antitumor activity in prostate cancers and showed promising results. Drugs that inhibit HIF-1 have therapeutic consequences and limit the proliferation of tumor cells. Puppo et al. demonstrated in neuroblastoma that topotecan blocks HIF-mediated VEGF production and angiogenesis (172). Similarly, Shin et al. recently reported that bortezomib increases FIH-mediated repression of HIF (173). Injection of EPO combined with chemotherapy was proposed to circumvent the detrimental effect of hypoxia on chemotherapy and radiotherapy but has had limited success. In tests it failed to reduce tumor burden, and thus does not appear to be useful for clinical application (174, 175). Drugs that mimic NO have shown an antitumor effect when combined with chemotherapy (176). Indeed, drugs for which the toxicity does not depend on O_2, such as mTOR inhibitors, are attractive therapies for hypoxic tumors (177). Finally, drugs that decrease the interstitial pressure of hypoxic tumor (e.g., paclitaxel) and allow normal blood flow and reoxygenation could potentiate chemotherapy or radiotherapy (178).

An increasing number of radiosensitizers have been proposed to improve the efficacy of radiotherapy for hypoxic tumors. Radiosensitizers mimic oxygen in hypoxic cells to allow DNA

damage and cell death. However, most of these radiosensitizers have limitations such as toxicity preventing the use of efficient doses, and poor sensitization to radiation. The therapeutic
value of new drugs such as nitroimidazoles (nimorazole) (179)
was validated in head and neck cancers (179–181) and showed
that combined with radiotherapy it improved the outcome of the
treatment. Another radiotherapeutic strategy, ARCON (accelerated radiotherapy, carbogen, nicotinamide), uses nicotinamide to
induce vasodilatation (decreased occlusion of blood vessel) and
carbogen to increase the oxygen pressure of the tumor mass (182)
in combination with radiotherapy. Clinical studies using ARCON
in head and neck cancers, glioma, bladder cancer, non-small-cell
lung cancers, and breast cancers have been reported (182–184).
A novel radiosensitizer, TX-1877 ((2-nitroimidazole-acetamide),
together with radiation, resulted in pancreatic tumor regression
in nude mice bearing subcutaneous (s.c.) or orthotopic human
tumors (185). Furthermore, Oshikawa et al. showed in a squamous cell carcinoma mouse model that TX1877 response is in
part mediated by anti-tumor CD8 T-cells (186). Stern et al.
have investigated the uses of immunoadjuvants (LPS or lipid-A)
and IFN-γ to stimulate inducible nitric oxide synthase (iNOS)
to produce NO for the purpose of increasing radiosensitization of hypoxic tumors and successfully control tumor progression (187, 188). Wilson et al. have investigated the efficacy of
radiation-activated prodrugs such as nitroarylmethyl quaternary
salts (NMQ), which are activated via reduction with ionizing radiation rather than by enzymes (189, 190). However, these appealing new drugs need further investigation. Alternatives such as
the use of hyperbaric oxygen breathing associated to radiotherapy have also been reported. In a phase II study, Sunh et al.
combined radiotherapy with an allosteric modifier of hemoglobin
(efaproxiral/RSR-13) and found a benefit for patients with brain
metastases (191). Hyperbaric oxygen (HBO) requires that the
patient inhale 100% oxygen at elevated pressure (greater than
1.5 atmospheres absolute), with oxygen then distributed to tissues in a passive way. This strategy has been investigated in head
and neck cancers, with the benefits being an increased level of
oxygen and reduced inflammation (192). However, side effects
resulting from this approach limit its clinical application. More
recently, Bennett et al. reported that HBO combined with radiotherapy controlled local tumors and increased the survival of
patients with head and neck cancer, and this combination also
controlled local cancers of the uterine cervix (193). Finally, hyperthermia has also been investigated; this therapy uses high temper-
atures as a treatment approach. In hypoxic cancers, blood vessels are not available to diffuse the heat generated by the therapy,
thus killing the cancer cells (194). Conversely, the presence of
blood vessels prevents damage of normal tissue by evacuating the

heat. It has been shown that hypothermia enhances the efficiency of radiotherapy as well as the effect of some drugs in hypoxic tumors (195).

Numerous gene therapy approaches to treating hypoxic tumors have been explored in the past few decades (196). Among them are approaches that use various hypoxia-regulated genes such as cytosine deamisase (197), nitroreductase suicide therapy (190, 198), hypoxia-regulated oncolytic viruses (199, 200), adenoviruses that encode hypoxia regulated thymidine kinase gene (HRE-HSK/TK) (201, 202), antisense HIF-1α plasmids, and siRNA targeting HIF and CAIX molecules. Bacteria such as Clostridium oncolyticum genetically modified with cytosine deaminase have also been reported as therapeutic tools against hypoxic tumors (203, 204). Many of these gene therapy approaches showed success and anticipate a bystander-effect, such that non-modified malignant cells would also respond to the therapy.

Antibodies targeting HIF or CAIX alone or in combination with radiotherapy or IL-2 have also been investigated and showed encouraging results in renal cell carcinoma (205, 206). Antibody-directed enzyme prodrug therapy allows an enzyme to be delivered into the tumor mass before a prodrug is administered (207). The targeted enzyme converts and activates the prodrug, which becomes toxic solely at the tumor. In human colorectal cancer, gene therapy using adenovirus encoding iNOS combined with radiotherapy has been explored (208).

Several studies have targeted tumor hypoxic areas using cell therapy. Griffiths et al. have engineered macrophages to deliver human cytochrome P4502B6 as an anticancer drug (209). Using a spheroid tumor model they showed that macrophages were able to deliver the drug to hypoxic tumors, and tumor cell death in the presence of cyclophosphamide. Unfortunately the limitation of this approach seem to be the restriction of specific homing of macrophages, and thus the potential for them to release the therapy in non-malignant tissues (57). We have engineered tumor specific T cells that express IL-2 in hypoxic tumors, and thus better survive the lack of oxygen, thereby improving tumor regression (121).

Another alternative approach utilizes an oxygen-dependent domain (ODD) attached to a therapeutic protein. The presence of oxygen targets these proteins for degradation, thus restricting their effects to hypoxic areas. One such example used a diphtheria toxin-A fusion containing the ODD (210, 211), and in a pre-clinical mouse model of Lewis lung carcinoma, Koshikaw et al. showed increased apoptosis of hypoxic tumor cells and retardation of tumor growth. In a similar pre-clinical study using capase-3 fused to ODD, Inoue et al. prolonged survival and cured 60% of rats with malignant ascites (81).

6. Conclusion

It is evident that hypoxic tumors are a major concern and should be targeted to improve the outcome of malignant diseases. The improvement and development of new tools to non-invasively detect and measure oxygen tension in vivo will ensure a better assessment and diagnosis of hypoxic tumors. As single/mono therapies have been proven inefficient in eradicating hypoxic tumors, combining multiple therapeutic approaches should circumvent current limitations and improve the overall efficacy of tumor treatment. The better understanding of the effects of hypoxia and the tumor microenvironment gained over the past decade will provide us with new strategies to tackle hypoxic tumors.

References

1. Crowther, M., Brown, N. J., Bishop, E. T., and Lewis, C. E. (2001) Microenvironmental influence on macrophage regulation of angiogenesis in wounds and malignant tumors. *J Leukoc Biol 70*, 478–490.
2. Espey, M. G. (2006) Tumor macrophage redox and effector mechanisms associated with hypoxia. *Free Radic Biol Med 41*, 1621–1628.
3. Lukashev, D., Ohta, A., and Sitkovsky, M. (2007) Hypoxia-dependent anti-inflammatory pathways in protection of cancerous tissues. *Cancer Metastasis Rev 26*, 273–279.
4. Semenza, G. L. (2001) Hypoxia-inducible factor 1: oxygen homeostasis and disease pathophysiology. *Trends Mol Med 7*, 345–350.
5. Zinkernagel, A. S., Johnson, R. S., and Nizet, V. (2007) Hypoxia inducible factor (HIF) function in innate immunity and infection. *J Mol Med 85*, 1339–1346.
6. Dayan, F., Mazure, N. M., Brahimi-Horn, M. C., and Pouyssegur, J. (2008) A Dialogue between the Hypoxia-Inducible Factor and the Tumor Microenvironment. *Cancer Microenviron 1*, 53–68.
7. Elas, M., Williams, B. B., Parasca, A., Mailer, C., Pelizzari, C. A., Lewis, M. A., River, J. N., Karczmar, G. S., Barth, E. D., and Halpern, H. J. (2003) Quantitative tumor oxymetric images from 4D electron paramagnetic resonance imaging (EPRI): methodology and comparison with blood oxygen level-dependent (BOLD) MRI. *Magn Reson Med 49*, 682–691.
8. Evans, S. M., Kachur, A. V., Shiue, C. Y., Hustinx, R., Jenkins, W. T., Shive, G. G., Karp, J. S., Alavi, A., Lord, E. M., Dolbier, W. R., Jr., and Koch, C. J. (2000) Noninvasive detection of tumor hypoxia using the 2-nitroimidazole [18F]EF1. *J Nucl Med 41*, 327–336.
9. Franco, M., Man, S., Chen, L., Emmenegger, U., Shaked, Y., Cheung, A. M., Brown, A. S., Hicklin, D. J., Foster, F. S., and Kerbel, R. S. (2006) Targeted antivascular endothelial growth factor receptor-2 therapy leads to short-term and long-term impairment of vascular function and increase in tumor hypoxia. *Cancer Res 66*, 3639–3648.
10. Komar, G., Seppanen, M., Eskola, O., Lindholm, P., Gronroos, T. J., Forsback, S., Sipila, H., Evans, S. M., Solin, O., and Minn, H. (2008) 18F-EF5: a new PET tracer for imaging hypoxia in head and neck cancer. *J Nucl Med 49*, 1944–1951.
11. Cairns, R. A., Kalliomaki, T., and Hill, R. P. (2001) Acute (cyclic) hypoxia enhances spontaneous metastasis of KHT murine tumors. *Cancer Res 61*(24), 8903–8908.
12. Chiche, j., llc, K., Laferriere, j., Trottier, E., Dayan, F., Mazure, N. M., Brahimi-Horn, M. C., and Pouyssegur, j. (2009) Hypoxia-inducible carbonic anhydrase IX and XII promote tumor cell growth by counteracting acidosis through the regulation of the intracellular pH. *Cancer Res 69*, 358–368.
13. Wykoff, C. C., Beasley, N. J., Watson, P. H., Turner, K. J., Pastorek, J., Sibtain, A., Wilson, G. D., Turley, H., Talks, K. L.,

Maxwell, P. H., Pugh, C. W., Ratcliffe, P. J., and Harris, A. L. (2000) Hypoxia-inducible expression of tumor-associated carbonic anhydrases. *Cancer Res 60*, 7075–7083.

14. Brahimi-Horn, M. C., Chiche, J., and Pouyssegur, J. (2007) Hypoxia signalling controls metabolic demand. *Curr Opin Cell Biol 19*, 223–229.

15. Chiche, J., Ilc, K., Laferriere, J., Trottier, E., Dayan, F., Mazure, N. M., Brahimi-Horn, M. C., and Pouyssegur, J. (2009) Hypoxia-inducible carbonic anhydrase IX and XII promote tumor cell growth by counteracting acidosis through the regulation of the intracellular pH. *Cancer Res 69*, 358–368.

16. Martinez-Zaguilan, R., Seftor, E. A., Seftor, R. E., Chu, Y. W., Gillies, R. J., and Hendrix, M. J. (1996) Acidic pH enhances the invasive behavior of human melanoma cells. *Clin Exp Metastasis 14*, 176–186.

17. Azad, M. B., Chen, Y., Henson, E. S., Cizeau, J., McMillan-Ward, E., Israels, S. J., and Gibson, S. B. (2008) Hypoxia induces autophagic cell death in apoptosis-competent cells through a mechanism involving BNIP3. *Autophagy 4*, 195–204.

18. Zhang, H., Bosch-Marce, M., Shimoda, L. A., Tan, Y. S., Baek, J. H., Wesley, J. B., Gonzalez, F. J., and Semenza, G. L. (2008) Mitochondrial autophagy is an HIF-1-dependent adaptive metabolic response to hypoxia. *J Biol Chem 283*, 10892–903.

19. Yen, W. L., and Klionsky, D. J. (2008) How to live long and prosper: autophagy, mitochondria, and aging. *Physiology (Bethesda) 23*, 248–262.

20. Mathew, R., Karantza-Wadsworth, V., and White, E. (2007) Role of autophagy in cancer. *Nat Rev Cancer 7*, 961–967.

21. Ceradini, D. J., Kulkarni, A. R., Callaghan, M. J., Tepper, O. M., Bastidas, N., Kleinman, M. E., Capla, J. M., Galiano, R. D., Levine, J. P., and Gurtner, G. C. (2004) Progenitor cell trafficking is regulated by hypoxic gradients through HIF-1 induction of SDF-1. *Nat Med 10*, 858–864.

22. Du, R., Lu, K. V., Petritsch, C., Liu, P., Ganss, R., Passegue, E., Song, H., Vandenberg, S., Johnson, R. S., Werb, Z., and Bergers, G. (2008) HIF1alpha induces the recruitment of bone marrow-derived vascular modulatory cells to regulate tumor angiogenesis and invasion. *Cancer Cell 13*, 206–220.

23. Sheng, H., Wang, Y., Jin, Y., Zhang, Q., Zhang, Y., Wang, L., Shen, B., Yin, S., Liu, W., Cui, L., and Li, N. (2008) A critical role of IFNgamma in priming MSC-mediated suppression of T cell proliferation through up-regulation of B7-H1. *Cell Res 18*, 846–857.

24. Sevick, E. M., and Jain, R. K. (1989) Viscous resistance to blood flow in solid tumors: effect of hematocrit on intratumor blood viscosity. *Cancer Res 49*, 3513–3519.

25. Sitkovsky, M., and Lukashev, D. (2005) Regulation of immune cells by local-tissue oxygen tension: HIF1 alpha and adenosine receptors. *Nat Rev Immunol 5*, 712–721.

26. Scortegagna, M., Martin, R. J., Kladney, R. D., Neumann, R. G., and Arbeit, J. M. (2009) Hypoxia-inducible factor-1alpha suppresses squamous carcinogenic progression and epithelial-mesenchymal transition. *Cancer Res 69*, 2638–2646.

27. Carmeliet, P. (2000) Mechanisms of angiogenesis and arteriogenesis. *Nat Med 6*, 389–395.

28. Helmlinger, G., Endo, M., Ferrara, N., Hlatky, L., and Jain, R. K. (2000) Formation of endothelial cell networks. *Nature 405*, 139–141.

29. Pepper, M. S. (1997) Transforming growth factor-beta: vasculogenesis, angiogenesis, and vessel wall integrity. *Cytokine Growth Factor Rev 8*, 21–43.

30. Suzuki, A., Kusakai, G., Shimojo, Y., Chen, J., Ogura, T., Kobayashi, M., and Esumi, H. (2005) Involvement of transforming growth factor-beta 1 signaling in hypoxia-induced tolerance to glucose starvation. *J Biol Chem 280*, 31557–31563.

31. Sanchez-Elsner, T., Botella, L. M., Velasco, B., Corbi, A., Attisano, L., and Bernabeu, C. (2001) Synergistic cooperation between hypoxia and transforming growth factor-beta pathways on human vascular endothelial growth factor gene expression. *J Biol Chem 276*, 38527–38535.

32. Bacac, M., and Stamenkovic, I. (2008) Metastatic cancer cell. *Annu Rev Pathol 3*, 221–247.

33. Esteban, M. A., Tran, M. G., Harten, S. K., Hill, P., Castellanos, M. C., Chandra, A., Raval, R., O'Brien T, S., and Maxwell, P. H. (2006) Regulation of E-cadherin expression by VHL and hypoxia-inducible factor. *Cancer Res 66*, 3567–3575.

34. Lash, G. E., Fitzpatrick, T. E., and Graham, C. H. (2001) Effect of hypoxia on cellular adhesion to vitronectin and fibronectin. *Biochem Biophys Res Commun 287*, 622–629.

35. Ide, T., Kitajima, Y., Miyoshi, A., Ohtsuka, T., Mitsuno, M., Ohtaka, K., and

Miyazaki, K. (2007) The hypoxic environment in tumor-stromal cells accelerates pancreatic cancer progression via the activation of paracrine hepatocyte growth factor/c-Met signaling. *Ann Surg Oncol 14*, 2600–2607.

36. Graeber, T. G., Osmanian, C., Jacks, T., Housman, D. E., Koch, C. J., Lowe, S. W., and Giaccia, A. J. (1996) Hypoxia-mediated selection of cells with diminished apoptotic potential in solid tumours. *Nature 379*, 88–91.

37. Vaupel, P., Mayer, A., and Hockel, M. (2004) Tumor hypoxia and malignant progression. *Methods Enzymol 381*, 335–354.

38. Vaupel, P., and Mayer, A. (2007) Hypoxia in cancer: significance and impact on clinical outcome. *Cancer Metastasis Rev 26*, 225–239.

39. Dong, Z., and Wang, J. (2004) Hypoxia selection of death-resistant cells. A role for Bcl-X(L). *J Biol Chem 279*, 9215–9221.

40. Bindra, R. S., and Glazer, P. M. (2007) Repression of RAD51 gene expression by E2F4/p130 complexes in hypoxia. *Oncogene 26*, 2048–2057.

41. Meng, A. X., Jalali, F., Cuddihy, A., Chan, N., Bindra, R. S., Glazer, P. M., and Bristow, R. G. (2005) Hypoxia down-regulates DNA double strand break repair gene expression in prostate cancer cells. *Radiother Oncol 76*, 168–176.

42. Bell, E. L., Klimova, T. A., Eisenbart, J., Schumacker, P. T., and Chandel, N. S. (2007) Mitochondrial reactive oxygen species trigger hypoxia-inducible factor-dependent extension of the replicative life span during hypoxia. *Mol Cell Biol 27*, 5737–5745.

43. Siemens, D. R., Hu, N., Sheikhi, A. K., Chung, E., Frederiksen, L. J., Pross, H., and Graham, C. H. (2008) Hypoxia increases tumor cell shedding of MHC class I chain-related molecule: role of nitric oxide. *Cancer Res 68*, 4746–4753.

44. Ohnishi, S., Yasuda, T., Kitamura, S., and Nagaya, N. (2007) Effect of hypoxia on gene expression of bone marrow-derived mesenchymal stem cells and mononuclear cells. *Stem Cells 25*, 1166–1177.

45. Bingle, L., Brown, N. J., and Lewis, C. E. (2002) The role of tumour-associated macrophages in tumour progression: implications for new anticancer therapies. *J Pathol 196*, 254–265.

46. Sica, A., Saccani, A., Bottazzi, B., Bernasconi, S., Allavena, P., Gaetano, B., Fei, F., LaRosa, G., Scotton, C., Balkwill, F., and Mantovani, A. (2000) Defective expression of the monocyte chemotactic protein-1 receptor CCR2 in macrophages associated with human ovarian carcinoma. *J Immunol 164*, 733–738.

47. Bosco, M. C., Reffo, G., Puppo, M., and Varesio, L. (2004) Hypoxia inhibits the expression of the CCR5 chemokine receptor in macrophages. *Cell Immunol 228*, 1–7.

48. Grimshaw, M. J., and Balkwill, F. R. (2001) Inhibition of monocyte and macrophage chemotaxis by hypoxia and inflammation--a potential mechanism. *Eur J Immunol 31*, 480–489.

49. Leeper-Woodford, S. K., and Mills, J. W. (1992) Phagocytosis and ATP levels in alveolar macrophages during acute hypoxia. *Am J Respir Cell Mol Biol 6*, 326–334.

50. Anand, R. J., Gribar, S. C., Li, J., Kohler, J. W., Branca, M. F., Dubowski, T., Sodhi, C. P., and Hackam, D. J. (2007) Hypoxia causes an increase in phagocytosis by macrophages in a HIF-1alpha-dependent manner. *J Leukoc Biol 82*, 1257–1265.

51. Lahat, N., Rahat, M. A., Ballan, M., Weiss-Cerem, L., Engelmayer, M., and Bitterman, H. (2003) Hypoxia reduces CD80 expression on monocytes but enhances their LPS-stimulated TNF-alpha secretion. *J Leukoc Biol 74*, 197–205.

52. Murata, Y., Ohteki, T., Koyasu, S., and Hamuro, J. (2002) IFN-gamma and pro-inflammatory cytokine production by antigen-presenting cells is dictated by intracellular thiol redox status regulated by oxygen tension. *Eur J Immunol 32*, 2866–2873.

53. Huang, C. J., Haque, I. U., Slovin, P. N., Nielsen, R. B., Fang, X., and Skimming, J. W. (2002) Environmental pH regulates LPS-induced nitric oxide formation in murine macrophages. *Nitric Oxide 6*, 73–78.

54. Murata, Y., Shimamura, T., and Hamuro, J. (2002) The polarization of T(h)1/T(h)2 balance is dependent on the intracellular thiol redox status of macrophages due to the distinctive cytokine production. *Int Immunol 14*, 201–212.

55. Onita, T., Ji, P. G., Xuan, J. W., Sakai, H., Kanetake, H., Maxwell, P. H., Fong, G. H., Gabril, M. Y., Moussa, M., and Chin, J. L. (2002) Hypoxia-induced, perinecrotic expression of endothelial Per-ARNT-Sim domain protein-1/hypoxia-inducible factor-2alpha correlates with tumor progression, vascularization, and

focal macrophage infiltration in bladder cancer. *Clin Cancer Res 8*, 471–480.

56. Koga, F., Kageyama, Y., Kawakami, S., Fujii, Y., Hyochi, N., Ando, N., Takizawa, T., Saito, K., Iwai, A., Masuda, H., and Kihara, K. (2004) Prognostic significance of endothelial Per-Arnt-sim domain protein 1/hypoxia-inducible factor-2alpha expression in a subset of tumor associated macrophages in invasive bladder cancer. *J Urol 171*, 1080–1084.

57. Burke, B., Giannoudis, A., Corke, K. P., Gill, D., Wells, M., Ziegler-Heitbrock, L., and Lewis, C. E. (2003) Hypoxia-induced gene expression in human macrophages: implications for ischemic tissues and hypoxia-regulated gene therapy. *Am J Pathol 163*, 1233–1243.

58. Yun, J. K., McCormick, T. S., Villabona, C., Judware, R. R., Espinosa, M. B., and Lapetina, E. G. (1997) Inflammatory mediators are perpetuated in macrophages resistant to apoptosis induced by hypoxia. *Proc Natl Acad Sci U S A 94*, 13903–13908.

59. Kuwabara, K., Ogawa, S., Matsumoto, M., Koga, S., Clauss, M., Pinsky, D. J., Lyn, P., Leavy, J., Witte, L., Joseph-Silverstein, J., and et al. (1995) Hypoxia-mediated induction of acidic/basic fibroblast growth factor and platelet-derived growth factor in mononuclear phagocytes stimulates growth of hypoxic endothelial cells. *Proc Natl Acad Sci U S A 92*, 4606–4610.

60. O'Sullivan, C., Lewis, C. E., Harris, A. L., and McGee, J. O. (1993) Secretion of epidermal growth factor by macrophages associated with breast carcinoma. *Lancet 342*, 148–149.

61. Leek, R. D., Hunt, N. C., Landers, R. J., Lewis, C. E., Royds, J. A., and Harris, A. L. (2000) Macrophage infiltration is associated with VEGF and EGFR expression in breast cancer. *J Pathol 190*, 430–436.

62. Sasaki, T., Nakamura, T., Rebhun, R. B., Cheng, H., Hale, K. S., Tsan, R. Z., Fidler, I. J., and Langley, R. R. (2008) Modification of the primary tumor microenvironment by transforming growth factor alpha-epidermal growth factor receptor signaling promotes metastasis in an orthotopic colon cancer model. *Am J Pathol 173*, 205–216.

63. Schmeisser, A., Marquetant, R., Illmer, T., Graffy, C., Garlichs, C. D., Bockler, D., Menschikowski, D., Braun–Dullaeus, R., Daniel, W. G., and Strasser, R. H. (2005) The expression of macrophage migration inhibitory factor 1alpha (MIF 1alpha) in human atherosclerotic plaques is induced by different proatherogenic stimuli and associated with plaque instability. *Atherosclerosis 178*, 83–94.

64. Compeau, C. G., Ma, J., DeCampos, K. N., Waddell, T. K., Brisseau, G. F., Slutsky, A. S., and Rotstein, O. D. (1994) In situ ischemia and hypoxia enhance alveolar macrophage tissue factor expression. *Am J Respir Cell Mol Biol 11*, 446–455.

65. Murdoch, C., Muthana, M., and Lewis, C. E. (2005) Hypoxia regulates macrophage functions in inflammation. *J Immunol 175*, 6257–6263.

66. Lewis, J. S., Landers, R. J., Underwood, J. C., Harris, A. L., and Lewis, C. E. (2000) Expression of vascular endothelial growth factor by macrophages is up-regulated in poorly vascularized areas of breast carcinomas. *J Pathol 192*, 150–158.

67. Harmey, J. H., Dimitriadis, E., Kay, E., Redmond, H. P., and Bouchier-Hayes, D. (1998) Regulation of macrophage production of vascular endothelial growth factor (VEGF) by hypoxia and transforming growth factor beta-1. *Ann Surg Oncol 5*, 271–278.

68. Mantovani, A., Schioppa, T., Porta, C., Allavena, P., and Sica, A. (2006) Role of tumor-associated macrophages in tumor progression and invasion. *Cancer Metastasis Rev 25*, 315–322.

69. Condeelis, J., and Pollard, J. W. (2006) Macrophages: obligate partners for tumor cell migration, invasion, and metastasis. *Cell 124*, 263–266.

70. Stojadinovic, A., Kiang, J., Smallridge, R., Galloway, R., and Shea-Donohue, T. (1995) Induction of heat-shock protein 72 protects against ischemia/reperfusion in rat small intestine. *Gastroenterology 109*, 505–515.

71. Colgan, S. P., Dzus, A. L., and Parkos, C. A. (1996) Epithelial exposure to hypoxia modulates neutrophil transepithelial migration. *J Exp Med 184*, 1003–1015.

72. Baggiolini, M. (1998) Chemokines and leukocyte traffic. *Nature 392*, 565–568.

73. Bosco, M. C., Puppo, M., Blengio, F., Fraone, T., Cappello, P., Giovarelli, M., and Varesio, L. (2008) Monocytes and dendritic cells in a hypoxic environment: Spotlights on chemotaxis and migration. *Immunobiology 213*, 733–749.

74. Mecklenburgh, K. I., Walmsley, S. R., Cowburn, A. S., Wiesener, M., Reed, B. J., Upton, P. D., Deighton, J., Greening, A. P., and Chilvers, E. R. (2002) Involvement of

a ferroprotein sensor in hypoxia-mediated inhibition of neutrophil apoptosis. *Blood* **100**, 3008–3016.

75. Walmsley, S. R., Print, C., Farahi, N., Peyssonnaux, C., Johnson, R. S., Cramer, T., Sobolewski, A., Condliffe, A. M., Cowburn, A. S., Johnson, N., and Chilvers, E. R. (2005) Hypoxia-induced neutrophil survival is mediated by HIF-1alpha-dependent NF-kappaB activity. *J Exp Med* **201**, 105–115.

76. Wood, J. G., Johnson, J. S., Mattioli, L. F., and Gonzalez, N. C. (1999) Systemic hypoxia promotes leukocyte-endothelial adherence via reactive oxidant generation. *J Appl Physiol* **87**, 1734–1740.

77. Ginis, I., Mentzer, S. J., and Faller, D. V. (1993) Oxygen tension regulates neutrophil adhesion to human endothelial cells via an LFA-1-dependent mechanism. *J Cell Physiol* **157**, 569–578.

78. Hannah, S., Mecklenburgh, K., Rahman, I., Bellingan, G. J., Greening, A., Haslett, C., and Chilvers, E. R. (1995) Hypoxia prolongs neutrophil survival in vitro. *FEBS Lett* **372**, 233–237.

79. Loeffler, D. A., Keng, P. C., Baggs, R. B., and Lord, E. M. (1990) Lymphocytic infiltration and cytotoxicity under hypoxic conditions in the EMT6 mouse mammary tumor. *Int J Cancer* **45**, 462–467.

80. Allen, D. B., Maguire, J. J., Mahdavian, M., Wicke, C., Marcocci, L., Scheuenstuhl, H., Chang, M., Le, A. X., Hopf, H. W., and Hunt, T. K. (1997) Wound hypoxia and acidosis limit neutrophil bacterial killing mechanisms. *Arch Surg* **132**, 991–996.

81. Araki, A., Inoue, T., Cragoe, E. J., Jr., and Sendo, F. (1991) Na+/H+ exchange modulates rat neutrophil mediated tumor cytotoxicity. *Cancer Res* **51**, 3212–3216.

82. Rotstein, O. D., Fiegel, V. D., Simmons, R. L., and Knighton, D. R. (1988) The deleterious effect of reduced pH and hypoxia on neutrophil migration in vitro. *J Surg Res* **45**, 298–303.

83. Martinez, D., Vermeulen, M., Trevani, A., Ceballos, A., Sabatte, J., Gamberale, R., Alvarez, M. E., Salamone, G., Tanos, T., Coso, O. A., and Geffner, J. (2006) Extracellular acidosis induces neutrophil activation by a mechanism dependent on activation of phosphatidylinositol 3-kinase/Akt and ERK pathways. *J Immunol* **176**, 1163–1171.

84. Qutub, A. A., and Popel, A. S. (2008) Reactive oxygen species regulate hypoxia-inducible factor 1alpha differentially in cancer and ischemia. *Mol Cell Biol* **28**, 5106–5119.

85. Gronert, K., Colgan, S. P., and Serhan, C. N. (1998) Characterization of human neutrophil and endothelial cell ligand-operated extracellular acidification rate by microphysiometry: impact of reoxygenation. *J Pharmacol Exp Ther* **285**, 252–261.

86. Eltzschig, H. K., Thompson, L. F., Karhausen, J., Cotta, R. J., Ibla, J. C., Robson, S. C., and Colgan, S. P. (2004) Endogenous adenosine produced during hypoxia attenuates neutrophil accumulation: coordination by extracellular nucleotide metabolism. *Blood* **104**, 3986–3992.

87. Eltzschig, H. K., Eckle, T., Mager, A., Kuper, N., Karcher, C., Weissmuller, T., Boengler, K., Schulz, R., Robson, S. C., and Colgan, S. P. (2006) ATP release from activated neutrophils occurs via connexin 43 and modulates adenosine-dependent endothelial cell function. *Circ Res* **99**, 1100–1108.

88. Rosenberger, P., Schwab, J. M., Mirakaj, V., Masekowsky, E., Mager, A., Morote-Garcia, J. C., Unertl, K., and Eltzschig, H. K. (2009) Hypoxia-inducible factor-dependent induction of netrin-1 dampens inflammation caused by hypoxia. *Nat Immunol* **10**, 195–202.

89. Ly, N. P., Komatsuzaki, K., Fraser, I. P., Tseng, A. A., Prodhan, P., Moore, K. J., and Kinane, T. B. (2005) Netrin-1 inhibits leukocyte migration in vitro and in vivo. *Proc Natl Acad Sci U S A* **102**, 14729–14734.

90. Welbourn, C. R., Goldman, G., Paterson, I. S., Valeri, C. R., Shepro, D., and Hechtman, H. B. (1991) Pathophysiology of ischaemia reperfusion injury: central role of the neutrophil. *Br J Surg* **78**, 651–655.

91. Nagorsen, D., Voigt, S., Berg, E., Stein, H., Thiel, E., and Loddenkemper, C. (2007) Tumor-infiltrating macrophages and dendritic cells in human colorectal cancer: relation to local regulatory T cells, systemic T-cell response against tumor-associated antigens and survival. *J Transl Med* **5**, 62.

92. Ohm, J. E., Shurin, M. R., Esche, C., Lotze, M. T., Carbone, D. P., and Gabrilovich, D. I. (1999) Effect of vascular endothelial growth factor and FLT3 ligand on dendritic cell generation in vivo. *J Immunol* **163**, 3260–3268.

93. Oyama, T., Ran, S., Ishida, T., Nadaf, S., Kerr, L., Carbone, D. P., and Gabrilovich, D. I. (1998) Vascular endothelial growth

factor affects dendritic cell maturation through the inhibition of nuclear factor-kappa B activation in hemopoietic progenitor cells. *J Immunol 160*, 1224–1232.

94. Ohm, J. E., and Carbone, D. P. (2001) VEGF as a mediator of tumor-associated immunodeficiency. *Immunol Res 23*, 263–272.

95. Jantsch, J., Chakravortty, D., Turza, N., Prechtel, A. T., Buchholz, B., Gerlach, R. G., Volke, M., Glasner, J., Warnecke, C., Wiesener, M. S., Eckardt, K. U., Steinkasserer, A., Hensel, M., and Willam, C. (2008) Hypoxia and hypoxia-inducible factor-1 alpha modulate lipopolysaccharide-induced dendritic cell activation and function. *J Immunol 180*, 4697–705.

96. Elia, A. R., Cappello, P., Puppo, M., Fraone, T., Vanni, C., Eva, A., Musso, T., Novelli, F., Varesio, L., and Giovarelli, M. (2008) Human dendritic cells differentiated in hypoxia down-modulate antigen uptake and change their chemokine expression profile. *J Leukoc Biol 84*, 1472–1482.

97. Adema, G. J., Hartgers, F., Verstraten, R., de Vries, E., Marland, G., Menon, S., Foster, J., Xu, Y., Nooyen, P., McClanahan, T., Bacon, K. B., and Figdor, C. G. (1997) A dendritic-cell-derived C-C chemokine that preferentially attracts naive T cells. *Nature 387*, 713–717.

98. Vulcano, M., Struyf, S., Scapini, P., Cassatella, M., Bernasconi, S., Bonecchi, R., Calleri, A., Penna, G., Adorini, L., Luini, W., Mantovani, A., Van Damme, J., and Sozzani, S. (2003) Unique regulation of CCL18 production by maturing dendritic cells. *J Immunol 170*, 3843–3849.

99. Carr, M. W., Roth, S. J., Luther, E., Rose, S. S., and Springer, T. A. (1994) Monocyte chemoattractant protein 1 acts as a T-lymphocyte chemoattractant. *Proc Natl Acad Sci U S A 91*, 3652–3656.

100. Angiolillo, A. L., Sgadari, C., Taub, D. D., Liao, F., Farber, J. M., Maheshwari, S., Kleinman, H. K., Reaman, G. H., and Tosato, G. (1995) Human interferon-inducible protein 10 is a potent inhibitor of angiogenesis in vivo. *J Exp Med 182*, 155–162.

101. Zhao, P., Li, X. G., Yang, M., Shao, Q., Wang, D., Liu, S., Song, H., Song, B., Zhang, Y., and Qu, X. (2008) Hypoxia suppresses the production of MMP-9 by human monocyte-derived dendritic cells and requires activation of adenosine receptor A2b via cAMP/PKA signaling pathway. *Mol Immunol 45*, 2187–2195.

102. Qu, X., Yang, M. X., Kong, B. H., Qi, L., Lam, Q. L., Yan, S., Li, P., Zhang, M., and Lu, L. (2005) Hypoxia inhibits the migratory capacity of human monocyte-derived dendritic cells. *Immunol Cell Biol 83*, 668–673.

103. Zhao, W., Darmanin, S., Fu, Q., Chen, J., Cui, H., Wang, J., Okada, F., Hamada, J., Hattori, Y., Kondo, T., Hamuro, J., Asaka, M., and Kobayashi, M. (2005) Hypoxia suppresses the production of matrix metalloproteinases and the migration of human monocyte-derived dendritic cells. *Eur J Immunol 35*, 3468–3477.

104. Mancino, A., Schioppa, T., Larghi, P., Pasqualini, F., Nebuloni, M., Chen, I. H., Sozzani, S., Austyn, J. M., Mantovani, A., and Sica, A. (2008) Divergent effects of hypoxia on dendritic cell functions. *Blood 112*, 3723–3734.

105. Gottfried, E., Kunz-Schughart, L. A., Ebner, S., Mueller-Klieser, W., Hoves, S., Andreesen, R., Mackensen, A., and Kreutz, M. (2006) Tumor-derived lactic acid modulates dendritic cell activation and antigen expression. *Blood 107*, 2013–2021.

106. Panther, E., Corinti, S., Idzko, M., Herouy, Y., Napp, M., la Sala, A., Girolomoni, G., and Norgauer, J. (2003) Adenosine affects expression of membrane molecules, cytokine and chemokine release, and the T-cell stimulatory capacity of human dendritic cells. *Blood 101*, 3985–3990.

107. Panther, E., Idzko, M., Herouy, Y., Rheinen, H., Gebicke-Haerter, P. J., Mrowietz, U., Dichmann, S., and Norgauer, J. (2001) Expression and function of adenosine receptors in human dendritic cells. *Faseb J 15*, 1963–1970.

108. Chen, L., Fredholm, B. B., and Jondal, M. (2008) Adenosine, through the A1 receptor, inhibits vesicular MHC class I cross-presentation by resting DC. *Mol Immunol 45*, 2247–2254.

109. Ricciardi, A., Elia, A. R., Cappello, P., Puppo, M., Vanni, C., Fardin, P., Eva, A., Munroe, D., Wu, X., Giovarelli, M., and Varesio, L. (2008) Transcriptome of hypoxic immature dendritic cells: modulation of chemokine/receptor expression. *Mol Cancer Res 6*, 175–185.

110. Vermeulen, M., Giordano, M., Trevani, A. S., Sedlik, C., Gamberale, R., Fernandez-Calotti, P., Salamone, G., Raiden, S., Sanjurjo, J., and Geffner, J. R. (2004) Acidosis improves uptake of antigens and MHC class I-restricted presentation by dendritic cells. *J Immunol 172*, 3196–3204.

111. Makino, Y., Nakamura, H., Ikeda, E., Ohnuma, K., Yamauchi, K., Yabe, Y., Poellinger, L., Okada, Y., Morimoto, C., and Tanaka, H. (2003) Hypoxia–inducible factor regulates survival of antigen receptor-driven T cells. *J Immunol* 171, 6534–6540.

112. Biju, M. P., Neumann, A. K., Bensinger, S. J., Johnson, R. S., Turka, L. A., and Haase, V. H. (2004) Vhlh gene deletion induces Hif-1-mediated cell death in thymocytes. *Mol Cell Biol* 24, 9038–9047.

113. Sitkovsky, M. V., Kjaergaard, J., Lukashev, D., and Ohta, A. (2008) Hypoxia-adenosinergic immunosuppression: tumor protection by T regulatory cells and cancerous tissue hypoxia. *Clin Cancer Res* 14, 5947–5952.

114. Atkuri, K. R., Herzenberg, L. A., and Herzenberg, L. A. (2005) Culturing at atmospheric oxygen levels impacts lymphocyte function. *Proc Natl Acad Sci U S A* 102, 3756–3759.

115. Conforti, L., Petrovic, M., Mohammad, D., Lee, S., Ma, Q., Barone, S., and Filipovich, A. H. (2003) Hypoxia regulates expression and activity of Kv1.3 channels in T lymphocytes: a possible role in T cell proliferation. *J Immunol* 170, 695–702.

116. Caldwell, C. C., Kojima, H., Lukashev, D., Armstrong, J., Farber, M., Apasov, S. G., and Sitkovsky, M. V. (2001) Differential effects of physiologically relevant hypoxic conditions on T lymphocyte development and effector functions. *J Immunol* 167, 6140–6149.

117. Neumann, A. K., Yang, J., Biju, M. P., Joseph, S. K., Johnson, R. S., Haase, V. H., Freedman, B. D., and Turka, L. A. (2005) Hypoxia inducible factor 1 alpha regulates T cell receptor signal transduction. *Proc Natl Acad Sci U S A* 102, 17071–17076.

118. Chandy, K. G., DeCoursey, T. E., Cahalan, M. D., McLaughlin, C., and Gupta, S. (1984) Voltage-gated potassium channels are required for human T lymphocyte activation. *J Exp Med* 160, 369–385.

119. Zuckerberg, A. L., Goldberg, L. I., and Lederman, H. M. (1994) Effects of hypoxia on interleukin-2 mRNA expression by T lymphocytes. *Crit Care Med* 22, 197–203.

120. Naldini, A., Carraro, F., Silvestri, S., and Bocci, V. (1997) Hypoxia affects cytokine production and proliferative responses by human peripheral mononuclear cells. *J Cell Physiol* 173, 335–342.

121. Kim, H., Peng, G., Hicks, J. M., Weiss, H. L., Van Meir, E. G., Brenner, M. K., and Yotnda, P. (2008) Engineering human tumor-specific cytotoxic T cells to function in a hypoxic environment. *Mol Ther* 16, 599–606.

122. Carraro, F., Pucci, A., Pellegrini, M., Pelicci, P. G., Baldari, C. T., and Naldini, A. (2007) p66Shc is involved in promoting HIF-1alpha accumulation and cell death in hypoxic T cells. *J Cell Physiol* 211, 439–447.

123. Kiang, J. G., Krishnan, S., Lu, X., and Li, Y. (2008) Inhibition of inducible nitric-oxide synthase protects human T cells from hypoxia-induced apoptosis. *Mol Pharmacol* 73, 738–747.

124. Heinzman, J. M., Brower, S. L., and Bush, J. E. (2008) Comparison of angiogenesis-related factor expression in primary tumor cultures under normal and hypoxic growth conditions. *Cancer Cell Int* 8, 11.

125. Lukashev, D., Klebanov, B., Kojima, H., Grinberg, A., Ohta, A., Berenfeld, L., Wenger, R. H., Ohta, A., and Sitkovsky, M. (2006) Cutting edge: hypoxia-inducible factor 1alpha and its activation-inducible short isoform I.1 negatively regulate functions of CD4+ and CD8+ T lymphocytes. *J Immunol* 177, 4962–4965.

126. Fischer, K., Hoffmann, P., Voelkl, S., Meidenbauer, N., Ammer, J., Edinger, M., Gottfried, E., Schwarz, S., Rothe, G., Hoves, S., Renner, K., Timischl, B., Mackensen, A., Kunz-Schughart, L., Andreesen, R., Krause, S. W., and Kreutz, M. (2007) Inhibitory effect of tumor cell-derived lactic acid on human T cells. *Blood* 109, 3812–3819.

127. Loeffler, D. A., Juneau, P. L., and Masserant, S. (1992) Influence of tumour physico-chemical conditions on interleukin-2-stimulated lymphocyte proliferation. *Br J Cancer* 66, 619–622.

128. Loeffler, D. A., Juneau, P. L., and Heppner, G. H. (1991) Natural killer-cell activity under conditions reflective of tumor microenvironment. *Int J Cancer* 48, 895–899.

129. Severin, T., Muller, B., Giese, G., Uhl, B., Wolf, B., Hauschildt, S., and Kreutz, W. (1994) pH-dependent LAK cell cytotoxicity. *Tumour Biol* 15, 304–310.

130. Muller, B., Fischer, B., and Kreutz, W. (2000) An acidic microenvironment impairs the generation of non-major histocompatibility complex-restricted killer cells. *Immunology* 99, 375–384.

131. Fischer, B., Muller, B., Fisch, P., and Kreutz, W. (2000) An acidic microenvironment inhibits antitumoral non-major histocompatibility complex-restricted cytotoxicity: implications for cancer immunotherapy. *J Immunother* 23, 196–207.

132. Valko, M., Izakovic, M., Mazur, M., Rhodes, C. J., and Telser, J. (2004) Role of oxygen radicals in DNA damage and cancer incidence. *Mol Cell Biochem* **266**, 37–56.

133. Allan, I. M., Lunec, J., Salmon, M., and Bacon, P. A. (1987) Reactive oxygen species selectively deplete normal T lymphocytes via a hydroxyl radical dependent mechanism. *Scand J Immunol* **26**, 47–53.

134. Hildeman, D. A. (2004) Regulation of T-cell apoptosis by reactive oxygen species. *Free Radic Biol Med* **36**, 1496–1504.

135. Kwon, J., Devadas, S., and Williams, M. S. (2003) T cell receptor-stimulated generation of hydrogen peroxide inhibits MEK-ERK activation and lck serine phosphorylation. *Free Radic Biol Med* **35**, 406–417.

136. Jackson, S. H., Devadas, S., Kwon, J., Pinto, L. A., and Williams, M. S. (2004) T cells express a phagocyte-type NADPH oxidase that is activated after T cell receptor stimulation. *Nat Immunol* **5**, 818–827.

137. Cauley, L. S., Miller, E. E., Yen, M., and Swain, S. L. (2000) Superantigen-induced CD4 T cell tolerance mediated by myeloid cells and IFN-gamma. *J Immunol* **165**, 6056–6066.

138. Hansson, M., Romero, A., Thoren, F., Hermodsson, S., and Hellstrand, K. (2004) Activation of cytotoxic lymphocytes by interferon-alpha: role of oxygen radical-producing mononuclear phagocytes. *J Leukoc Biol* **76**, 1207–1213.

139. Schmielau, J., and Finn, O. J. (2001) Activated granulocytes and granulocyte-derived hydrogen peroxide are the underlying mechanism of suppression of t-cell function in advanced cancer patients. *Cancer Res* **61**, 4756–4760.

140. Fulton, A. M., and Chong, Y. C. (1992) The role of macrophage-derived TNFa in the induction of sublethal tumor cell DNA damage. *Carcinogenesis* **13**, 77–81.

141. Nambiar, M. P., Fisher, C. U., Enyedy, E. J., Warke, V. G., Kumar, A., and Tsokos, G. C. (2002) Oxidative stress is involved in the heat stress-induced downregulation of TCR zeta chain expression and TCR/CD3-mediated [Ca(2+)](i) response in human T-lymphocytes. *Cell Immunol* **215**, 151–161.

142. Nindl, G., Peterson, N. R., Hughes, E. F., Waite, L. R., and Johnson, M. T. (2004) Effect of hydrogen peroxide on proliferation, apoptosis and interleukin-2 production of Jurkat T cells. *Biomed Sci Instrum* **40**, 123–128.

143. Gringhuis, S. I., Papendrecht-van der Voort, E. A., Leow, A., Nivine Levarht, E.

W., Breedveld, F. C., and Verweij, C. L. (2002) Effect of redox balance alterations on cellular localization of LAT and downstream T-cell receptor signaling pathways. *Mol Cell Biol* **22**, 400–411.

144. Takahashi, A., Hanson, M. G., Norell, H. R., Havelka, A. M., Kono, K., Malmberg, K. J., and Kiessling, R. V. (2005) Preferential cell death of CD8+ effector memory (CCR7-CD45RA-) T cells by hydrogen peroxide-induced oxidative stress. *J Immunol* **174**, 6080–6087.

145. Huang, S., Apasov, S., Koshiba, M., and Sitkovsky, M. (1997) Role of A2a extracellular adenosine receptor-mediated signaling in adenosine-mediated inhibition of T-cell activation and expansion. *Blood* **90**, 1600–1610.

146. Hoskin, D. W., Mader, J. S., Furlong, S. J., Conrad, D. M., and Blay, J. (2008) Inhibition of T cell and natural killer cell function by adenosine and its contribution to immune evasion by tumor cells (Review). *Int J Oncol* **32**, 527–535.

147. Ohta, A., Gorelik, E., Prasad, S. J., Ronchese, F., Lukashev, D., Wong, M. K., Huang, X., Caldwell, S., Liu, K., Smith, P., Chen, J. F., Jackson, E. K., Apasov, S., Abrams, S., and Sitkovsky, M. (2006) A2A adenosine receptor protects tumors from antitumor T cells. *Proc Natl Acad Sci U S A* **103**, 13132–13137.

148. Sitkovsky, M. V., and Ohta, A. (2005) The 'danger' sensors that STOP the immune response: the A2 adenosine receptors? *Trends Immunol* **26**, 299–304.

149. Ohta, A., Kjaergaard, J., Sharma, S., Mohsin, M., Goel, N., Madasu, M., Fradkov, E., Ohta, A., and Sitkovsky, M. (2009) In vitro induction of T cells that are resistant to A2 adenosine receptor-mediated immunosuppression. *Br J Pharmacol* **156**, 297–306.

150. Raskovalova, T., Huang, X., Sitkovsky, M., Zacharia, L. C., Jackson, E. K., and Gorelik, E. (2005) Gs protein-coupled adenosine receptor signaling and lytic function of activated NK cells. *J Immunol* **175**, 4383–4391.

151. Lokshin, A., Raskovalova, T., Huang, X., Zacharia, L. C., Jackson, E. K., and Gorelik, E. (2006) Adenosine-mediated inhibition of the cytotoxic activity and cytokine production by activated natural killer cells. *Cancer Res* **66**, 7758–7765.

152. Raskovalova, T., Lokshin, A., Huang, X., Jackson, E. K., and Gorelik, E. (2006) Adenosine-mediated inhibition of cytotoxic activity and cytokine production by IL-2/

NKp46-activated NK cells: involvement of protein kinase A isozyme I (PKA I). *Immunol Res 36*, 91–99.

153. Sitkovsky, M. V. (2009) T regulatory cells: hypoxia-adenosinergic suppression and re-direction of the immune response. *Trends Immunol 30*, 102–108.

154. Ben-Shoshan, J., Maysel-Auslender, S., Mor, A., Keren, G., and George, J. (2008) Hypoxia controls CD4+CD25+ regulatory T-cell homeostasis via hypoxia-inducible factor-1alpha. *Eur J Immunol 38*, 2412–2418.

155. Eltzschig, H. K., Ibla, J. C., Furuta, G. T., Leonard, M. O., Jacobson, K. A., Enjyoji, K., Robson, S. C., and Colgan, S. P. (2003) Coordinated adenine nucleotide phospho-hydrolysis and nucleoside signaling in posthypoxic endothelium: role of ectonu-cleotidases and adenosine A2B receptors. *J Exp Med 198*, 783–796.

156. Mrena, J., Wiksten, J. P., Thiel, A., Kokkola, A., Pohjola, L., Lundin, J., Nordling, S., Ristimaki, A., and Haglund, C. (2005) Cyclooxygenase-2 is an indepen-dent prognostic factor in gastric cancer and its expression is regulated by the messenger RNA stability factor HuR. *Clin Cancer Res 11*, 7362–7368.

157. Su, Y., Huang, X., Raskovalova, T., Zacharia, L., Lokshin, A., Jackson, E., and Gorelik, E. (2008) Cooperation of adenosine and prostaglandin E2 (PGE2) in amplification of cAMP-PKA signaling and immunosuppression. *Cancer Immunol Immunother 57*, 1611–1623.

158. Kundu, N., Walser, T. C., Ma, X., and Fulton, A. M. (2005) Cyclooxygenase inhibitors modulate NK activities that con-trol metastatic disease. *Cancer Immunol Immunother 54*, 981–987.

159. Kojima, H., Gu, H., Nomura, S., Cald-well, C. C., Kobata, T., Carmeliet, P., Semenza, G. L., and Sitkovsky, M. V. (2002) Abnormal B lymphocyte devel-opment and autoimmunity in hypoxia-inducible factor 1alpha -deficient chimeric mice. *Proc Natl Acad Sci U S A 99*, 2170–2174.

160. Kojima, H., Jones, B. T., Chen, J., Cascalho, M., and Sitkovsky, M. V. (2004) Hypoxia-inducible factor 1alpha-deficient chimeric mice as a model to study abnormal B lymphocyte development and autoimmunity. *Methods Enzymol 381*, 218–229.

161. Piovan, E., Tosello, V., Indraccolo, S., Masiero, M., Persano, L., Esposito, G., Zamarchi, R., Ponzoni, M., Chieco-Bianchi, L., Dalla-Favera, R., and Amadori, A. (2007) Differential regulation of hypoxia-induced CXCR4 triggering during B-cell development and lymphomagenesis. *Cancer Res 67*, 8605–8614.

162. Goda, N., Ryan, H. E., Khadivi, B., McNulty, W., Rickert, R. C., and John-son, R. S. (2003) Hypoxia-inducible factor 1alpha is essential for cell cycle arrest during hypoxia. *Mol Cell Biol 23*, 359–369.

163. Hockel, M., and Vaupel, P. (2001) Tumor hypoxia: definitions and current clinical, biologic, and molecular aspects. *J Natl Cancer Inst 93*, 266–276.

164. Isa, A. Y., Ward, T. H., West, C. M., Slevin, N. J., and Homer, J. J. (2006) Hypoxia in head and neck cancer. *Br J Radiol 79*, 791–798.

165. Albertoni, M., Shaw, P. H., Nozaki, M., Godard, S., Tenan, M., Hamou, M. F., Fair-lie, D. W., Breit, S. N., Paralkar, V. M., de Tribolet, N., Van Meir, E. G., and Hegi, M. E. (2002) Anoxia induces macrophage inhibitory cytokine-1 (MIC-1) in glioblas-toma cells independently of p53 and HIF-1. *Oncogene 21*, 4212–4219.

166. Erler, J. T., Cawthorne, C. J., Williams, K. J., Koritzinsky, M., Wouters, B. G., Wil-son, C., Miller, C., Demonacos, C., Strat-ford, I. J., and Dive, C. (2004) Hypoxia-mediated down-regulation of Bid and Bax in tumors occurs via hypoxia-inducible fac-tor 1-dependent and -independent mech-anisms and contributes to drug resistance. *Mol Cell Biol 24*, 2875–2889.

167. Comerford, K. M., Wallace, T. J., Karhausen, J., Louis, N. A., Montalto, M. C., and Colgan, S. P. (2002) Hypoxia-inducible factor-1-dependent regulation of the multidrug resistance (MDR1) gene. *Cancer Res 62*, 3387–3394.

168. Reichert, M., Steinbach, J. P., Supra, P., and Weller, M. (2002) Modulation of growth and radiochemosensitivity of human malig-nant glioma cells by acidosis. *Cancer 95*, 1113–1119.

169. Le, Q. T., Taira, A., Budenz, S., Jo Dorie, M., Goffinet, D. R., Fee, W. E., Goode, R., Bloch, D., Koong, A., Martin Brown, J., and Pinto, H. A. (2006) Mature results from a randomized Phase II trial of cis-platin plus 5-fluorouracil and radiotherapy with or without tirapazamine in patients with resectable Stage IV head and neck squamous cell carcinomas. *Cancer 106*, 1940–1949.

170. Steward, W. P., Middleton, M., Benghiat, A., Loadman, P. M., Hayward, C., Waller, S., Ford, S., Halbert, G., Patterson, L. H.,

and Talbot, D. (2007) The use of pharmacokinetic and pharmacodynamic end points to determine the dose of AQ4N, a novel hypoxic cell cytotoxin, given with fractionated radiotherapy in a phase I study. *Ann Oncol* **18**, 1098–1103.

171. Albertella, M. R., Loadman, P. M., Jones, P. H., Phillips, R. M., Rampling, R., Burnet, N., Alcock, C., Anthoney, A., Vjaters, E., Dunk, C. R., Harris, P. A., Wong, A., Lalani, A. S., and Twelves, C. J. (2008) Hypoxia-selective targeting by the bioreductive prodrug AQ4N in patients with solid tumors: results of a phase I study. *Clin Cancer Res* **14**, 1096–1104.

172. Puppo, M., Battaglia, F., Ottaviano, C., Delfino, S., Ribatti, D., Varesio, L., and Bosco, M. C. (2008) Topotecan inhibits vascular endothelial growth factor production and angiogenic activity induced by hypoxia in human neuroblastoma by targeting hypoxia-inducible factor-1alpha and -2alpha. *Mol Cancer Ther* **7**, 1974–1984.

173. Shin, D. H., Chun, Y. S., Lee, D. S., Huang, L. E., and Park, J. W. (2008) Bortezomib inhibits tumor adaptation to hypoxia by stimulating the FIH-mediated repression of hypoxia-inducible factor-1. *Blood* **111**, 3131–3136.

174. Hirst, D. G. (1986) Anemia: a problem or an opportunity in radiotherapy? *Int J Radiat Oncol Biol Phys* **12**, 2009–2017.

175. Bokemeyer, C., Aapro, M. S., Courdi, A., Foubert, J., Link, H., Osterborg, A., Repetto, L., and Soubeyran, P. (2007) EORTC guidelines for the use of erythropoietic proteins in anaemic patients with cancer: 2006 update. *Eur J Cancer* **43**, 258–270.

176. Frederiksen, L. J., Sullivan, R., Maxwell, L. R., Macdonald-Goodfellow, S. K., Adams, M. A., Bennett, B. M., Siemens, D. R., and Graham, C. H. (2007) Chemosensitization of cancer in vitro and in vivo by nitric oxide signaling. *Clin Cancer Res* **13**, 2199–2206.

177. Thomas, G. V., Tran, C., Mellinghoff, I. K., Welsbie, D. S., Chan, E., Fueger, B., Czernin, J., and Sawyers, C. L. (2006) Hypoxia-inducible factor determines sensitivity to inhibitors of mTOR in kidney cancer. *Nat Med* **12**, 122–127.

178. Taghian, A. G., Abi-Raad, R., Assaad, S. I., Casty, A., Ancukiewicz, M., Yeh, E., Molokhia, P., Attia, K., Sullivan, T., Kuter, I., Boucher, Y., and Powell, S. N. (2005) Paclitaxel decreases the interstitial fluid pressure and improves oxygenation in breast cancers in patients treated with neoadjuvant chemotherapy: clinical implications. *J Clin Oncol* **23**, 1951–1961.

179. Overgaard, J., Hansen, H. S., Overgaard, M., Bastholt, L., Berthelsen, A., Specht, L., Lindelov, B., and Jorgensen, K. (1998) A randomized double-blind phase III study of nimorazole as a hypoxic radiosensitizer of primary radiotherapy in supraglottic larynx and pharynx carcinoma. Results of the Danish Head and Neck Cancer Study (DAHANCA) Protocol 5-85. *Radiother Oncol* **46**, 135–146.

180. Overgaard, J., Eriksen, J. G., Nordsmark, M., Alsner, J., and Horsman, M. R. (2005) Plasma osteopontin, hypoxia, and response to the hypoxia sensitiser nimorazole in radiotherapy of head and neck cancer: results from the DAHANCA 5 randomised double-blind placebo-controlled trial. *Lancet Oncol* **6**, 757–764.

181. Overgaard, J. (1994) Clinical evaluation of nitroimidazoles as modifiers of hypoxia in solid tumors. *Oncol Res* **6**, 509–518.

182. van Laarhoven, H. W., Kaanders, J. H., Lok, J., Peeters, W. J., Rijken, P. F., Wiering, B., Ruers, T. J., Punt, C. J., Heerschap, A., and van der Kogel, A. J. (2006) Hypoxia in relation to vasculature and proliferation in liver metastases in patients with colorectal cancer. *Int J Radiat Oncol Biol Phys* **64**, 473–482.

183. Hoogsteen, I. J., Pop, L. A., Marres, H. A., Merkx, M. A., van den Hoogen, F. J., van der Kogel, A. J., and Kaanders, J. H. (2006) Oxygen-modifying treatment with ARCON reduces the prognostic significance of hemoglobin in squamous cell carcinoma of the head and neck. *Int J Radiat Oncol Biol Phys* **64**, 83–89.

184. Bernier, J., Denekamp, J., Rojas, A., Minatel, E., Horiot, J., Hamers, H., Antognoni, P., Dahl, O., Richaud, P., van Glabbeke, M., and Pierart, M. (2000) ARCON: accelerated radiotherapy with carbogen and nicotinamide in head and neck squamous cell carcinomas. The experience of the Co-operative group of radiotherapy of the european organization for research and treatment of cancer (EORTC). *Radiother Oncol* **55**, 111–119.

185. Miyake, K., Shimada, M., Nishioka, M., Sugimoto, K., Batmunkh, E., Uto, Y., Nagasawa, H., and Hori, H. (2008) The novel hypoxic cell radiosensitizer, TX-1877 has antitumor activity through suppression of angiogenesis and inhibits liver metastasis on xenograft model of pancreatic cancer. *Cancer Lett* **272**, 325–335.

186. Oshikawa, T., Okamoto, M., Ahmed, S. U., Furuichi, S., Tano, T., Sasai, A., Kan, S., Kasai, S., Uto, Y., Nagasawa, H., Hori, H., and Sato, M. (2005) TX-1877, a bifunctional hypoxic cell radiosensitizer, enhances anticancer host response: immune cell migration and nitric oxide production. *Int J Cancer* 116, 571–578.

187. De Ridder, M., Jiang, H., Van Esch, G., Law, K., Monsaert, C., Van den Berge, D. L., Verellen, D., Verovski, V. N., and Storme, G. A. (2008) IFN-gamma+ CD8+ T lymphocytes: possible link between immune and radiation responses in tumor-relevant hypoxia. *Int J Radiat Oncol Biol Phys* 71, 647–651.

188. Janssens, M. Y., Van den Berge, D. L., Verovski, V. N., Monsaert, C., and Storme, G. A. (1998) Activation of inducible nitric oxide synthase results in nitric oxide-mediated radiosensitization of hypoxic EMT-6 tumor cells. *Cancer Res* 58, 5646–5648.

189. Wilson, W. R., Tercel, M., Anderson, R. F., and Denny, W. A. (1998) Radiation-activated prodrugs as hypoxia-selective cytotoxins: model studies with nitroarylmethyl quaternary salts. *Anticancer Drug Des* 13, 663–685.

190. Kriste, A. G., Tercel, M., Anderson, R. F., Ferry, D. M., and Wilson, W. R. (2002) Pathways of reductive fragmentation of heterocyclic nitroarylmethyl quaternary ammonium prodrugs of mechlorethamine. *Radiat Res* 158, 753–762.

191. Suh, J. H., Stea, B., Nabid, A., Kresl, J. J., Fortin, A., Mercier, J. P., Senzer, N., Chang, E. L., Boyd, A. P., Cagnoni, P. J., and Shaw, E. (2006) Phase III study of efaproxiral as an adjunct to whole-brain radiation therapy for brain metastases. *J Clin Oncol* 24, 106–114.

192. Mayer, R., Hamilton-Farrell, M. R., van der Kleij, A. J., Schmutz, J., Granstrom, G., Sicko, Z., Melamed, Y., Carl, U. M., Hartmann, K. A., Jansen, E. C., Ditri, L., and Sminia, P. (2005) Hyperbaric oxygen and radiotherapy. *Strahlenther Onkol* 181, 113–123.

193. Bennett, M., Feldmeier, J., Smee, R., and Milross, C. (2008) Hyperbaric oxygenation for tumour sensitisation to radiotherapy: a systematic review of randomised controlled trials. *Cancer Treat Rev* 34, 577–591.

194. Zaffaroni, N., Fiorentini, G., and De Giorgi, U. (2001) Hyperthermia and hypoxia: new developments in anticancer chemotherapy. *Eur J Surg Oncol* 27, 340–342.

195. Kuemmerle, A., Decosterd, L. A., Buclin, T., Lienard, D., Stupp, R., Chassot, P. G., Mosimann, F., and Lejeune, F. (2009) A phase I pharmacokinetic study of hypoxic abdominal stop-flow perfusion with gemcitabine in patients with advanced pancreatic cancer and refractory malignant ascites. *Cancer Chemother Pharmacol* 63, 331–341.

196. Trinh, Q. T., Austin, E. A., Murray, D. M., Knick, V. C., and Huber, B. E. (1995) Enzyme/prodrug gene therapy: comparison of cytosine deaminase/5-fluorocytosine versus thymidine kinase/ganciclovir enzyme/prodrug systems in a human colorectal carcinoma cell line. *Cancer Res* 55, 4808–4812.

197. Dachs, G. U., Patterson, A. V., Firth, J. D., Ratcliffe, P. J., Townsend, K. M., Stratford, I. J., and Harris, A. L. (1997) Targeting gene expression to hypoxic tumor cells. *Nat Med* 3, 515–520.

198. Shibata, T., Giaccia, A. J., and Brown, J. M. (2002) Hypoxia-inducible regulation of a prodrug-activating enzyme for tumor-specific gene therapy. *Neoplasia* 4, 40–48.

199. Post, D. E., Devi, N. S., Li, Z., Brat, D. J., Kaur, B., Nicholson, A., Olson, J. J., Zhang, Z., and Van Meir, E. G. (2004) Cancer therapy with a replicating oncolytic adenovirus targeting the hypoxic microenvironment of tumors. *Clin Cancer Res* 10, 8603–8612.

200. Hernandez-Alcoceba, R., Pihalja, M., Qian, D., and Clarke, M. F. (2002) New oncolytic adenoviruses with hypoxia- and estrogen receptor-regulated replication. *Hum Gene Ther* 13, 1737–1750.

201. Binley, K., Askham, Z., Martin, L., Spearman, H., Day, D., Kingsman, S., and Naylor, S. (2003) Hypoxia-mediated tumour targeting. *Gene Ther* 10, 540–549.

202. Koshikawa, N., Takenaga, K., Tagawa, M., and Sakiyama, S. (2000) Therapeutic efficacy of the suicide gene driven by the promoter of vascular endothelial growth factor gene against hypoxic tumor cells. *Cancer Res* 60, 2936–2941.

203. Liu, S. C., Minton, N. P., Giaccia, A. J., and Brown, J. M. (2002) Anticancer efficacy of systemically delivered anaerobic bacteria as gene therapy vectors targeting tumor hypoxia/necrosis. *Gene Ther* 9, 291–296.

204. Li, Z., Fallon, J., Mandeli, J., Wetmur, J., and Woo, S. L. (2008) A genetically enhanced anaerobic bacterium for oncopathic therapy of pancreatic cancer. *J Natl Cancer Inst* 100, 1389–400.

205. Brouwers, A. H., van Eerd, J. E., Frielink, C., Oosterwijk, E., Oyen, W. J., Corstens, F. H., and Boerman, O. C. (2004) Optimization of radioimmunotherapy of renal cell carcinoma: labeling of monoclonal antibody cG250 with 131I, 90Y, 177Lu, or 186Re. *J Nucl Med* **45**, 327–337.

206. Bleumer, I., Oosterwijk, E., Oosterwijk-Wakka, J. C., Voller, M. C., Melchior, S., Warnaar, S. O., Mala, C., Beck, J., and Mulders, P. F. (2006) A clinical trial with chimeric monoclonal antibody WX-G250 and low dose interleukin-2 pulsing scheme for advanced renal cell carcinoma. *J Urol* **175**, 57–62.

207. Martin, J., Stribbling, S. M., Poon, G. K., Begent, R. H., Napier, M., Sharma, S. K., and Springer, C. J. (1997) Antibody-directed enzyme prodrug therapy: pharmacokinetics and plasma levels of prodrug and drug in a phase I clinical trial. *Cancer Chemother Pharmacol* **40**, 189–201.

208. Wang, Z., Cook, T., Alber, S., Liu, K., Kovesdi, I., Watkins, S. K., Vodovotz, Y., Billiar, T. R., and Blumberg, D. (2004) Adenoviral gene transfer of the human inducible nitric oxide synthase gene enhances the radiation response of human colorectal cancer associated with alterations in tumor vascularity. *Cancer Res* **64**, 1386–1395.

209. Griffiths, L., Binley, K., Iqball, S., Kan, O., Maxwell, P., Ratcliffe, P., Lewis, C., Harris, A., Kingsman, S., and Naylor, S. (2000) The macrophage – a novel system to deliver gene therapy to pathological hypoxia. *Gene Ther* **7**, 255–262.

210. Koshikawa, N., and Takenaga, K. (2005) Hypoxia-regulated expression of attenuated diphtheria toxin A fused with hypoxia-inducible factor-1alpha oxygen-dependent degradation domain preferentially induces apoptosis of hypoxic cells in solid tumor. *Cancer Res* **65**, 11622–11630.

211. Harada, H., Hiraoka, M., and Kizaka-Kondoh, S. (2002) Antitumor effect of TAT-oxygen-dependent degradation-caspase-3 fusion protein specifically stabilized and activated in hypoxic tumor cells. *Cancer Res* **62**, 2013–2018.

Chapter 2

Characterization of Regulatory T Cells in Tumor Suppressive Microenvironments

Guangyong Peng

Abstract

Increasing evidence suggests that immunotherapy is a promising strategy for treating patients with invasive and metastatic cancers, but clinical trails are discouraging so far. Recent studies showed that several subsets of regulatory tumor-infiltrating lymphocytes (TILs), such as naturally occurring $CD4^+CD25^+$ regulatory T cells (Treg), and adaptively induced Treg cells of Tr1, Th3, $CD8^+$, as well as $\gamma\delta$ Treg cells, have been identified in human cancers. These Treg-cell subsets form a tumor suppressive microenvironment that presents a major barrier to successful anti-tumor immunotherapy. Thus, how to modulate the Treg-cell function in tumor microenvironments is essential for cancer treatment and elimination. To date, there is no unique and selective marker for all subsets of Treg cells, and a combination of assays for Treg-associated markers and suppressive activity is still the most common way used to define these tumor-associated Treg cells. In this chapter, we describe protocols to purify and characterize tumor-associated Treg cells from peripheral blood and TILs of cancer patients, which is critical for predicting clinical outcomes and monitoring the effects of tumor immunotherapy.

Key words: Regulatory T cells, tumor suppressive microenvironment, $CD4^+CD25^+$ T cells, Tr1 cells, Th3 cells, $\gamma\delta$ T cells, FoxP3, CFSE.

1. Introduction

Over the past several years, regulatory T cells (Treg) have been extensively studied in both physiological and pathological conditions in the human immune system. It is now widely accepted that Treg cells have a broad immunosuppressive capacity on different lineages of immune cells and play a central role in controlling immune tolerance and homeostasis of the immune system

P. Yotnda (ed.), *Immunotherapy of Cancer*, Methods in Molecular Biology 651,
DOI 10.1007/978-1-60761-786-0_2, © Springer Science+Business Media, LLC 2010

(1–3). Furthermore, Treg-cell research brings a new view into current tumor immunology and has become one of the most important issues in anti-tumor immunity (4–7). A large body of studies revealed elevated levels of Treg cells among total T-cell populations isolated from tumor tissues or peripheral blood in patients with various cancers, including lung cancer (8), colorectal cancer (9), breast cancer (10), ovarian cancer (11), melanoma (12–14), gastric cancer (15, 16), and lymphoma (16). More importantly, studies in some types of human cancers, including ovarian cancer, renal cell carcinoma, lung cancer and gastric cancer, identified correlations between Treg cells and tumor progression, and poorer patient prognosis (11, 17–20). Recent studies also demonstrated that tumor-associated Treg cells are heterogeneous, existing as subsets including the following: naturally occurring Treg cells and adaptively induced Treg cells of Tr1, Th3, CD8+, as well as γδ Treg cell subsets, which have all been identified in human cancers (21–26). It is now clear that these tumor-associated Treg cells form a tumor-suppressive microenvironment and inhibit immune responses against cancer, which is a major obstacle for successful tumor immunotherapy (3, 4, 6, 7, 18). Tumor-associated Treg-cell concept prompts us to rethink the current immunotherapeutic strategies against cancer. It is now widely acknowledged that modulating Treg-cell functions in tumor microenvironments is essential for cancer treatment and elimination. Actually, several strategies, including depletion, blocking development, trafficking, or suppressive activities, have been proposed to manage Treg-cell function to treat cancers (5, 7, 26–28), and some of them have already been integrated into the clinical trials and have returned promising results (29, 30).

Detection and characterization of these tumor-associated Treg cells in peripheral blood and TILs from cancer patients are critical for predicting clinical outcome and monitoring the effects of cancer immunotherapy. Since highly heterogeneous populations of Treg cells exist with multiple suppressive mechanisms, including cell–cell contact dependent effects and/or soluble factor(s), it is impossible to distinguish different subsets of Treg cells, or distinguish tumor-associated Treg cells from other Treg cells based on a single phenotypic marker or some other property. A combination of assays for Treg-associated markers and suppressive activity is still the most common strategy used to define these cells (3, 6, 31, 32). In addition, the most studied Treg-cell population in tumor microenvironments is CD4+CD25+ naturally occurring Treg cells, and commercial availability of isolation kits and detection antibodies facilitate the basic and clinical studies on the role of this population in anti-tumor immunity.

2. Materials

2.1. Cell Culture and Maintenance

Cells and suitable medium, serum, and other relevant supplements are varied depending on the cell types under investigation.

1. Human T-cell growth medium: RPMI 1640 containing 10% human heat-inactivated serum type AB (supplemented with 2 mM L-glutamine, 2-mercaptoethanol, and 50 U/ml of IL-2.

2. Human tumor cell growth medium: RPMI 1640 medium with 10% fetal calf serum (FCS) or fetal bovine serum (FBS). Some epithelial-derived tumor cells (such as breast cancer and prostate cancer cells) are established and maintained in the keratinocyte medium (Invitrogen, Inc.) containing 25 μg/ml bovine pituitary extract, 5 ng/ml epidermal growth factor, 2 mM L-glutamine, 10 mM HEPES buffer, 2% heat-inactivated FCS, and 100 U/ml penicillin–streptomycin.

2.2. Purification of Peripheral Blood Mononuclear Cells (PBMCs)

1. RPMI 1640.

2. Ficoll separation solution: Ficoll-Paque Plus, density 1.077 g/ml, store in the dark.

3. Freezing medium: 10% DMSO in FCS, freshly prepare and keep at 4°C.

2.3. Generation of Tumor-Infiltrating T Cells

1. T-cell growth medium: *see* **Section 2.1**.

2. 10× enzyme digestion medium (100 ml, store at −80°C, dilute with RPMI 1640, and filter before use): Collagenase type IV (5 mg), deoxyribonuclease type IV (150,000 units), hyaluronidase type V (500 mg) (Sigma), RPMI 1640 medium, gentamicin (50 mg/ml), penicillin (10,000 u/ml)/streptomycin (10,000 μg/ml), Fungizone (250 μg/ml), and L-glutamine (200 mM).

3. 24-well plates.

4. Cell strainer, 100 μm nylon.

5. Autoclaved scissors and forceps.

2.4. T-Cell Subset Purification

1. CD4[+] and CD8[+] T-cell purification: Human CD4 and CD8 microbeads for positive selection (Miltenyi Biotec).

2. CD4[+]CD25[+] Treg-cell purification: CD4[+]CD25[+] regulatory T cell isolation kit, or CD4[+]CD25[+]CD127[dim/−] regulatory T cell isolation kit (Miltenyi Biotec).

3. MS or LS columns and adapters (Miltenyi Biotec).

4. Buffer: pH 7.2 PBS containing 2% FCS (or 0.5% BSA) and 2 mM EDTA. Keep the buffer at 4°C.

2.5. Flow Cytometry Analysis

1. A panel of antibodies specific for T-cell markers, either directly conjugated to a fluorochrome or non-conjugated. These antibodies include anti-CD4, anti-CD25, anti-GITR, anti-CTLA4, anti-FoxP3, anti-CD127, anti-CCR5, anti-CCR7, anti-CD62L, anti-CD45RA, and anti-CD45RO.

2. Staining buffer: pH 7.4 PBS containing 2% FCS, filter and store at 4°C.

3. Permeabilization Kit (BD Bioscience): Cytofix/ Cytoperm™ solution and Perm/Wash™ solution.

4. Fixation buffer: Paraformaldeyhde (4%) in PBS.

5. Phorbol myristate acetate (PMA) and ionomycin (sigma).

6. GolgiStop (BD Bioscience).

7. Flow cytometer: FACScaliburTM, FACScanTM, and FACSSort, etc.

2.6. Cytokine Production Profile

1. Anti-CD3 antibody (clone OKT3).

2. T-cell assay medium: RPMI 1640 medium containing 2% human heat-inactivated serum type AB supplemented with 2 mM L-glutamine and 2-mercaptoethanol.

3. Cytokine detection kits of ELISA kits or Bio-Plex Chemokine Assay kits.

2.7. Suppressive Function Assays

2.7.1. ^{3}H-Thymidine Incorporation Assay

1. Anti-CD3 antibody (clone OKT3).

2. Purified CD4$^+$ responding cells and monocyte-derived dendritic cells.

3. U-bottom 96-well plates.

4. ^{3}H-thymidine: 1 mCi/ml, 1:100 diluted in RPMI 1640 (1 μCi/well).

5. MicroScint™-20 scintillation fluid (Packard Instruments).

6. A liquid scintillation counter (ß-counter; Beckmann Instruments).

7. T-cell assay medium: RPMI 1640 medium containing 2% human heat-inactivated serum type AB supplemented with 2 mM L-glutamine and 2-mercaptoethanol.

2.7.2. Carboxyfluorescein Succinimidyl Ester (CFSE) Dilution Assay

1. 5 μM CFSE (Molecular Probes, concentration stock 1000× in DMSO at –80°C).

2. Reaction buffer: 1% FCS in PBS.

3. Stop buffer: 100% FCS or FBS.

4. Wash buffer: 1% FCS in PBS.

5. Flow cytometer: FACScaliburTM, FACScanTM, FAC-SSort, etc.

2.7.3. Suppression Assay for IL-2 and IFN-γ Release from Effector T Cells

1. Anti-CD3 antibody (clone OKT3).

2. CD4+ or CD8+ effector T cells, monocyte-derived dendritic cells.

3. U-bottom 96-well plates.

4. Effector T-cell-specific peptide and a control non-specific peptide.

5. ELISA kits for IL-2 and IFN-γ detection.

6. T-cell assay medium: RPMI 1640 medium containing 2% human heat-inactivated serum type AB supplemented with 2 mM L-glutamine and 2-mercaptoethanol.

2.8. Transwell Assay

1. Anti-CD3 antibody (clone OKT3).

2. Purified CD4+ responding cells; APCs or monocyte-derived dendritic cells.

3. 24-well plates with pore size 0.4 μm; U-bottom 96-well plates.

4. ^{3}H-thymidine: 1 mCi/ml, 1:100 diluted in RPMI 1640 (1 μCi/well).

5. A liquid scintillation counter.

6. T-cell assay medium: RPMI 1640 medium containing 2% human heat-inactivated serum type AB supplemented with 2 mM L-glutamine and 2-mercaptoethanol.

3. Methods

CD25 has been used as a highly expressed Treg-specific cell surface marker to isolate CD4+CD25+ naturally occurring Treg cells, but CD25 is not selectively expressed on Treg cells, as it is also expressed on activated effector T cells (33). Lack of specificity also occurs with other Treg markers such as glucocorticoid-induced TNFR family related gene (GITR) and cytotoxic T lymphocyte antigen-4 (CTLA-4), which have enriched expression on Treg cells as well as activated effector T cells. Foxp3, which was recently identified as essential to Treg differentiation, is the best Treg-cell marker to date (34–36). However, FoxP3 is an intracellular molecule that requires cell fixation and permeabilization for detection; thus, it can not be used as a marker for purification.

More recently, cell surface IL-7 receptor α chain (CD127) has been identified as a relatively specific marker for Treg cells, and the T-cell population with lacking or lower expression of CD127 population was considered as functional Treg cells (37, 38). In addition, CD127 expression can discriminate FoxP3$^+$ Treg cells from activated CD25$^+$ T cells and be used as a purification marker (39). Besides CD4$^+$CD25$^+$ naturally occurring Treg cells generated in the thymus, there are other CD4$^+$ Treg-cell populations of Tr1 and Th3 cells, which are exclusively generated in the periphery (40–42). These two adaptively induced Treg cells have a unique feature in that they can secrete a large amount of IL-10 and/or TGF-β, which can be used as characterization markers. Taken together there is no specific and selective marker for Treg cells, and the definition and purification of CD4$^+$ Treg cells are still based on the combination of several Treg-associated markers. In addition, the assays for suppressive activity are the most important methods for further defining CD4$^+$ Treg-cell population as well as other subsets of Treg cells, including inhibition of naïve T-cell proliferation and cytokine production by effector T cells.

3.1. Purification of PBMCs from Whole Blood

Peripheral blood samples are collected from healthy donors or cancer patients by leukapheresis, and PBMCs are further purified from the blood samples based on ficoll-sodium metrizoate density gradients.

1. Warm RPMI 1640 to 37°C.

2. Pour the heparinized blood samples or buffy coats (15 ml) into a 50-ml Falcon tube and dilute with an equal volume of RPMI 1640 (15 ml:15 ml).

3. Aliquot 20 ml of Ficoll-Paque Plus separation solution into new 50-ml Falcon tubes.

4. Carefully lay the diluted whole blood/RPMI 1640 or buffy coat/RPMI 1640 mixture (30 ml) on the top of the ficoll layer with a 10-ml pipette.

5. Spin the tubes for 20 min at a speed of 1100 × g without brake.

6. Collect the interface comprising of mononuclear cells layer into new 50-ml Falcon tubes, and add RPMI 1640 with volume up to 50 ml and mix thoroughly (**Note 1**).

7. Spin at 180 × g for 8 min and then aspirate the supernatant and gently resuspend cell pellet with 50 ml RPMI 1640 medium.

8. Spin at 625 × g for 7 min and then aspirate the supernatant and resuspend cells with 20 ml of RPMI 1640.

9. Spin at 625 × g for 5 min, aspirate the supernatants, freeze cells at 10 × 10^6/ml/vial in the freeze medium, and store the cells in liquid nitrogen.

3.2. Generation of Tumor-Infiltrating T Cells (TILs)

Fresh tumor tissues are collected from different stages of identified primary types of tumors obtained from hospitalized cancer patients who undergo surgery, and TILs will be generated from these tumor tissues. Tissue-infiltrating lymphocytes can also be generated from the tumor-matched normal tissues using the same generation protocol as TILs (13, 23).

1. Prepare enzyme digestion medium. Add the following components into RPMI 1640 and then filter the mixture to make it sterile. The final concentrations of the components are as follows: DNase (30 U/ml), hyaluronidase (0.1 mg/ml), collagenase (1 mg/ml), L-glutamine (2 mM), penicillin (50 U/ml) (optional), streptomycin (50 μg/ml) (optional), gentamicin (10 μg/ml), and Fungizone (1.25 μg/ml) (optional). Medium can be store at 4°C up to 1 month.

2. Prepare T-cell growth medium (2.1.1).

3. Wash the fresh tumor pieces twice in RPMI 1640.

4. Remove fatty, connective, and/or necrotic tissues from the tumor mass in a 10-cm dish. Then, cut the tissue into 1- to 2-mm pieces in the RPMI 1640 (**Note 2**).

5. Transfer the minced tumor pieces into a 15-ml or a 50-ml conical tube and incubate them with the triple enzyme digestion medium for 2 h at room temperature with gentle shaking.

6. Wash the digested tissue twice with RPMI 1640; centrifuge at 1500 rpm for 5 min.

7. Resuspend tissue in 10 ml RPMI 1640 and filter through a 100-μm cell strainer.

8. Collect the tissue trapped on the strainer and put them into several wells containing 1 ml of T-cell growth medium in a 24-well plate, and culture for 5–10 days to generate TILs.

3.3. Isolation of CD4⁺ or CD4⁺ CD25⁺ Treg Cells from PBMCs and/or TILs

CD4⁺CD25⁺ T cells can be purified from PBMCs and/or TILs of cancer patients. The purification can be performed either through FACS sorting after double staining the cells with anti-human CD4 and CD25 antibodies conjugated to PE or FITC, or using microbeads conjugated to the antibodies.

Currently, two relatively specific Treg-cell markers CD25 and CD127 are used for the purification of CD4⁺ Treg cells. The following procedures are based on the CD4⁺CD25⁺ regulatory T cell isolation kit from Miltenyi Biotec Inc. The isolation is performed in a two-step procedure. First, CD4⁺ T cells are purified by negative selection. Non-CD4⁺ cells are indirectly magnetically labeled with a cocktail of biotin-conjugated antibodies and anti-biotin microbeads. The labeled cells are subsequently depleted by separation over a MACS column. In the second step, CD4$^+$CD25$^+$ T cells are directly labeled with CD25 microbeads and isolated by positive selection from the pre-enriched CD4$^+$ T-cell fraction.

1. Determine the cell numbers of PBMCs or TILs.

2. Wash the cells once with the buffer and centrifuge the cell suspension at $300 \times g$ for 10 min. Pipette off supernatant completely.

3. Resuspend cell pellet in 90 µl of buffer per 10^7 cells and add 10 µl of Biotin-Antibody Cocktail per 10^7 cells. Mix well and incubate for 10 min at 4–8°C.

4. Add 20 µl of Anti-Biotin MicroBeads per 10^7 cells and mix well and incubate for an additional 15 min at 4–8°C.

5. Wash the cells by adding 1–2 ml of buffer and centrifuge at $300 \times g$ for 10 min at 4–8°C. Pipette off supernatant completely and resuspend up to 10^8 cells in 500 µl of buffer.

6. Place LS column in the magnetic field of a suitable MACS separator and prepare the column by rinsing with 2 ml of buffer (**Note 3**).

7. Apply the cell suspension to the column.

8. Collect unlabeled cells that pass through and wash the column with 2×1 ml of buffer. Collect total effluent, which contains the unlabeled pre-enriched CD4$^+$ T-cell fraction (**Note 4**).

9. Centrifuge cells at $300 \times g$ for 10 min. Pipette off supernatant completely and resuspend cell pellet in 90 µl of buffer.

10. Add 10 µl of CD25 Microbeads, mix well, and incubate for 15 min at 4–8°C.

11. Wash the cells by adding 10–20× labeling volume of buffer and centrifuge at $300 \times g$ for 10 min. Pipette off supernatant completely and resuspend up to 10^8 cells in 500 µl of buffer.

12. Place MS column in the magnetic field of a suitable MACS separator and prepare the column by rinsing with 500 µl of buffer (**Note 3**).

13. Apply cell suspension onto the column. Collect unlabeled cells that pass through and wash the column with $3 \times$ 500 ml of the buffer.

14. Remove column from the separator and place it on a suitable collection tube.

15. Pipette 1 ml of buffer onto the column. Immediately flush out the fraction with magnetically labeled cells by firmly applying the plunger supplied with the column.

16. Check the purity by FACS staining before proceeding to functional assays (**Note 5**).

3.4. FACS Analysis of Treg-Cell-Associated Markers

Since there is no specific marker to distinguish human Treg cells from other subsets of T cells, the definition of human CD4$^+$ Treg cells needs a combination of several associated markers, including CD25, GITR, CTLA4, FoxP3, CD127$^{dim/-}$, CCR5, CCR7, and CD45RA. Some markers require intracellular staining for detection. To characterize adaptive CD4$^+$ Treg cells, the intracellular cytokines of IL-10 and/or TGF-β can also be analyzed as definitive markers.

3.4.1. Surface Staining

1. Prepare and count the cells, and then suspend cells in ice-cold staining buffer (50 μl for each test /1–2×10^6 cells) in plastic tubes or microwell plates (**Note 6**).

2. Add a pre-titrated optimal concentration of a fluorochrome-conjugated anti-human monoclonal antibody specific for a Treg-cell-associated marker. Mix well and incubate for 15–30 min on ice or at 4°C in dark (**Note 7**).

3. Wash the cells twice with 1 ml staining buffer/wash (150 μl staining buffer/wash with microwell plates), spin at 250 × g, and discard the supernatant.

4. Add 500 μl FACS staining buffer to each tube to resuspend cell pellet and analyze the cells on a flow cytometer, such as FACScalibur^{TM} (**Note 8**).

3.4.2. Intracellular Staining

1. Prepare and count the cells, spin at 250 × g, and discard the supernatant (**Note 9**).

2. Thoroughly resuspend cells in 100 μl of Cytofix/Cytoperm^{TM} solution for 10–20 min at 4°C.

3. Wash the cells twice in Perm/Wash^{TM} solution (1 ml/wash for staining in tubes), spin, and remove the supernatant.

4. Thoroughly resuspend fixed/permeabilized cells in 50 μl of Perm/Wash^{TM} solution containing a predetermined optimal concentration of fluorochrome-conjugated anti-human monoclonal antibody specific for a Treg-cell-associated marker. Mix well and incubate for 15–30 min on ice or at 4°C in dark (**Note 10**).

5. Wash the cells twice with 1 ml Perm/Wash^{TM} solution/wash (150 μl staining buffer/wash with microwell plates), spin at 250 × g, and discard the supernatant.

6. Add 500 μl FACS staining buffer to each tube to resuspend the cell pellet, and analyze the cells on a flow cytometer.

3.5. Detection of Cytokine Production from Treg Cells

Treg cells have a common characteristic, that is, they do not secrete IL-2 upon TCR-mediated stimulation. In addition, CD4$^+$CD25$^+$ naturally occurring Treg cells also fail to produce other cytokines such as IL-4, IL-5, and IFN-γ, although Tr1, Th3, and some tumor antigen-specific Treg cells can produce a large amount of IL-10 and/or TGF-β.

1. Culture Treg cells in T-cell medium with low concentration of IL-2 (5 U/ml) for 2–3 days.

2. Prepare 2 μg/ml of anti-CD3 antibody (OKT3) in pH 7.4 PBS and add 100 μl/well to 96-well U-bottom plates, and keep the plates overnight at 4°C.

3. Wash CD4$^+$ Treg cells twice with T-cell assay medium (without IL-2), resuspend with T-cell assay medium (without IL-2), and adjust the number at 1×10^6/ml.

4. Add 100 μl/well of Treg cells into an anti-CD3-precoated 96-well plate and incubate the cells at 37°C in 5% CO2 for 24 h.

5. Collect the supernatants and test the production of cytokines using ELISA kits or Bio-Plex Chemokine Assay kits (**Note 11**).

3.6. Determination of Suppressive Activity of Treg Cells

Possession of a potent suppressive activity is the common feature for different subsets of human Treg cells. The suppressive activity of Treg cells can be determined by assays of inhibition of naïve/effector T-cell proliferation and cytokine secretion (IFN-γ and IL-2) by effector T cells (13, 26). The T-cell proliferation can be determined either by a ^{3}H-thymidine incorporation assay or by a CFSE dilution assay (28).

3.6.1. Inhibition of Naïve T-cell Proliferation Using a ^{3}H-Thymidine Incorporation Assay

The proliferation of naïve CD4$^+$ T cells can be measured by two assay approaches: (a) with antigen-presenting cell (APC) involvement. This assay system includes APCs and soluble anti-CD3 antibody (at a final concentration of 100 ng/ml). (b) Without APC involvement. This assay system needs plate-bound anti-CD3 (2 μg/ml) antibody (28). The following procedure is based on the approach of non-APC involvement (**Fig. 2.1**).

1. Culture Treg cells in T-cell medium with low concentration of IL-2 (5 U/ml) for 2–3 days.

2. Prepare naïve CD4$^+$ T cells (positive selection or negative selection using microbeads; procedure described in **Section 3.3**) and culture in T-cell medium (**Note 12**).

3. Prepare 2 μg/ml of anti-CD3 antibody in pH 7.4 PBS and add 100 μl/well to 96-well U-bottom plates, and keep the plates overnight at 4°C.

4. Wash naïve CD4$^+$ T cells and Treg cells twice with T-cell assay medium and pellet the cells.

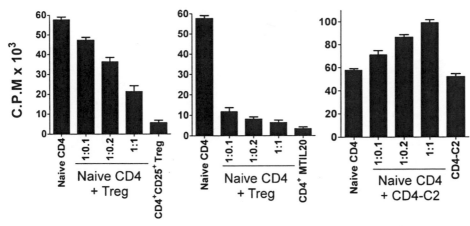

Fig. 2.1. Suppression of naïve CD4$^+$ T-cell proliferation by Treg cells. The proliferative activity of freshly prepared naïve CD4$^+$ (responding) T cells (1 × 10^5) was inhibited by different numbers of CD4$^+$CD25$^+$ naturally occurring Treg cells and CD4$^+$ MTIL20 Treg cells in the presence of anti-CD3 antibody. Proliferation of naïve CD4$^+$ T cells was assayed by adding ^{3}H-thymidine during the last 16 h of culture. In contrast, CD4-C2 T cells enhanced rather than suppressed the proliferative activity of responding CD4$^+$ T cells. MTIL20: a melanoma-derived CD4$^+$ Treg cell line. CD4-C2 T cells: an effector T cell line. Results represent one of three independent experiments.

5. Resuspend naïve CD4$^+$ T cells with T-cell assay medium and adjust the number at 1×10^6/ml.

6. Resuspend Treg cells with T-cell assay medium and adjust the number at 1×10^6/ml, 2×10^5/ml, and 1×10^5/ml.

7. Add 100 μl/well of naïve CD4$^+$ T cells and 100 μl/well different concentrations of Treg cells in the following combinations: (a) naïve CD4$^+$ T cell alone (1×10^5/well); (b) naïve CD4$^+$ T cells plus Treg cells (1:1); (c) naïve CD4$^+$ T cells plus Treg cells (1:1/5); (d) naïve CD4$^+$ T cells plus Treg cells (1:1/10); and (e) Treg cells alone (1×10^5/well). Each group includes triplicate wells.

8. Incubate the cells at 37°C in 5% CO_2 for 56 h.

9. Prepare ^{3}H-thymidine (add 100 μl ^{3}H-thymidine of 1 mCi/ml into 0.9 ml of T-cell assay medium for each 96 well-plate) and add 10 μl to each well at a final concentration of 1 μCi/well.

10. Harvest cells after an additional 16 h of culture to a 96-well format filter film and dry the film at room temperature.

11. Add 30 μl/well of scintillation fluid to the dried film and measure the incorporation of ^{3}H-thymidine using a liquid scintillation counter.

3.6.2. Inhibition of Naïve T-cell Proliferation Using a CFSE Dilution Assay

CFSE is a fluorescent cell staining dye. CFSE can diffuse freely inside the cells and is retained by the cell in the cytoplasm, but it does not adversely affect cellular function. During each round of cell division, relative fluorescence intensity of the CFSE is decreased by half. The CFSE staining allows us to examine specific

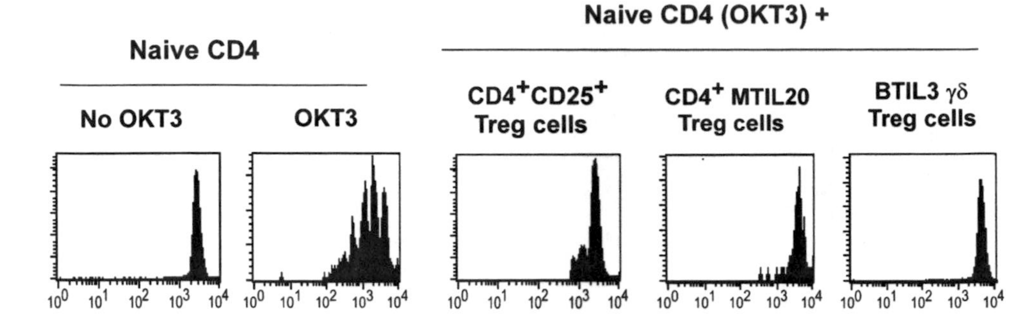

Fig. 2.2. Suppression of CFSE-labeled naïve CD4+ T-cell division by Treg cells. Naïve CD4+ T cells alone proliferated well and exhibited several divisions after stimulation by OKT3. However, different types of Treg cells of CD4+CD25+ Treg cells, CD4+ MTIL20 Treg cells, and BTIL3 γδ Treg cells significantly inhibited the proliferation of naïve CD4+ T cells. CFSE-labeled naïve CD4+ T cells were co-cultured with different types of Treg cells at a 1:1 ratio in OKT3-coated 24-well plates. After 3 days of culture, cells were harvested and analyzed for cell divisions by FACS gated on the CFSE-labeled cells. CFSE-labeled naïve CD4+ T cells alone stimulated with or without OKT3 served as controls. MTIL20: a melanoma-derived CD4+ Treg cell line. BTIL3 γδ Treg cells: a breast cancer-derived γδ Treg cell line. Data are one of three independent experiments.

populations of proliferating cells and identify the successive cell generations (26, 28) (**Fig. 2.2**).

1. Prepare naïve CD4+ T cells and suspend with concentration of 1×10^7 cells per ml in PBS with 1% FBS.

2. Add CFSE to a final concentration of 5 μM (stock 1000× in DMSO), vortex gently, and incubate at 37°C for 10–15 min (**Notes 13 and 14**).

3. Add an equal volume of pre-warmed FBS (100%) to stop labeling, and incubate cells in a 37°C water bath for 20 min for the efflux of excessive CFSE.

4. Wash the stained cells twice in PBS with 1% FBS and resuspend cells in T-cell culture medium (**Note 15**).

5. For the suppressive assay, the stained naïve CD4+ T cells (1×10^6/well) are cultured in an anti-CD3 (2 μg/ml)-precoated 24-well plate with or without Treg cells at different ratios of 1:1, 1:1/5, and 1:1/10.

6. Harvest the cells after 3 days of culture, wash the cells twice with 1 ml staining buffer per wash, spin at 250 × *g*, and discard the supernatants.

7. Add 500 μl of FACS staining buffer to each tube to resuspend cell pellet and then analyze the cells on a flow cytometer gating on the CFSE-positive population.

3.6.3. Suppression Assay for IL-2 and IFN-γ Release from CD4+ and CD8+ Effector T Cells

1. Culture Treg cells in T-cell medium with low concentration of IL-2 (5 U/ml) for 2–3 days.

2. Prepare effector CD4+ or CD8+ T cells and anti-CD3-activated Treg cells, and culture them in the T-cell growth medium (**Note 16**).

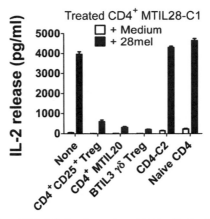

Fig. 2.3. Treg cells inhibited IL-2 release from CD4$^+$ effector T cells. CD4$^+$CD25$^+$ Treg cells, CD4$^+$ MTIL20, and BTIL3 $\gamma\delta$ Treg cells strongly inhibited the ability of CD4$^+$ MTIL28-C1 helper T cells to secret IL-2. By contrast, naïve CD4$^+$ T cells and CD4-C2 effector T cell line did not affect the ability of CD4$^+$ MTIL28-C1 helper T cells to secret IL-2. Anti-CD3 antibody-activated, tumor-derived different types of Treg cells or control CD4$^+$ T cells were co-cultured with CD4$^+$ MTIL28-C1 helper T cells for 24 h. After washing, 28 mel tumor cells were added to the mixture. IL-2 secretion in the culture supernatants were determined by ELISA after 18 h of incubation. Results are representative of three independent experiments. CD4$^+$ MTIL28-C1: a melanoma-derived CD4$^+$ T helper cell line. 28 mel: a melanoma cell line.

3. Wash effector CD4$^+$ T cells and the anti-CD3-activated Treg cells twice with T-cell assay medium and then resuspend and co-culture them at a 1:1 ratio in T-cell growth medium containing 10 U/ml IL-2 for 24 h.

4. After washing, the treated effector T cells (1×10^5/well) are co-cultured with autologous DCs (2×10^4/well) pulsed with the effector T-cell-specific peptide or a control peptide for another 24 h in a 96-well plate in T-cell assay medium (without IL-2) (**Note 17**).

5. Harvest culture supernatants and determine IL-2 and IFN-γ secretion by ELISA (**Fig. 2.3**).

3.7. Determination of Suppressive Mechanisms of Treg Cells Using a Transwell Assay

Transwell experiments are performed in 24-well plates with a pore size of 0.4 μm, which can distinguish whether the suppressive activity mediated by Treg cells is through soluble factor(s) or through a cell–cell contact manner (**Fig. 2.4**).

1. Culture Treg cells in T-cell medium with low concentration of IL-2 (5 U/ml) for 2–3 days.

2. Prepare naïve CD4$^+$ T cells (positive selection or negative selection using microbeads; described in **Section 3.3**) and APCs (PBMCs depleted CD4$^+$ and CD8$^+$ T cells using the depletion microbeads).

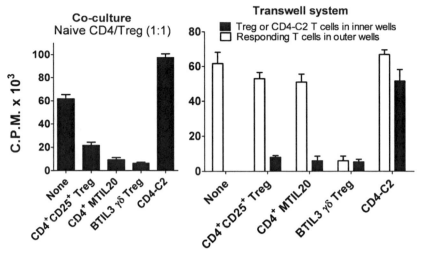

Fig. 2.4. The suppressive mechanisms of tumor-associated Treg cells. In the co-culture system, different types of Treg cells including CD4+CD25+ Treg, CD4+ MTIL20 Treg, and BTIL3 γδ Treg cells strongly suppressed the proliferation of naïve CD4+ T cells, whereas control CD4-C2 T cells did not inhibit the proliferation of naïve CD4+ T cells. In the transwell system, cell–cell contact is required for T-cell suppression of CD4+CD25+ Treg cells and CD4+ MTIL20 Treg cells; however, the suppressive activity of BTIL3 γδ Treg cells was mediated through soluble factor(s). In contrast, CD4-C2 T cells in the inner wells did not inhibit the proliferation of the naïve CD4+ T cells in the outer wells. Equal numbers of naïve CD4+ T cells were cultured in outer wells, and Treg cells or control CD4-C2 T cells were cultured in inner wells. Culture conditions were identical between inner and outer wells. The OKT3-stimulated proliferation of naïve CD4+ T cells was determined by ^{3}H-thymidine incorporation assays. Results shown are mean ± SD from three independent experiments.

3. Wash naïve CD4+ T cells, APCs, and Treg cells twice with T-cell assay medium, and resuspend these cells in T-cell assay medium.

4. Add 2×10^5 freshly purified naïve CD4+ T cells together with 2×10^5 APCs in the outer wells of 24-well plates in medium containing 0.5 μg/ml of anti-CD3 antibody.

5. Add equal number of Treg cells or control effector T cells into the inner wells in the same medium containing 0.5 μg/ml anti-CD3 antibody and 2×10^5 APCs.

6. After 56 h of culture, the cells in the outer and inner wells are harvested separately and transferred to 96-well plates. The cells in each 24-well plate will be divided into two wells in a 96-well plate.

7. Prepare ^{3}H-thymidine (take 100 μl ^{3}H-thymidine of 1 mCi/ml into 0.9 ml of T-cell assay medium for each plate) and add 10 μl to each well at a final concentration of 1 μCi/well.

8. Harvest cells after an additional 16 h of culture to a 96-well format filter film and dry the film at room temperature.

9. Add 30 μl/well of scintillation fluid to the dried film and measure the incorporation of ^{3}H-thymidine using a liquid scintillation counter.

4. Notes

1. When you collect the white layer of the cells with a 10-ml pipette, you should be careful to avoid contamination with too much plasma above this layer and ficoll underneath this layer, and avoid touching the bottom red layer of cells.

2. Do not let the tissue dry out.

3. You may choose different sizes of columns based on the number of labeled cells.

4. Perform washing steps by adding buffer successively once the column reservoir is empty.

5. To increase the purity of $CD4^+CD25^+$ cells, you should not overload the cells in the columns, and you can also repeat the magnetic separation procedure as described in steps 12–15 using a new column.

6. All of the staining procedures must be performed on resting cells.

7. PI can be used to exclude dead cells and it can also be mixed with the surface antibodies concomitantly with the surface staining.

8. If you want to perform double staining with a surface marker and an intracellular marker at the same time, it is recommended that staining of cell surface antigen be done with live, unfixed cells prior to fixation/permeabilization and staining of intracellular cytokines.

9. Intracellular staining for some suppressive cytokines, such as IL-4 and IL-10, requires cell activation using PMA and ionomycin in the presence of GolgiStop for 5 h before the staining.

10. To reduce non-specific immunofluorescent staining, the FC receptors on human $CD4^+$ T cells can be pre-blocked by incubating cells with an excess of irrelevant purified human Ig or by incubation with 10% FCS in PBS.

11. To determine the cytokines released from tumor-specific Treg cell lines, you may co-culture the isolated Treg cell lines with autologous tumor cells or peptide-pulsed autologous DCs for 24 h and then measure cytokines in the culture supernatants.

12. Responder cells may either be naïve $CD4^+$ T cells or $CD4^+CD25^-$ T cells, and may be autologous or allogeneic.

13. CFSE should be prepared in DMSO and stored in small aliquots at $-80°C$. CFSE decays quickly, and yellow

discoloration indicates that the CFSE will no longer conjugate to proteins.

14. Do not label the cells with CFSE at a high concentration if you want to look at cell division in a short time period. For the investigation at longer time points, you can increase the CFSE concentration for the labeling.

15. At this time point, you may take a day zero CSFE-staining samples to determine initial labeling, and run cells immediately by FACS analysis or fix in 1–4% paraformaldehyde.

16. Treg cells can be cultured and activated in OKT-3 (2 μg/ml)-coated plates for 24 h.

17. DCs are derived from the monocytes in culture with IL-4, GM-CSF, and TNF-α (26). If you do not know the specific antigen recognized by the effector cells, you can also determine IL-2 and IFN-γ secretion from the effector T cells with a non-specific stimulation by OKT3.

References

1. Sakaguchi, S. (2004) Naturally arising CD4$^+$ regulatory T cells for immunologic self-tolerance and negative control of immune responses. *Annu Rev Immunol 22*, 531–562.
2. Sakaguchi, S., Wing, K., and Miyara, M. (2007) Regulatory T cells – a brief history and perspective. *Eur J Immunol 37* Suppl *1*, S116–123.
3. Shevach, E. M. (2002) CD4$^+$ CD25$^+$ suppressor T cells: more questions than answers. *Nat Rev Immunol 2*, 389–400.
4. Curiel, T. J. (2007) Tregs and rethinking cancer immunotherapy. *J Clin Invest 117*, 1167–1174.
5. Curiel, T. J. (2008) Regulatory T cells and treatment of cancer. *Curr Opin Immunol 20*, 241–246.
6. Zou, W. (2006) Regulatory T cells, tumour immunity and immunotherapy. *Nature reviews 6*, 295–307.
7. Wang, H. Y., and Wang, R. F. (2007) Regulatory T cells and cancer. *Current opinion in immunology 19*, 217–223.
8. Woo, E. Y., Chu, C. S., Goletz, T. J., Schlienger, K., Yeh, H., Coukos, G., Rubin, S. C., Kaiser, L. R., and June, C. H. (2001) Regulatory CD4$^{(+)}$CD25$^{(+)}$ T cells in tumors from patients with early-stage non-small cell lung cancer and late-stage ovarian cancer. *Cancer Res 61*, 4766–4772.
9. Somasundaram, R., Jacob, L., Swoboda, R., Caputo, L., Song, H., Basak, S., Monos, D., Peritt, D., Marincola, F., Cai, D., Birebent, B., Bloome, E., Kim, J., Berencsi, K., Mastrangelo, M., and Herlyn, D. (2002) Inhibition of cytolytic T lymphocyte proliferation by autologous CD4$^+$/CD25$^+$ regulatory T cells in a colorectal carcinoma patient is mediated by transforming growth factor-beta. *Cancer Res 62*, 5267–5272.
10. Liyanage, U. K., Moore, T. T., Joo, H. G., Tanaka, Y., Herrmann, V., Doherty, G., Drebin, J. A., Strasberg, S. M., Eberlein, T. J., Goedegebuure, P. S., and Linehan, D. C. (2002) Prevalence of regulatory T cells is increased in peripheral blood and tumor microenvironment of patients with pancreas or breast adenocarcinoma. *J Immunol 169*, 2756–2761.
11. Curiel, T. J., Coukos, G., Zou, L., Alvarez, X., Cheng, P., Mottram, P., Evdemon-Hogan, M., Conejo-Garcia, J. R., Zhang, L., Burow, M., Zhu, Y., Wei, S., Kryczek, I., Daniel, B., Gordon, A., Myers, L., Lackner, A., Disis, M. L., Knutson, K. L., Chen, L., and Zou, W. (2004) Specific recruitment of regulatory T cells in ovarian carcinoma fosters immune privilege and predicts reduced survival. *Nature medicine 10*, 942–949.
12. Wang, H. Y., Peng, G., Guo, Z., Shevach, E. M., and Wang, R. F. (2005) Recognition of a new ARTC1 peptide ligand uniquely expressed in tumor cells by antigen-specific CD4$^+$ regulatory T cells. *J Immunol 174*, 2661–2670.
13. Wang, H. Y., Lee, D. A., Peng, G., Guo, Z., Li, Y., Kiniwa, Y., Shevach, E. M., and Wang, R. F. (2004) Tumor-specific human

CD4$^+$ regulatory T cells and their ligands: implications for immunotherapy. *Immunity* **20**, 107–118.

14. Viguier, M., Lemaitre, F., Verola, O., Cho, M. S., Gorochov, G., Dubertret, L., Bachelez, H., Kourilsky, P., and Ferradini, L. (2004) Foxp3 expressing CD4$^+$CD25(high) regulatory T cells are overrepresented in human metastatic melanoma lymph nodes and inhibit the function of infiltrating T cells. *J Immunol* **173**, 1444–1453.

15. Kawaida, H., Kono, K., Takahashi, A., Sugai, H., Mimura, K., Miyagawa, N., Omata, H., Ooi, A., and Fujii, H. (2005) Distribution of CD4$^+$CD25high regulatory T-cells in tumor-draining lymph nodes in patients with gastric cancer. *The Journal of surgical research* **124**, 151–157.

16. Yang, Z. Z., Novak, A. J., Stenson, M. J., Witzig, T. E., and Ansell, S. M. (2006) Intratumoral CD4$^+$CD25$^+$ regulatory T-cell-mediated suppression of infiltrating CD4$^+$ T cells in B-cell non-Hodgkin lymphoma. *Blood* **107**, 3639–3646.

17. Wolf, D., Wolf, A. M., Rumpold, H., Fiegl, H., Zeimet, A. G., Muller-Holzner, E., Deibl, M., Gastl, G., Gunsilius, E., and Marth, C. (2005) The expression of the regulatory T cell-specific forkhead box transcription factor FoxP3 is associated with poor prognosis in ovarian cancer. *Clin Cancer Res* **11**, 8326–8331.

18. Knutson, K. L., Disis, M. L., and Salazar, L. G. (2007) CD4 regulatory T cells in human cancer pathogenesis. *Cancer Immunol Immunother* **56**, 271–285.

19. Siddiqui, S. A., Frigola, X., Bonne-Annee, S., Mercader, M., Kuntz, S. M., Krambeck, A. E., Sengupta, S., Dong, H., Cheville, J. C., Lohse, C. M., Krco, C. J., Webster, W. S., Leibovich, B. C., Blute, M. L., Knutson, K. L., and Kwon, E. D. (2007) Tumor-infiltrating Foxp3-CD4$^+$CD25$^+$ T cells predict poor survival in renal cell carcinoma. *Clin Cancer Res* **13**, 2075–2081.

20. Kono, K., Kawaida, H., Takahashi, A., Sugai, H., Mimura, K., Miyagawa, N., Omata, H., and Fujii, H. (2006) CD4$^{(+)}$CD25 high regulatory T cells increase with tumor stage in patients with gastric and esophageal cancers. *Cancer Immunol Immunother* **55**, 1064–1071.

21. Roncarolo, M. G., Gregori, S., Battaglia, M., Bacchetta, R., Fleischhauer, K., and Levings, M. K. (2006) Interleukin-10-secreting type 1 regulatory T cells in rodents and humans. *Immunological reviews* **212**, 28–50.

22. Gajewski, T. F. (2007) The expanding universe of regulatory T cell subsets in cancer. *Immunity* **27**, 185–187.

23. Kiniwa, Y., Miyahara, Y., Wang, H. Y., Peng, W., Peng, G., Wheeler, T. M., Thompson, T. C., Old, L. J., and Wang, R. F. (2007) CD8$^+$ Foxp3$^+$ Regulatory T Cells Mediate Immunosuppression in Prostate Cancer. *Clin Cancer Res* **13**, 6947–6958.

24. Shevach, E. M. (2006) From vanilla to 28 flavors: multiple varieties of T regulatory cells. *Immunity* **25**, 195–201.

25. Wei, S., Kryczek, I., Zou, L., Daniel, B., Cheng, P., Mottram, P., Curiel, T., Lange, A., and Zou, W. (2005) Plasmacytoid dendritic cells induce CD8$^+$ regulatory T cells in human ovarian carcinoma. *Cancer research* **65**, 5020–5026.

26. Peng, G., Wang, H. Y., Peng, W., Kiniwa, Y., Seo, K. H., and Wang, R. F. (2007) Tumor-infiltrating gammadelta T cells suppress T and dendritic cell function via mechanisms controlled by a unique toll-like receptor signaling pathway. *Immunity* **27**, 334–348.

27. Colombo, M. P., and Piconese, S. (2007) Regulatory-T-cell inhibition versus depletion: the right choice in cancer immunotherapy. *Nat Rev Cancer* **7**, 880–887.

28. Peng, G., Guo, Z., Kiniwa, Y., Voo, K. S., Peng, W., Fu, T., Wang, D. Y., Li, Y., Wang, H. Y., and Wang, R. F. (2005) Toll-like receptor 8-mediated reversal of CD4$^+$ regulatory T cell function. *Science* **309**, 1380–1384.

29. Powell, D. J., Jr., Felipe-Silva, A., Merino, M. J., Ahmadzadeh, M., Allen, T., Levy, C., White, D. E., Mavroukakis, S., Kreitman, R. J., Rosenberg, S. A., and Pastan, I. (2007) Administration of a CD25-directed immunotoxin, LMB-2, to patients with metastatic melanoma induces a selective partial reduction in regulatory T cells in vivo. *J Immunol* **179**, 4919–4928.

30. Molenkamp, B. G., van Leeuwen, P. A., Meijer, S., Sluijter, B. J., Wijnands, P. G., Baars, A., van den Eertwegh, A. J., Scheper, R. J., and de Gruijl, T. D. (2007) Intradermal CpG-B activates both plasmacytoid and myeloid dendritic cells in the sentinel lymph node of melanoma patients. *Clin Cancer Res* **13**, 2961–2969.

31. Sakaguchi, S., and Powrie, F. (2007) Emerging challenges in regulatory T cell function and biology. *Science (New York, N.Y* **317**, 627–629.

32. Dieckmann, D., Plottner, H., Berchtold, S., Berger, T., and Schuler, G. (2001) Ex vivo isolation and characterization of

CD4$^{(+)}$)CD25$^{(+)}$ T cells with regulatory properties from human blood. *J Exp Med* **193**, 1303–1310.

33. Baecher-Allan, C., Brown, J. A., Freeman, G. J., and Hafler, D. A. (2001) CD4$^+$CD25high regulatory cells in human peripheral blood. *J Immunol* **167**, 1245–1253.

34. Fontenot, J. D., Gavin, M. A., and Rudensky, A. Y. (2003) Foxp3 programs the development and function of CD4$^+$CD25$^+$ regulatory T cells. *Nat Immunol* **4**, 330–336.

35. Walker, M. R., Kasprowicz, D. J., Gersuk, V. H., Benard, A., Van Landeghen, M., Buckner, J. H., and Ziegler, S. F. (2003) Induction of FoxP3 and acquisition of T regulatory activity by stimulated human CD4$^+$CD25- T cells. *J Clin Invest* **112**, 1437–1443.

36. Hori, S., Nomura, T., and Sakaguchi, S. (2003) Control of regulatory T cell development by the transcription factor Foxp3. *Science* **299**, 1057–1061.

37. Liu, W., Putnam, A. L., Xu-Yu, Z., Szot, G. L., Lee, M. R., Zhu, S., Gottlieb, P. A., Kapranov, P., Gingeras, T. R., Fazekas de St Groth, B., Clayberger, C., Soper, D. M., Ziegler, S. F., and Bluestone, J. A. (2006) CD127 expression inversely correlates with FoxP3 and suppressive function of human CD4$^+$ T reg cells. *J Exp Med* **203**, 1701–1711.

38. Seddiki, N., Santner-Nanan, B., Martinson, J., Zaunders, J., Sasson, S., Landay, A., Solomon, M., Selby, W., Alexander, S. I., Nanan, R., Kelleher, A., and Fazekas de St Groth, B. (2006) Expression of interleukin (IL)-2 and IL-7 receptors discriminates between human regulatory and activated T cells. *J Exp Med* **203**, 1693–1700.

39. Banham, A. H. (2006) Cell-surface IL-7 receptor expression facilitates the purification of FOXP3$^{(+)}$ regulatory T cells. *Trends Immunol* **27**, 541–544.

40. Lohr, J., Knoechel, B., Nagabhushanam, V., and Abbas, A. K. (2005) T-cell tolerance and autoimmunity to systemic and tissue-restricted self-antigens. *Immunol Rev* **204**, 116–127.

41. Battaglia, M., Gregori, S., Bacchetta, R., and Roncarolo, M. G. (2006) Tr1 cells: from discovery to their clinical application. *Semin Immunol* **18**, 120–127.

42. Levings, M. K., Gregori, S., Tresoldi, E. Cazzaniga, S., Bonini, C., and Roncarolo, M. G. (2005) Differentiation of Tr1 cells by immature dendritic cells requires IL-10 but not CD25$^+$CD4$^+$ Tr cells. *Blood* **105**, 1162–1169.

Chapter 3

Generation of Cytotoxic T Lymphocytes for Immunotherapy of EBV-Associated Malignancies

Corey Smith and Rajiv Khanna

Abstract

Current approaches for the treatment of tumours typically employ broad acting radiotherapeutic and chemotherapeutic approaches, which have led to high success rates but can be associated with unwanted side-effects. Cytotoxic T cell (CTL)-based immunotherapy offers an alternative approach that is designed to specifically target protein antigens expressed in malignant cells and is thus likely to limit any adverse side-effects. Defining tumour-specific antigens is therefore critical for the successful application of CTL-based therapy. Epstein-Barr virus (EBV)-associated malignancies offer an attractive target for CTL-based immunotherapy due to presence of virally encoded antigens in the malignant cells. Recent success in treating Epstein-Barr virus (EBV)-associated post-transplant lymphoproliferative disorder (PTLD) using cytotoxic T cell (CTL)-based immunotherapy has led to interest in the development of CTL-based immunotherapy to treat other EBV-associated malignancies in which antigen expression patterns are well defined but limited to a restricted number of proteins.

Key words: CTL, immunotherapy, EBV, LCL, adenoviral vector, polyepitope.

1. Introduction

Infection with Epstein-Barr virus typically leads to an asymptomatic latent infection in most individual. However, EBV can be associated with malignancies that arise in both immunocompetent and immunocompromised individuals (1). EBV therefore offers an attractive target for the development of CTL-based immunotherapy for the treatment of these malignancies and has been successfully applied to treat post-transplant lymphoproliferative diseases (PTLD) that occur in both stem cell and solid organ transplant patients (2, 3). PTLD display a latency type 3

P. Yotnda (ed.), *Immunotherapy of Cancer*, Methods in Molecular Biology 651,
DOI 10.1007/978-1-60761-786-0_3, © Springer Science+Business Media, LLC 2010

gene expression profile characterised by the expression of all of the EBV latent genes. This therapy is based on the use of EBV-transformed lymphoblastoid cell lines (LCL) to generate CTL primarily directed against the immunodominant latent antigens, EBV nuclear antigens (EBNA) (3–6).

A number of studies have employed LCL-based expansion to generate CTL to treat EBV-associated latency type 2 malignancies (4, 5). However, these malignancies express a limited array of typically subdominant antigens, the Latent membrane proteins (LMP) 1 and 2 and EBNA1, suggesting that strategies aimed at optimising the generation of CTL to target these antigens would maximise the potential effectiveness of any CTL-based therapy. The strategy we have developed to produce CTL to treat EBV-associated latency type 2 malignancies, the AdE1-LMPpoly vector, encodes a polyepitope of CTL epitopes from LMP1 and 2 fused to a truncated EBNA1 gene in a replication deficient adenoviral expression vector (6). This strategy allows for the rapid generation of CTL following stimulation of PBMC with autologous PBMC infected with AdE1-LMPpoly for 14 days.

This chapter will outline current methods being employed to generate CTL specific for EBV antigens expressed in different malignancies and T-cell assays to determine the functionality of CTL cultures.

2. Materials

2.1. Purification of Peripheral Blood Mononuclear Cells (PBMC)

1. RPMI-1640 with L-glutamine (Gibco Invitrogen, Carlsbad, CA, USA) is supplemented with gentamicin alone (referred to as RPMI).

2. Lymphoprep (GE Healthcare).

3. Trypan Blue (Sigma-Aldrich) is supplied as a 0.4% solution and is stored at room temperature.

2.2. Generation of Lymphoblastoid Cell Lines (LCL)

1. RPMI and RPMI supplemented with 10% foetal bovine serum (Sigma-Aldrich) (referred to as RPMI/10% FBS).

2. B95.8 strain of EBV.

3. Cyclosporin A is stored at −20°C.

2.3. Generation of CTL Lines

1. RPMI and RPMI/10% FBS.

2. Autologous LCL for the generation of CTL using LCL.

3. Replication-incompetent adenovirus for the generation of CTL using recombinant adenoviral-based vectors. The replication-incompetent adenovirus used in our laboratory is produced at the Centre for Cell and Gene Therapy, Baylor College of Medicine, Houston, TX, USA. Refer to Smith et al. for construction of the AdE1-LMPpoly vector used in our studies (6).

4. Recombinant interleukin-2 (IL-2) (Norvatis, Basel, Switzerland) is dissolved at 60,000 IU/ml and stored at −80°C.

5. Trypan Blue.

6. Albumex 4 (CSL Limited, Parkville, VIC, Australia) containing 4% (w/v) human albumin.

7. Dimethyl sulfoxide (DMSO) is supplied by Sigma-Aldrich.

8. 1.8 ml Cryovials (Nunc, Roskilde, Denmark).

2.4. Generation of Phytohaemagglu-tanin (PHA)-Blast Cells

1. PBMC.
2. RPMI/10% FBS.
3. PHA is stored at −20°C at a stock concentration of 2 mg/ml.
4. IL-2.

2.5. CTL Assay

1. PHA-blasts.

2. CTL peptide epitopes (Mimotopes, Clayton, VIC, Australia) derived from EBV antigens are dissolved at 2 mg/ml in 10% DMSO and stored at −80°C. Working stocks are diluted to 200 μg/ml in RPMI and stored at −20°C (*see* **Notes 1** and **2**).

3. Sodium dodecyl sulphate (SDS) (Sigma-Aldrich) is dissolved in distilled water to a final concentration of 10% (w/v).

4. Chromium 51 (^{51}Cr) is supplied by Perkin Elmer (Waltham, MA, USA) and stored at 4°C.

5. LumaPlates are supplied by Perkin Elmer.

2.6. Intracellular Cytokine Staining

1. PBS supplemented with 2% FBS.

2. CTL peptide epitopes; see ^{51}Cr release assay.

3. Phorbol 12-myristate 13-acetate (PMA) (Sigma-Aldrich) is dissolved in DMSO and stored at 5 μg/ml.

4. Ionomycin calcium salt (Sigma-Aldrich) is stored at 100 μg/ml.

5. APC-conjugated anti-human CD3, PerCP-conjugated anti-human CD8, FITC-conjugated anti-human CD4 and PE-conjugated anti-human IFN-γ are supplied by BD Biosciences, San Jose, CA, USA.

6. The BD Cytofix/Cytoperm Plus Fixation/Permeabilization Kit with BD GolgiPlug protein transport inhibitor containing brefeldin A is supplied by BD Biosciences.

7. Paraformaldehyde (Sigma-Aldrich) is dissolved in PBS to a final concentration of 2% (w/v) and stored at 4°C.

3. Methods

3.1. Purification of Peripheral Blood Mononuclear Cells (PBMC)

1. Dilute the blood sample 1:1 with room temperature RPMI and carefully layer 25 ml of blood into 50-ml tubes, each containing 10–15 ml of Lymphoprep.

2. Centrifuge the sample at 800 g for 20–30 min at room temperature with the centrifuge brake switched off.

3. Remove the mononuclear cell interface and transfer into 50-ml tubes containing 30-ml aliquots of RPMI (*see* **Note 3**). Adjust volume of each tube to 50 ml with RPMI.

4. Centrifuge at 311 g (1200 rpm) for 10 min at room temperature with the brake on. Aspirate and discard the supernatant.

5. Resuspend the cell pellets in RPMI and combine into one or two tubes at a final volume of 50 ml per tube. Centrifuge at room temperature, 216 g (1000 rpm), for 10 min.

6. Discard the supernatant and resuspend the pellet(s) in a final volume of 50 ml of RPMI. Remove 50 µl from the tube, dilute 1:1 with Trypan Blue and determine the number of viable cells using a Haemocytometer (*see* **Note 4**).

7. The PBMC cell suspension can now be used immediately or prepared for storage in liquid N_2 (*see* **Sections 3.4.7 and 3.4.8**).

8. For storage in liquid N_2, centrifuge the cells at 216 g (1000 rpm) for 10 min. Wash the cells twice by adding 20 ml of Albumex. Resuspend in an appropriate volume of Albumex + 10% DMSO and aliquot into cryovials.

9. Lower temperature of T cells using a controlled rate freezer. Then transfer to a vapour phase liquid N_2 storage tank.

3.2. Generation of Lymphoblastoid Cell Lines (LCL)

1. Resuspend 2–5×10⁶ PBMC in 500 µl RPMI. Add 500 µl of RPMI containing 100–500 infectious units of EBV. Incubate for 1 hr at 37°C in a CO_2 incubator.

2. Add 9 ml of RPMI/10% FBS and centrifuge at 1000 rpm for 5 min. Resuspend cells in RPMI/10% FBS containing

10 μg/ml of Cyclosporin A. Perform 6–8 twofold serial dilutions of infected cells in a 24-well plate (*see* **Note 5**).

3. Incubate at 37°C in a CO_2 incubator. Replenish media weekly for up to 4 weeks by discarding half and adding fresh RPMI/10% FBS with 10 μg/ml of Cyclosporin A.

4. Three to four weeks post-infection, LCL colony formation should be evident in the lower dilutions. When confluent, harvest the lowest dilution containing evidence of colony formation and transfer to a T25 flask containing RPMI/10% FBS.

5. LCL can now be expanded and used to generate CTL (*see* **Note 6**).

3.3. Generation of CTL Using LCL

This method is used to generate CTL cultures that predominately recognise the immunodominant latent antigens of EBV, EBNA3–6. PBMC for this method are prepared prior to use and stored in liquid N_2.

1. Thaw PBMC (between 2×10^6 and 3×10^6 PBMC are required per culture) as quickly as possible. Transfer into 9 ml of RPMI/10% FBS and centrifuge at 1000 rpm for 10 min. Resuspend in 10 ml RPMI+10% FBS. Incubate for 1 h.

2. Determine the number of viable cells using the trypan blue exclusion method. Resuspend at $2–3 \times 10^6$ PBMC/ml and add 1 ml per well of a 24-well plate.

3. Harvest $1–2 \times 10^6$ autologous LCL and gamma irradiate at 8000 rads to prepare stimulator cells. Wash and resuspend the stimulator cells in 10 ml of RPMI/10% FBS.

4. Determine the number of viable LCL using the trypan blue exclusion method. Resuspend stimulator cells at 6.7×10^4 to 1×10^5 cells/ml and add 1 ml per well of PBMC to give a final ratio of 30 PBMC to 1 LCL.

5. On day 3 or 4 discard half of the culture supernatant and add 1 ml of RPMI/10% FBS containing IL-2 to generate a final concentration of 120 IU/ml. Additional IL-2 is added every 3–4 days until the end of the culture period.

6. On day 7 discard half of the culture supernatant and gently resuspend the cells. Determine the remaining volume and the number of viable cells using the trypan blue exclusion method. Prepare LCL stimulators (as for steps 3 and 4) and add to give a ratio of 30 cultured cells to 1 LCL. If the total cell number is greater than 3×10^6, split cells into two wells and add RPMI/10% FBS and IL-2 to a total volume of 2 ml per well.

7. On day 10 or 11, repeat as for day 3 or 4.

8. On day 14, repeat as for day 7. If the total cell number is greater than 10×10^6 transfer the cells into a T25 flask standing upright and add RPMI/10% FBS and IL-2 to a total volume of 12 ml. Lay the flask down flat if the total cell number is greater than 15×10^6.

9. On day 17 or 18, repeat as for day 3 or 4.

10. On day 21, remove the cells from the incubator and transfer cell suspension to a tube. Determine the number of viable cells using the trypan blue exclusion method. Remove an appropriate number of cells for analysis of T-cell function and store the remaining cells as outlined in **Section 3.1** (*see* **Note 7**).

3.4. Generation of CTL Using Recombinant Adenoviral-Based Vectors

This method is used in our laboratory to generate CTL that predominately target the subdominant latent EBV antigens, LMP1 and 2 and EBNA1.

1. Harvest 100 million PBMC per T75 tissue culture flask to be used. Divide PBMC into two at a ratio of 3 (stimulators):7 (responders). Centrifuge cells at room temperature, 216 g (1000 rpm), for 10 min.

2. Resuspend responder cells in 10 ml of RPMI/10% FBS. Transfer responder cells into a T75 tissue culture flask and place these cells into a CO_2 incubator while the stimulator cells are prepared.

3. Resuspend stimulator PBMC at 2×10^7 ml^{-1} in RPMI and add the recombinant adenovirus at a multiplicity of infection (MOI) of 10:1. Incubate for 1 h at 37°C in a CO_2 incubator.

4. Wash stimulator cells three times by resuspending in 10 ml of RPMI/10% FBS and centrifuge at 216 g (1000 rpm) for 10 min. Resuspend cells in 1 ml of RPMI/10% FBS and gamma irradiate for 2000 rads.

5. Resuspend the stimulator cells in 10 ml of RPMI/10% FBS. Add to the T75 flask containing the responder cells. Transfer the flask standing upright into the incubator. On days 3, 7 and 10 add 10 ml of RPMI/10% FBS containing IL-2 to generate a final concentration of 120 IU/ml. Lay the flask down flat in the incubator on day 3.

6. On day 14 remove the flask from the incubator and transfer the T-cell suspension to a tube. Determine the number of viable cells using the trypan blue exclusion method. Remove an appropriate number of cells for analysis of T-cell function, typically between 5×10^5 and 1×10^6 cells per test, and store the remaining cells as outlined in **Section 3.1** (*see* **Note 8**).

3.5. Generation of Phytohaemag glutanin (PHA) Blast Cells

1. Resuspend PBMC at 1×10^6 cells/ml in RPMI/10% FBS. Add PHA to a final concentration of 20 μg/ml. Dispense 2 ml of cells per well on a 24-well plate. Incubate at 37°C in a CO_2 Incubator.

2. On Day 3, carefully remove half of the supernatant and add RPMI/10% FCS to a final volume of 2 ml. Add IL-2 to a final concentration of 120 IU/ml.

3. On Day 7, resuspend cells and transfer into a tube. Centrifuge at 1000 rpm for 5 min. Resuspend in10 ml of RPMI/10% FBS + 120 IU/ml IL-2 and transfer into a T25 flask.

4. Maintain cells twice weekly with fresh IL-2 supplemented media. Expand into a T75 flask when confluent and store after 1–2 weeks. Cells should remain viable for up to 8 weeks in culture.

3.6. CTL Assay

1. Incubate donor-derived PHA-blasts (target cells) with 1 μg/ml of the appropriate HLA-matched peptides in RPMI for 1 h at 37°C. Wash cells three times with 10 ml of RPMI and centrifuge at 1000 rpm for 5 min.

2. Label target cells with 50 μCi of ^{51}Cr. Incubate cells for 1 h at 37°C. Wash cells three times with 10 ml of RPMI/10% FBS and centrifuge at 1000 rpm for 5 min.

3. Determine the number of viable cells using the trypan blue exclusion method. Adjust target cell concentration to 10^5 cells/ml. Dispense 100 μl of target cells to the appropriate wells of a 96-well round bottom plate.

4. Resuspend cultured T cells (effector cells) to a final concentration of $1–2\times10^6$ cells/ml. Dispense 100 μl of effector cells into the appropriate wells of the 96-well round bottom plate to generate effector to target ratios of between 20:1 and 10:1. In six control wells containing target cells alone, add 100 μl of RPMI/10% FBS (spontaneous release) and in another six wells add 10% SDS (maximal release). Centrifuge plates at 500 rpm/5 min and incubate at 37°C for 5 h.

5. Centrifuge plates at 500 rpm for 5 min. Transfer 25 μl of supernatant from each well into a LumaPlate. Allow plate to dry overnight at room temperature.

6. Determine total counts using the Perkin Elmer Top-Count NXT.

7. Determine the percentage lysis based on ^{51}Cr release compared to spontaneous and maximal release. An example of CTL activity using AdE1-LMPpoly-stimulated T cells is shown in **Fig. 3.1**.

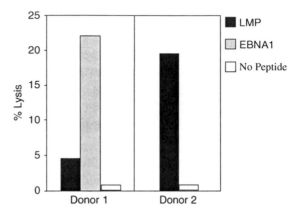

Fig 3.1. CTL assay of AdE1-LMPpoly-stimulated T cells. PBMC from two EBV-positive donors were stimulated with AdE1-LMPpoly. Following stimulation T cells were assessed for cytolytic activity against LMP or EBNA1 peptide-pulsed targets. Data represent specific lysis at an effector: target ratio of 20:1.

3.7. Intracellular IFN-γ Staining

1. Dilute the appropriate HLA matched peptide epitopes to 2 μg/ml in RPMI1640-10% FBS (final concentration in the assay will be 1 μg/ml). Dilute PMA to 100 ng/ml and Ionomycin to 2 μg/ml in a single tube in RPMI1640-10% FBS (*see* **Note 9**). Add 100 μl of the appropriate CTL epitope, 100 μl PMA/Ionomycin or 100 μl RPMI1640-10% FBS (no peptide control) to the appropriate wells of a 96-well V-bottom plate.

2. Dilute T cells to between 5×10^6 and 1×10^7 cells/ml in RPMI1640-10% FBS. Add GolgiPlug to a concentration of 2 μl/ml of cells (final concentration of GolgiPlug in the assay will be 1 μl/ml). Add 100 μl of cell suspension (5×10^5 to 1×10^6 cells) per well to the required wells of the 96-well V-bottom plate. Incubate for 4–5 h at 37°C in a CO_2 incubator.

3. Centrifuge the plate at 2300 rpm for 2 min. Wash cells twice by adding 200 μl of PBS-2% FBS per well and centrifuge the plate at 2300 rpm for 2 min.

4. Resuspend cells in 50 μl/well of PBS-2% FBS containing 2 μl of APC-conjugated anti-CD3, 8 μl of PerCP-conjugated anti-CD8 and 1 μl of FITC-conjugated anti-CD4 per 10^6 cells. Incubate for 30 min at 4°C. Wash the cells as in step 3.

5. Resuspend cells in 100 μl per well of cytofix/cytoperm solution and incubate at 4°C for 20 min. Centrifuge the plate at 2300 rpm for 2 min. Wash the cells twice by adding 200 μl of Perm/Wash per well and centrifuge.

6. Resuspend fixed/permeabilised cells in 50 μl/well of Perm/Wash solution containing 0.25 μl of PE-conjugated

anti-IFNγ per 10^6 cells. Incubate for 30 min at 4°C. Wash the cells as in step 5.

7. Resuspend the cells in 200 μl of PBS-2% paraformalde-hyde and store at 4°C. Analyse the percentage of antigen-specific CD3+CD8+ using a flow cytometer. Calculate the percentage of CD3+CD8+ lymphocytes producing IFN-γ in response to each CTL peptide, no peptide (neg-ative control) and PMA/Ionymycin (positive control). Representative FACS data following generation of CTL following stimulation with recombinant adenovirus com-pared to the response detected in PBMC are shown in **Fig. 3.2**.

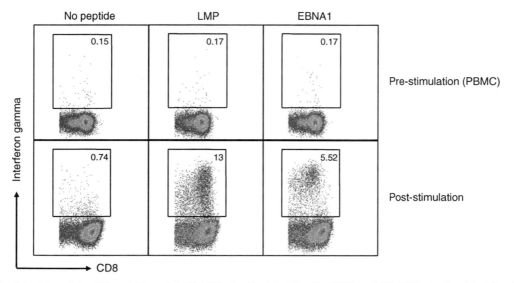

Fig. 3.2. Intracellular IFN-γ staining of AdE1-LMPpoly-stimulated T cells. PBMC or AdE1-LMPpoly-stimulated T cells from an EBV-positive donor were stimulated with LMP or EBNA-encoded peptides and assessed for intracellular IFN-γ production. Data represent the percentage of IFN-γ-producing CD8+ T cells.

4. Notes

1. Prior to commencement of either preparation of functional assays, establishment of the HLA-type of the donor is required to determine the appropriate peptide epitopes to be used.

2. See Hislop et al. for a list of known EBV-derived CTL epi-topes and corresponding HLA restriction (7).

3. The mononuclear cell interface is the whitish layer at the interface between the yellowish-coloured uppermost plasma and the clear Lymphoprep.

4. PBMC yields typically between 0.5×10^6 and 2×10^6 cells/ml of blood. However, lower yields are often evident from patient donors, which need to be taken into account when a particular number of cells are required for the generation of CTL.

5. Add 2 ml of cells to the first well and transfer 1 ml into subsequent wells containing 1 ml of RPMI/10% FBS with 10 μg/ml of Cyclosporin A. Add an additional 1 ml of RPMI/10% FBS with 10 μg/ml of Cyclosporin A to each well to produce a final volume of 2 ml per well.

6. Once established, LCL are typically maintained by passage every 3–4 days with fresh RPMI/10% FCS to maintain cell viability.

7. Depending upon the size of the pre-existing memory CTL pool and the HLA-type of the donor, expansion of T cells with LCL will generate a five- to tenfold expansion in absolute cell number.

8. Depending upon the size of the pre-existing memory CTL pool and the HLA type of the donor, expansion with our recombinant AdE1-LMPpoly vector typically generates a one- to threefold expansion in absolute cell number after 14 days, and up to a 200-fold expansion in the number of antigen-specific cells. However, specific CTL cannot be generated from all donors, despite the fact that donors are HLA-matched to epitopes encoded for by AdE1-LMPpoly. This is likely due to an absence of specific memory CTL in the peripheral blood.

9. PMA and Ionymycin act as a strong positive control and should induce IFN-γ from a high proportion of cultured cells. They should be aliquoted for storage as freezing/thawing reduces function.

References

1. Khanna, R., Moss, D., Gandhi, M. (2005) Technology insight: applications of emerging immunotherapeutic strategies for Epstein-Barr virus-associated malignancies. *Nat Clin Pract Oncol* 2, 138–149.

2. Rooney, C. M., Smith, C. A., Ng, C. Y., et al. (1995) Use of gene-modified virus-specific T lymphocytes to control Epstein-Barr-virus-related lymphoproliferation. *Lancet* 345, 9–13.

3. Khanna, R., Bell, S., Sherritt, M., et al. (1999) Activation and adoptive transfer of Epstein-Barr virus-specific cytotoxic T cells in solid organ transplant patients with posttransplant lymphoproliferative disease. *Proc Natl Acad Sci USA* 96, 10391–10396.

4. Comoli, P., Pedrazzoli, P., Maccario, R., et al. (2005) Cell therapy of stage IV nasopharyngeal carcinoma with autologous Epstein-

Barr virus-targeted cytotoxic T lymphocytes. *J Clin Oncol 23*, 8942–8949.

5. Straathof, K. C., Bollard, C. M., Popat, U., et al. (2005) Treatment of nasopharyngeal carcinoma with Epstein-Barr virus--specific T lymphocytes. *Blood 105*, 1898–1904.

6. Smith, C., Cooper, L., Burgess, M., et al. (2006) Functional reversion of antigen-specific CD8[+] T cells from patients with Hodgkin lymphoma following in vitro stimulation with recombinant polyepitope. *J Immunol 177*, 4897–4906.

7. Hislop, A. D., Taylor, G. S., Sauce, D., Rickinson, A. B. (2007) Cellular responses to viral infection in humans: lessons from Epstein-Barr virus. *Annu Rev Immunol 25*, 587–617.

Chapter 4

Acquisition, Preparation, and Functional Assessment of Human NK Cells for Adoptive Immunotherapy

Dean A. Lee, Michael R. Verneris, and Dario Campana

Abstract

Human natural killer (NK) cells, a subset of peripheral blood lymphocytes that lack a T- or B-cell receptor, play a crucial role in the innate immune response to viruses and malignant cells. NK cells differentiate infected or malignant cells from normal cells by a complex balance between activating and inhibitory receptor–ligand interactions. Unlike T cells, NK cells do not proliferate in vitro in response to simple crosslinking of a single activating receptor. While many methods to study T-cell function and phenotype can also be applied to NK cells, this chapter addresses methods that are unique to the preparation and assessment of human NK cells for immunotherapy.

Key words: Natural killer cell, lymphokine-activated killer, antibody-dependent cell cytotoxicity, degranulation, depletion, flow cytometry, calcein, NK-cell expansion.

1. Introduction

It has been known for over 30 years that some lymphocytes have the ability to recognize and lyse a variety of human malignancies to which they have not previously been sensitized (1). Human natural killer (NK) cells are a subset of peripheral blood $CD2^+$ lymphocytes that lack a T-cell receptor complex (and are therefore $CD3^-$) but express the neural cell adhesion molecule (NCAM, CD56), the low-affinity immunoglobulin Fc-receptor III (FcγRIII, CD16), or both (2). NK cells display a variety of activating receptors, including NKp30, NKp44, NKp46, NKG2D, 2B4, and DNAM-1 (3). NK-cell activation is regulated by heterogeneous expression of killer inhibitory receptors (KIR),

P. Yotnda (ed.), *Immunotherapy of Cancer*, Methods in Molecular Biology 651,
DOI 10.1007/978-1-60761-786-0_4, © Springer Science+Business Media, LLC 2010

which interact with various dimorphic HLA class I epitope families (4). Thus, NK-cell diversity and specificity results from a wide variety of germline-encoded activating and inhibitory receptors that are non-clonally rearranged and whose expression is antigen independent.

NK cells play a crucial role in the innate immune response to viruses and tumors, differentiating infected or malignant cells from normal cells through a complex balance between activating and inhibitory receptor–ligand interactions (5). NK cell-mediated lysis correlates with the surface expression of these receptors on NK cells and of the corresponding ligands on tumor cells.

Early recognition that IL-2 activation of NK cells increased their cytotoxicity toward resistant targets (6, 7) led to clinical trials of in vitro activated autologous or haploidentical NK cells (8–10). Thus, adoptive transfer of NK cells has been tested in early-phase clinical trials and has emerged as a safe and potentially efficacious immunotherapy for cancer (10), but development of this therapeutic approach has been hampered by low numbers of NK cells available from donors. The most common strategy for obtaining sufficient numbers of NK cells for adoptive immunotherapy is leukapheresis followed by immunomagnetic selection (11).

High numbers of NK cells in allogeneic hematopoietic cell grafts are associated with improved transplant-associated outcomes. Recipients of allografts with high NK-cell content have significantly faster neutrophil recovery (12, 13), a lower incidence of non-relapse mortality (13, 14), fewer bacterial and viral infections, faster immune reconstitution (13), and less acute (15) and chronic (12) graft-versus-host disease (GVHD). Rapid recovery of NK cells after allogeneic hematopoietic stem cell transplantation (HSCT) is associated with a reduction in the rates of relapse, non-relapse mortality, and acute GVHD (16). Therefore, augmenting NK-cell dose and reconstitution with peritransplant adoptive transfer of donor NK cells might further improve transplant outcomes via these mechanisms.

Because NK cells constitute a small percentage of peripheral blood mononuclear cells, generating them in numbers sufficient to exert measurable clinical effects is problematic. Hence, the outcome of NK-cell-based therapies might be substantially improved by methods to produce large numbers of NK cells ex vivo. Receptor crosslinking in vitro does not result in significant sustained proliferation of NK cells, unlike T lymphocytes, and their proliferative responses to cytokines (with or without coculture with other accessory cells) have been modest and transient (17–20). Nevertheless, some expansion of NK cells (five- to tenfold over 1–2 weeks) can be achieved through high-dose IL-2 alone (21, 22). Activation of autologous T cells can also mediate NK-cell expansion, presumably through release of local cytokines (23, 24). Support with mesenchymal stroma (25), EBV-transformed lymphoblastoid cell lines (26), or genetically modified K562 cells (27–29) can promote the expansion of NK cells from both peripheral blood and cord blood.

2. Materials

2.1. NK Cell Purification

2.1.1. Magnetic Purification of NK Cells by CD3/CD14/CD20 Depletion or CD56 Positive Selection

1. Peripheral blood mononuclear cells (PBMC) obtained by density-gradient isolation from whole blood, normal donor buffy coat from blood bank red cell donation, or leukapheresis
2. RPMI-1640 medium, 4°C
3. Magnetic beads conjugated to antibodies against human CD56, or CD3, CD14, and CD20 (Dynal, Invitrogen, Miltenyi, Biotec)
4. Strong magnet for cell sorting
5. Conical tubes designed to fit the magnet

2.1.2. Purification of NK Cells Using RosetteSep Antibody Complexes

1. Whole blood or normal donor buffy coat from blood bank red cell donation (*see* **Note 1**)
2. RPMI-1640 medium, room temperature (*see* **Note 2**)
3. RosetteSep Human NK Cell Enrichment Cocktail (StemCell Technologies)
4. Ficoll-Paque or similar density-gradient separation medium, room temperature

2.2. NK Cell Activation

1. Purified NK cells
2. NK-cell activation medium: RPMI-1640 supplemented with 10% fetal calf serum, 2 mM L-glutamine, and 1000 IU/ml recombinant human IL-2 (*see* **Note 13**)

2.3. Ex Vivo Expansion of NK Cells with Genetically Modified K562 Cells (K562-mb15-41BBL)

1. Peripheral blood mononuclear cells (PBMC) obtained by density-gradient isolation from whole blood, normal donor buffy coat from blood bank red cell donation, or leukapheresis.
2. K562 gene-modified to express 41BBL and membrane-bound IL-15 (K562-mb15-41BBL), growing in log phase.

3. NK-cell growth medium: RPMI-1640 supplemented with 10% fetal calf serum, 2 mM L-glutamine, and 10 IU/ml recombinant human IL-2.

2.4. Assessing NK Activity

2.4.1. Direct Cytotoxicity of Calcein-Loaded Targets

1. NK cells to be assessed
2. Target cells (*see* **Note 21**) growing in log phase with viability >95%
3. Calcein-AM, 2.5 mM (1.6 mg/ml) in DMSO (Molecular Probes, BD Biosciences, Biotium) (*see* **Notes 22 and 23**)
4. Lysis buffer: 1% Triton X-100 in water
5. NK-cell assay medium: RPMI-1640 supplemented with 2% fetal calf serum and 10 IU/ml recombinant human IL-2
6. 96-well U-bottom plates
7. 96-well fluorescent plate reader

2.4.2. Flow Cytometry to Assess Target Cell Killing

1. NK cells to be assessed
2. Target cells growing in log phase with viability >95%
3. NK-cell assay medium: RPMI-1640 supplemented with 2% fetal calf serum and 10 IU/ml recombinant human IL-2
4. 12-well tissue culture plates
5. Fluorophore-labeled (not FL-3) antibodies specific for target cells (e.g., CD22 for B-lineage acute lymphoblastic leukemia, CD33 for acute myeloid leukemia)
6. 7-AAD (BD Biosciences)
7. Flow cytometry buffer: PBS, 1% fetal calf serum

2.4.3. Flow Cytometry to Assess NK-Cell Activation and Degranulation

1. NK cells to be assessed
2. Target cells growing in log phase with viability >95%
3. NK-cell assay medium: RPMI-1640 supplemented with 2% fetal calf serum and 10 IU/ml recombinant human IL-2
4. 12-well tissue culture plates
5. Fluorophore-labeled antibodies specific for CD107a and CD56
6. Fluorophore-labeled isotype control antibodies
7. Flow cytometry buffer: PBS, 1% fetal calf serum
8. Paraformaldehyde 0.5% in PBS

3. Methods

3.1. NK-Cell Purification

3.1.1. Magnetic Purification of NK Cells by CD3/CD14/CD20 Depletion or CD56 Positive Selection

1. Resuspend PBMC (*see* **Note 1**) in 4°C RPMI-1640 (*see* **Note 2**) at a concentration of 10^8 cells/ml.

2. Prepare magnetic beads sufficient for the starting number of PBMC. This will vary depending on manufacturer, but is most often in the range of 1–2 μL/10^6 cells. For CD3/CD14/CD20 depletion (*see* **Note 3**), an equal volume of each bead should be mixed together. In a tube(s) designed to fit in the magnet you are using, add the beads to at least twice their volume of RPMI-1640 (1 ml minimum), vortex lightly, and place next to the magnet. Wait at least 1 min until the beads are attracted to the side of the tube next to the magnet. Repeat the process, and then resuspend the beads in the same volume of RPMI-1640 used in step 1.

3. Mix the cells with the beads and incubate at 4°C for 15–30 min, with gentle resuspension every 5 min (*see* **Note 4**).

4. Place the tube next to the magnet for 3 min. If performing depletion, carefully aspirate the cells in suspension and transfer to another tube, discarding the magnetic cell pellet. If performing CD56 positive selection (*see* **Note 5**), carefully aspirate and discard the cells in suspension, and resuspend the cell pellet in twice the volume of fresh RPMI-1640 used in step 1.

5. Repeat step 4.

6. Centrifuge the cells at 400 g for 5 min. Resuspend cells as indicated for intended use.

3.1.2. Purification of NK Cells Using RosetteSep Antibody Complexes

1. Transfer whole blood or buffy coat (*see* **Note 6, 7**) to conical tubes, filling each tube no more than half full (**Fig. 4.1**).

2. Add RosetteSep 50 μL/ml for whole blood or 10 μL/ml for buffy coat, and mix by vortexing lightly (*see* **Note 8**).

3. Incubate for 20 min at room temperature (*see* **Note 9**).

4. Dilute the cells with an equal volume of RPMI-1640 and mix gently by inverting the tube several times. Do not vortex.

5. Place Ficoll-Paque in the bottom of a clean tube—use one-third of the tube volume (e.g., 5 ml for 15 ml tube, 15 ml for 50 ml tube) (*see* **Note 10**).

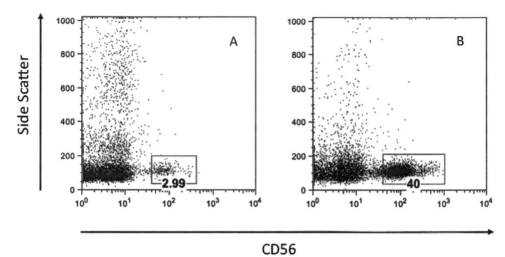

Fig 4.1. Enrichment of NK cells from blood bank normal donor buffy coat using RosetteSep. NK cells from a buffy coat unit were quantified by flow cytometry using anti-CD56-FITC before (**A**) and after (**B**) enrichment using RosetteSep as indicated in the protocol. Total NK cells recovered is typically $1–2 \times 10^7$.

6. Carefully layer the cell/RosetteSep suspension over the Ficoll-Paque (*see* **Note 9**).

7. Centrifuge at 1200 *g* (*see* **Note 11**) for 20 min, using slow acceleration and no deceleration (brake off) (*see* **Note 9**).

8. Aspirate the cells at the RPMI-Ficoll interface (*see* **Note 12**).

9. Wash the cells and resuspend as indicated for intended use.

3.2. NK Cell Activation (see Note 14)

1. Resuspend purified NK cells at 10^6 cells/ml in NK-cell activation medium.

2. Transfer cells to a tissue culture plate or flask sufficient to result in approximately 1 cm depth of culture medium (2 ml/well in a 24-well plate, 10–15 ml in a 25 cm² flask, etc. (*see* **Note 15**)).

3. Incubate for 24–48 h at 37°C in humidified 5% CO_2.

3.3. Ex Vivo Expansion of NK Cells with Genetically Modified K562 Cells (K562-mb15-41BBL)

1. Perform cell counts of viable PBMCs to be expanded.

2. Obtain sufficient K562-mb15-41BBL cells as needed for a PBMC:K562-mb15-41BBL ratio of 1.5:1.

3. Expose the K562-mb15-41BBL cells to 10,000 cGy γ-irradiation (*see* **Note 16**).

4. Wash the K562-mb15-41BBL cells once and resuspend at 1×10^6 cells/ml in NK-cell expansion medium.

5. Wash PBMC and resuspend at 1.5×10^6 cells/ml in NK-cell expansion medium.

6. Transfer cells to a tissue culture plate or flask sufficient to result in approximately 1 cm depth of culture medium (e.g., 30 ml in a 75-cm^2 flask).

7. Incubate at 37°C in humidified 5% CO_2.

8. On days 2, 4, and 6, remove half of the medium from the culture and replace it with an equal volume of fresh NK-cell expansion medium (*see* **Notes 17** and **18**).

9. On day 7, count the cells (*see* **Notes 19** and **20**). If further expansion is required repeat steps 2–9, replacing PBMC with expanded NK cells and changing the NK cell:K562-mb15-41BBL ratio to 1:10 for step 2 (*see* **Note 18**).

3.4. Assessing NK Activity

3.4.1. Direct Cytotoxicity of Calcein-Loaded Targets (see **Notes 21–23***)*

1. Determine the number of NK-cell sources, conditions, E:T ratios, and replicates needed for the experiment. Include one replicate set of target cells only to determine spontaneous release, and another to determine maximum release (**Fig. 4.2**). Calculate the number of target cells (*see* **Note 21**) needed for the experiment. Typically 10^4 target cells/well are ideal for 96-well plates.

2. Resuspend the target cells at 10^6 cells/ml in NK-cell assay medium.

3. Add 10 µL of stock calcein-AM solution to each milliliter of cells and incubate for 1 h at 37°C with gentle resuspension every 10–15 min.

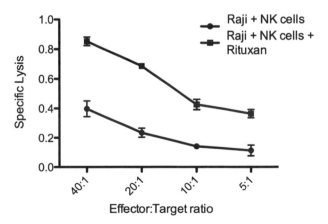

Fig. 4.2. Lysis of NK-resistant Raji cells with or without ADCC as assessed by the calcein assay. Raji cells were loaded with calcein as indicated in the protocol. Loaded cells were then incubated with control IgG (**A**) or rituximab (**B**) and then cultured with NK cells at indicated E:T ratios. Percent specific lysis was calculated as indicated in the protocol.

4. While target cells are incubating, count the NK cells and resuspend twice the number of cells needed for the highest E:T ratio at 4×10^6 cells/ml in NK-cell assay medium.

5. Perform three serial twofold dilutions by transferring half of the resuspended NK cells to a clean tube with an equal volume of NK-cell assay medium, and repeating this process for as many E:T ratios as you have determined to perform.

6. Wash the target cells twice and resuspend at 10^5 cells/ml in NK-cell assay medium (*see* **Note 24**).

7. Add 100 µl (10^4) target cells to each well of a 96-well U-bottom plate.

8. Add 100 µl of diluted NK cells to appropriate wells to achieve an E:T ratio ranging from 40:1 to 5:1. Add 100 µl of NK-cell assay medium to the wells designated for spontaneous release, and add 100 µl of Triton X-100 to the wells designated for maximum release.

9. Incubate for 4 h at 37°C and 21% CO_2.

10. After incubation, transfer 100 µl of the supernatant to a new plate.

11. Assess the fluorescence of each well (excitation filter at 485 nm, emission filter at 530 nm (*see* **Note 25**)).

12. Calculate percent specific lysis according to the formula:

$$\text{Percent Specific Lysis} = \frac{\left(\text{Fluorescence}_{\text{Experimental}} - \text{Fluorescence}_{\text{Spontaneous}}\right)}{\left(\text{Fluorescence}_{\text{Maximum}} - \text{Fluorescence}_{\text{Spontaneous}}\right)} \times 100$$

3.4.2. Flow Cytometry to Assess Target Cell Killing

Using flow-based assays to determine cytotoxicity requires the ability to separate NK cells from both dead and live targets using flow cytometric parameters. If the NK-cell population is sufficiently pure, the two populations may be distinguishable on the basis of side scatter and forward scatter characteristics alone (*see* **Note 26**). More often, labeled antibodies specific for the target cell are required to clearly distinguish the cell populations (*see* **Note 27**), particularly when cell lysis of a large target results in a small, granular dead cell that overlies the NK-cell population. There are many different methods published for determining cell cytotoxicity by flow cytometry. This method is based on the publication by Imai et al. (28).

1. Determine the number of NK-cell sources, conditions, E:T ratios, and replicates needed for the experiment. Include one set of target cells only to assess baseline cell death. Calculate the number of target cells (*see* **Note 26**) needed for the experiment. Typically 5×10^4 target cells/well are ideal.

2. Resuspend the target cells at 10^6 cells/ml in NK-cell assay medium.

3. Count the NK cells and resuspend twice the number of cells needed for the highest E:T ratio at 4×10^6 cells/ml in NK-cell assay medium.

5. Perform three serial twofold dilutions by transferring half of the resuspended NK cells to a clean tube with an equal volume of NK-cell assay medium, and repeat this process for as many E:T ratios as you have determined to perform.

6. Wash the target cells twice and resuspend at 10^5 cells/ml in NK-cell assay medium.

7. Add 500 μl (5×10^4) target cells to each well of a 12-well plate.

8. Add 500 μl of diluted NK cells to appropriate wells to achieve an E:T ratio ranging from 40:1 to 5:1. Add 100 μl of NK-cell assay medium to the wells designated as baseline cell death.

9. Incubate for 4 h at 37°C and 21% CO_2.

10. After 4 h, collect all of the cells from each well and transfer to a 12 mm × 75 mm flow cytometry tube.

11. Wash once with flow cytometry buffer and resuspend each cell pellet in 100 μl of buffer. Add 10 μl of labeled antibody recognizing the target cells. Incubate the cells on ice for 30 min. Wash once and resuspend in 0.5 ml of flow cytometry buffer.

12. Add 10 μl of 7-AAD. Incubate at room temperature for 10 min, then add 0.5 ml of 0.5% paraformaldehyde.

13. Assess the cells by flow cytometry. Set side scatter, forward scatter, and fluorescence gates to identify a population of live target cells. Acquire events and count the number of viable cells recorded by the instrument in 30 seconds.

14. Calculate Percent Specific Lysis according to the formula:

$$\text{Percent Specific Lysis} = \frac{\left(\text{Dead targets}_{\text{Experimental}} - \text{Dead targets}_{\text{Target cells only}}\right)}{\left(\text{Viable targets}_{\text{Target cells only}}\right)} \times 100$$

3.4.3. Flow Cytometry to Assess NK-Cell Activation and Degranulation

Several surface and intracellular markers have been used to assess for activation and/or degranulation of NK cells. The most widely used of these is CD107a, which identifies the expression of lysosomal proteins (LAMP1) that are transiently displayed on the NK-cell surface following degranulation (*see* **Note 28**) (**Fig. 4.3**).

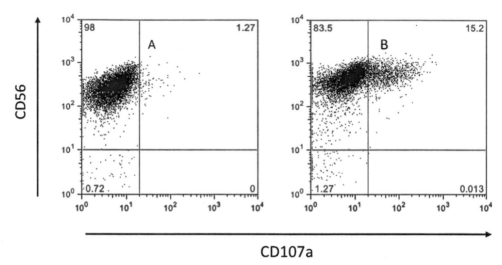

CD107a

Fig. 4.3. Functional assessment of NK-cell degranulation. CD107a expression on NK cells was quantified by flow cytometry using anti-CD56-FITC and anti-CD107a-PE. NK cells isolated from peripheral blood and activated overnight with IL-2 were cultured for 4 h alone (**A**) or with OS187 sarcoma cells as targets (**B**).

1. Determine the number of NK-cell sources, conditions, and replicates needed for the experiment. For the assessment of NK-cell degranulation, lower E:T ratios are more effective at stimulating degranulation. Add two wells of NK cells alone.

2. Prepare the cytotoxicity assay with targets as in steps 2–9 of **Section 3.4.2**.

3. Add 100 μl of CD107a antibody to each well (*see* **Note 29**), except to one of the wells having NK cells alone. To this well add 100 μl of the corresponding isotype control antibody.

4. After 4 h, collect all of the cells from each well. Split the sample equally into two flow cytometry tubes.

5. Wash once with flow cytometry buffer and resuspend each cell pellet in 100 μl of buffer. Add 10 μl of each labeled antibody. In tube 1 add the isotype control antibody for CD56. In tube 2, add the CD56 antibody (*see* **Note 30**).

6. Incubate the cells on ice for 30 min. Wash once and resuspend in 0.5 ml of flow cytometry buffer.

7. Add 10 μl of 7-AAD. Incubate at room temperature for 10 min, then add 0.5 ml of 0.5% paraformaldehyde.

8. Assess the cells by flow cytometry. Set side scatter, forward scatter, and fluorescence gates on the isotype-labeled NK cells that did not have targets. Then set the gates identifying NK cells on the CD56-labeled cells from this well. Acquire an equal number of viable events from each sample.

9. The CD107a-labeled NK cells cultured alone establish the baseline degranulation of NK cells in the absence of targets.

4. Notes

4.1. NK Cell Purification

4.1.1. Magnetic Purification of NK Cells by CD3/CD14/CD20 Depletion or CD56 Selection

1. NK cells can be purified with this method from whole peripheral blood, density-isolated PBMCs, blood bank buffy coat, cord blood, or leukapheresis products, but reagent concentrations must be optimized for each source. Several companies have marketed bead preparations pre-optimized for these different sources.

2. The product insert and many published protocols for leukocyte separation suggest using PBS or HBSS during wash and incubation steps. For the protocols described in this chapter, we have found that RPMI-1640 is often the same price or cheaper than these buffered salt solutions and provides a nutrient source that helps maintain viability.

3. Negative selection of NK cells by depleting PBMC of contaminating T cells (CD3), B cells (CD20), and monocytes (CD14) results in a product that is 70–90% NK cells as assessed for CD3$^-$/CD56$^+$ cells by flow cytometry. In clinical practice, most trials have used an NK-cell-enriched product by depletion of CD3 cells only, as removal of T cells is necessary to avoid development of GVHD. These products are typically 20–50% NK cells (30). If NK-cell enriched products are to be delivered to patients receiving highly immunosuppressed HSCT (haploidentical donors, T-cell-depleted grafts, or Campath therapy), additional B-cell depletion of the NK-cell product is recommended to reduce the risk of EBV-associated B-cell lymphomas (11).

4. A wide variety of kits are available from several manufacturers for either positive or negative selection. Some are based on an initial antibody binding step using purified unconjugated or streptavidin-conjugated mAb, with a second step using species-specific anti-IgG or biotin-conjugated magnetic beads. These two-stage products will require additional steps here prior to the magnetic separation.

5. Positive selection of NK cells using anti-CD56-conjugated magnetic beads has been performed (30, 31). Recovery using this method was poor and although initial reports suggested good NK-cell function, anecdotal reports have suggested that NK cells positively selected in this manner have reduced function. In addition, it should be noted that there are a variable number of CD3$^+$CD56$^+$ T cells present in the peripheral blood, and using a single CD56$^+$ selection step

will result in the isolation of CD3⁺CD56⁺ T cells in addition to the CD3⁻CD56⁺ NK cells. An alternative approach is to perform both CD3 depletion and CD56 positive selection.

4.1.2. Purification of NK Cells Using RosetteSep Antibody Complexes

6. The RosetteSep product requires sufficient red blood cells (RBC) in the cell source in order to bind to the unwanted leukocytes and carry them through the Ficoll-Paque to the bottom of the tube. Thus, this method does not work well for recovering NK cells directly from leukapheresis products or leukocyte reduction filters (*see* **Note 7**).

7. Adapting the methods of Warren et al. NK cells can be purified from fresh or cryopreserved PBMC with a significant reduction in the amount of RosetteSep reagent required for separation (32).

8. The product insert for RosetteSep includes volumes recommended for recovery of NK cells from whole blood. We have titrated the RosetteSep NK reagent for recovery from blood buffy coat products and found 10 µl of the reagent for each ml of buffy coat to provide optimal recovery and purity (**Fig. 4.1**).

9. As with other density-gradient methods, temperature, careful layering, transport, and centrifugation are essential in obtaining a clean separation of cells at the interface. Slow acceleration and deceleration (no brake) are essential in not disrupting the interface. We also find that layering the cells over the Ficoll-Paque, rather than underlaying the cells with Ficoll-Paque, results in a better interface. Cells, medium, and Ficoll-Paque should all be kept at room temperature, as this maintains the appropriate density of the medium and avoids convection currents that disrupt the interface.

10. Note that more Ficoll-Paque is recommended in this procedure than what is typically used for separation of PBMC from whole blood. As cells move through the Ficoll-Paque, the membrane-associated liquid dilutes the Ficoll-Paque and reduces the density. With RosetteSep, leukocytes conjugated to the red cells increase this effect.

11. RosetteSep crosslinks unwanted leukocytes to the more dense red blood cells. These large complexes have much greater resistance while sedimenting through the Ficoll-Paque and therefore require centrifugation at much higher g forces than for usual PBMC separation from whole blood.

12. As mentioned in **Note 2**, we use RPMI-1640 for all steps. In this procedure, we also find that the phenol

red in the RPMI-1640 aids in distinguishing the interface, particularly with the much smaller number of cells obtained than when using Ficoll-Paque for total PBMC recovery.

4.2. NK Cell Activation

13. IL-2 has been the standard cytokine used to generate activated NK cells. IL-12, IL-15, IL-21, and others may also be effective. IL-2 concentrations reported in the literature for NK-cell activation have ranged from 100 to 6000 IU/ml.

14. It is not known whether IL-2 activation needs to be performed ex vivo prior to administration, or if adoptively transferred NK cells can be activated sufficiently in vivo by administering high doses of IL-2. In practice, IL-2 has been used both in vivo and for ex vivo activation in most clinical trials.

15. Like other lymphocytes, NK-cell function and viability are optimized when cultured at cell densities that allow regular cell–cell contact. Therefore, it is important to choose a plate or flask with an appropriate surface area for the volume of cells being cultured.

4.3. Ex Vivo Expansion of NK Cells with Genetically Modified K562 Cells (K562-mb15-41BBL)

16. The genetically modified K562 must be irradiated before coculture with peripheral blood mononuclear cells. If an irradiator is not available, the genetically modified K562 cells can be treated with mitomycin C or another antimitotic to prevent cell division.

17. It is important to monitor the cells daily during expansion and change the medium earlier than described above if the medium is becoming acidic (yellow). Typically, changing the medium every 2 days is sufficient.

18. Proliferation of NK cells in these cultures starts on days 4–5 and continues thereafter. After 2–3 weeks, NK-cell proliferation reaches a plateau but can be restimulated by the addition of genetically modified K562 cells.

19. After 7 days of culture, genetically modified K562 should no longer be present in the cultures owing to the combined effect of irradiation (or anti-mitotic treatment) and NK-cell cytotoxicity.

20. T cells do not expand in these cultures. Their percentage should progressively decrease due to the expansion of NK cells.

4.4. Assessing NK Activity

21. A variety of cell lines have been used as targets for determining NK cell-activity. These cell lines are referred to as NK-cell sensitive, meaning they can be killed by freshly

isolated NK cells, or NK-cell resistant, meaning they can only be killed by IL-2-activated NK cells. The most commonly used cell lines for detecting human NK-cell activity are K562 and 721.221 (sensitive) and Daudi and Raji (resistant). Daudi and Raji are useful for assessing ADCC as described below, typically with anti-CD20 mAb.

4.4.1. Direct Cytotoxicity of Calcein-Loaded Targets

22. The calcein assay is validated as a non-radioactive substitute for Chromium[51] cytotoxicity assay, with similar sensitivity and specificity (33, 34). The principle and process are nearly identical—target cells are loaded with an intracellular marker that is released following lysis by the effector cells and can be detected with high sensitivity and specificity in the supernatant. The unlysed cells can be further analyzed using flow cytometric methods (35, 36).

23. In our experience, viability-based (e.g., formazan, CytoTox 96) and LDH-based assays, both of which require assessment of proteins or function endogenous to the target cell, are not useful assays for measuring NK-cell cytotoxicity. NK cells have some degree of autolysis during degranulation, which results in high levels of LDH released from the NK cells themselves. Likewise, the viable NK cells in high E:T ratios overshadow the relatively smaller number of target cells when assessing formazan degradation.

24. The additional role of ADCC in target cell lysis can be assessed using this method by pre-incubation of the targets with an excess of antibody specific for the target cell. For assessing ADCC in Raji or Daudi cells, we preincubate the target cells for 30 min with 1–10 μg/ml of anti-CD20 (rituximab) and wash the cells prior to adding them to the 96-well plate (**Fig. 4.2**).

25. Some fluorescent plate readers allow both direct (detection on the same side of the plate as the excitation beam) and indirect (detection on the opposite side of the plate as the excitation beam) fluorescence measurements. We have found that indirect measurement is much more reliable, being less sensitive to variation caused by bubbles, well alignment, meniscus variation, and absorption/autofluorescence of the medium.

4.4.2. Flow Cytometry to Assess Target Cell Killing

26. Using flow-based assays to determine cytotoxicity requires the ability to separate NK cells from both dead and live targets using flow cytometry parameters of light scatter or fluorescence.

27. As mentioned in **Note 24**, ADCC can be assessed using this method by pre-incubation of the targets with an excess

of antibody specific for the target cell. However, care must be taken not to use antibodies for ADCC that recognize the same epitope used to identify the target cells by flow cytometry.

4.4.3. Flow Cytometry
to Assess NK Cell
Activation
and Degranulation

28. NK-cell killing of target cells is mediated by the release of granules containing granzymes and perforin that are lined with lysosomal-associated membrane protein-1 (LAMP-1, CD107a). Exocytosis of these granules results in neo-expression of CD107a on the NK-cell surface, indicating that degranulation has occurred. CD137, CD69, and intracellular IFN-γ have also been used. These are activation markers that increase in most NK cells independent of degranulation and may be helpful in identifying responses of non-cytotoxic cytokine-releasing NK cells.

29. Presence of the antibody to CD107a during the entire culture period greatly increases the sensitivity of the assay. CD107a may be recycled rapidly from the NK-cell surface after degranulation, resulting in accumulation of the fluorescent probe within degranulating NK cells.

30. NK cells may also be identified using CD16. However, following engagement with targets, NK cells can lose or downregulate CD16 expression in a matrix metalloproteinase dependent fashion (37).

References

1. Kiessling, R., Klein, E., and Wigzell, H. (1975) "Natural" killer cells in the mouse. I. Cytotoxic cells with specificity for mouse Moloney leukemia cells. Specificity and distribution according to genotype. *Eur J Immunol 5*, 112–117.
2. Farag, S. S., Fehniger, T. A., Ruggeri, L., Velardi, A., and Caligiuri, M. A. (2002) Natural killer cell receptors: new biology and insights into the graft-versus-leukemia effect. *Blood 100*, 1935–1947.
3. Moretta, A., Bottino, C., Vitale, M., Pende, D., Cantoni, C., Mingari, M. C., Biassoni, R., and Moretta, L. (2001) Activating receptors and coreceptors involved in human natural killer cell-mediated cytolysis. *Annu Rev Immunol 19*, 197–223.
4. Raulet, D. H., and Held, W. (1995) Natural killer cell receptors: the offs and ons of NK cell recognition. *Cell 82*, 697–700.
5. Lanier, L. L. (2005) NK cell recognition. *Annu Rev Immunol 23*, 225–274.
6. Phillips, J. H., and Lanier, L. L. (1986) Dissection of the lymphokine-activated killer phenomenon. Relative contribution of peripheral blood natural killer cells and T lymphocytes to cytolysis. *J Exp Med 164*, 814–825.
7. Grimm, E. A., Mazumder, A., Zhang, H. Z., and Rosenberg, S. A. (1982) Lymphokine-activated killer cell phenomenon. Lysis of natural killer-resistant fresh solid tumor cells by interleukin 2-activated autologous human peripheral blood lymphocytes. *J Exp Med 155*, 1823–1841.
8. Benyunes, M. C., Massumoto, C., York, A., Higuchi, C. M., Buckner, C. D., Thompson, J. A., Petersen, F. B., and Fefer, A. (1993) Interleukin-2 with or without lymphokine-activated killer cells as consolidative immunotherapy after autologous bone marrow transplantation for acute myelogenous leukemia. *Bone Marrow Transplant 12*, 159–163.
9. Leemhuis, T., Wells, S., Scheffold, C., Edinger, M., and Negrin, R. S. (2005) A phase I trial of autologous cytokine-induced killer cells for the treatment of relapsed

Hodgkin disease and non-Hodgkin lymphoma. *Biol Blood Marrow Transplant 11*, 181–187.

10. Miller, J. S., Soignier, Y., Panoskaltsis-Mortari, A., McNearney, S. A., Yun, G. H., Fautsch, S. K., McKenna, D., Le, C., Defor, T. E., Burns, L. J., Orchard, P. J., Blazar, B. R., Wagner, J. E., Slungaard, A., Weisdorf, D. J., Okazaki, I. J., and McGlave, P. B. (2005) Successful adoptive transfer and in vivo expansion of human haploidentical NK cells in patients with cancer. *Blood 105*, 3051–3057.

11. Grzywacz, B., Miller, J. S., and Verneris, M. R. (2008) Use of natural killer cells as immunotherapy for leukaemia. *Best Pract Res Clin Haematol 21*, 467–483.

12. Larghero, J., Rocha, V., Porcher, R., Filion, A., Ternaux, B., Lacassagne, M. N., Robin, M., Peffault de Latour, R., Devergie, A., Biscay, N., Ribaud, P., Benbunan, M., Gluckman, E., Marolleau, J. P., and Socie, G. (2007) Association of bone marrow natural killer cell dose with neutrophil recovery and chronic graft-versus-host disease after HLA identical sibling bone marrow transplants. *Br J Haematol 138*, 101–109.

13. Kim, D. H., Won, D. I., Lee, N. Y., Sohn, S. K., Suh, J. S., and Lee, K. B. (2006) Non-CD34+ cells, especially CD8+ cytotoxic T cells and CD56+ natural killer cells, rather than CD34 cells, predict early engraftment and better transplantation outcomes in patients with hematologic malignancies after allogeneic peripheral stem cell transplantation. *Biol Blood Marrow Transplant 12*, 719–728.

14. Kim, D. H., Sohn, S. K., Lee, N. Y., Baek, J. H., Kim, J. G., Won, D. I., Suh, J. S., Lee, K. B., and Shin, I. H. (2005) Transplantation with higher dose of natural killer cells associated with better outcomes in terms of non-relapse mortality and infectious events after allogeneic peripheral blood stem cell transplantation from HLA-matched sibling donors. *Eur J Haematol 75*, 299–308.

15. Yamasaki, S., Henzan, H., Ohno, Y., Yamanaka, T., Iino, T., Itou, Y., Kuroiwa, M., Maeda, M., Kawano, N., Kinukawa, N., Miyamoto, T., Nagafuji, K., Shimoda, K., Inaba, S., Hayashi, S., Taniguchi, S., Shibuya, T., Gondo, H., Otsuka, T., and Harada, M. (2003) Influence of transplanted dose of CD56+ cells on development of graft-versus-host disease in patients receiving G-CSF-mobilized peripheral blood progenitor cells from HLA-identical sibling donors. *Bone Marrow Transplant 32*, 505–510.

16. Savani, B. N., Mielke, S., Adams, S., Uribe, M., Rezvani, K., Yong, A. S., Zeilah, J., Kurlander, R., Srinivasan, R., Childs, R., Hensel, N., and Barrett, A. J. (2007) Rapid natural killer cell recovery determines outcome after T-cell-depleted HLA-identical stem cell transplantation in patients with myeloid leukemias but not with acute lymphoblastic leukemia. *Leukemia 21*, 2145–2152.

17. Miller, J. S., Oelkers, S., Verfaillie, C., and McGlave, P. (1992) Role of monocytes in the expansion of human activated natural killer cells. *Blood 80*, 2221–2229.

18. Perussia, B., Ramoni, C., Anegon, I., Cuturi, M. C., Faust, J., and Trinchieri, G. (1987) Preferential proliferation of natural killer cells among peripheral blood mononuclear cells cocultured with B lymphoblastoid cell lines. *Nat Immun Cell Growth Regul 6*, 171–188.

19. Robertson, M. J., Cameron, C., Lazo, S., Cochran, K. J., Voss, S. D., and Ritz, J. (1996) Costimulation of human natural killer cell proliferation: role of accessory cytokines and cell contact-dependent signals. *Nat Immun 15*, 213–226.

20. Carson, W. E., Fehniger, T. A., Haldar, S., Eckhert, K., Lindemann, M. J., Lai, C. F., Croce, C. M., Baumann, H., and Caligiuri, M. A. (1997) A potential role for interleukin-15 in the regulation of human natural killer cell survival. *J Clin Invest 99*, 937–943.

21. Koehl, U., Esser, R., Zimmermann, S., Tonn, T., Kotchetkov, R., Bartling, T., Sorensen, J., Gruttner, H. P., Bader, P., Seifried, E., Martin, H., Lang, P., Passweg, J. R., Klingebiel, T., and Schwabe, D. (2005) Ex vivo expansion of highly purified NK cells for immunotherapy after haploidentical stem cell transplantation in children. *Klinische Padiatrie 217*, 345–350.

22. Klingemann, H. G., and Martinson, J. (2004) Ex vivo expansion of natural killer cells for clinical applications. *Cytotherapy 6*, 15–22.

23. Ayello, J., van de Ven, C., Fortino, W., Wade-Harris, C., Satwani, P., Baxi, L., Simpson, L. L., Sanger, W., Pickering, D., Kurtzberg, J., and Cairo, M. S. (2006) Characterization of cord blood natural killer and lymphokine activated killer lymphocytes following ex vivo cellular engineering. *Biol Blood Marrow Transplant 12*, 608–622.

24. Carlens, S., Gilljam, M., Chambers, B. J., Aschan, J., Guven, H., Ljunggren, H. G., Christensson, B., and Dilber, M. S. (2001) A new method for in vitro expansion of cytotoxic human CD3-CD56+ natural killer cells. *Hum Immunol 62*, 1092–1098.

25. Boissel, L., Tuncer, H. H., Betancur, M., Wolfberg, A., and Klingemann, H. (2008) Umbilical cord mesenchymal stem cells increase expansion of cord blood natural killer cells. *Biol Blood Marrow Transplant 14*, 1031–1038.

26. Berg, M., Lundqvist, A., McCoy, P., Jr., Samsel, L., Fan, Y., Tawab, A., and Childs, R. (2009) Clinical-grade ex vivo-expanded human natural killer cells up-regulate activating receptors and death receptor ligands and have enhanced cytolytic activity against tumor cells, *Cytotherapy 11*, 341–355.

27. Fujisaki, H., Kakuda, H., Imai, C., Mullighan, C. G., and Campana, D. (2009) Replicative potential of human natural killer cells, *Br J Haematol 145*, 606–613.

28. Imai, C., Iwamoto, S., and Campana, D. (2005) Genetic modification of primary natural killer cells overcomes inhibitory signals and induces specific killing of leukemic cells. *Blood 106*, 376–383.

29. Fujisaki, H., Kakuda, H., Shimasaki, N., Imai, C., Ma, J., Lockey, T., Eldridge, P., Leung, W. H., and Campana, D. (2009) Expansion of highly cytotoxic human natural killer cells for cancer cell therapy, *Cancer Res 69*, 4010–4017.

30. McKenna, D. H., Jr., Sumstad, D., Bostrom, N., Kadidlo, D. M., Fautsch, S., McNearney, S., Dewaard, R., McGlave, P. B., Weisdorf, D. J., Wagner, J. E., McCullough, J., and Miller, J. S. (2007) Good manufacturing practices production of natural killer cells for immunotherapy: a six-year single-institution experience. *Transfusion 47*, 520–528.

31. Lang, P., Pfeiffer, M., Handgretinger, R., Schumm, M., Demirdelen, B., Stanojevic, S., Klingebiel, T., Kohl, U., Kuci, S., and Niethammer, D. (2002) Clinical scale isolation of T cell-depleted CD56+ donor lymphocytes in children. *Bone Marrow Transplant 29*, 497–502.

32. Warren, H. S., and Rana, P. M. (2003) An economical adaptation of the Rosette-Sep procedure for NK cell enrichment from whole blood, and its use with liquid nitrogen stored peripheral blood mononuclear cells. *J Immunol Methods 280*, 135–138.

33. Lichtenfels, R., Biddison, W. E., Schulz, H., Vogt, A. B., and Martin, R. (1994) CARE-LASS (calcein-release-assay), an improved fluorescence-based test system to measure cytotoxic T lymphocyte activity. *J Immunol Methods 172*, 227–239.

34. Cholujova, D., Jakubikova, J., Kubes, M., Arendacka, B., Sapak, M., Robert, I., and Sedlak, J. (2008) Comparative study of four fluorescent probes for evaluation of natural killer cell cytotoxicity assays. *Immunobiology 213*, 629–640.

35. Roden, M. M., Lee, K. H., Panelli, M. C., and Marincola, F. M. (1999) A novel cytolysis assay using fluorescent labeling and quantitative fluorescent scanning technology. *J Immunol Methods 226*, 29–41.

36. Neri, S., Mariani, E., Meneghetti, A., Cattini, L., and Facchini, A. (2001) Calcein-acetoxymethyl cytotoxicity assay: standardization of a method allowing additional analyses on recovered effector cells and supernatants. *Clin Diagn Lab Immunol 8*, 1131–1135.

37. Grzywacz, B., Kataria, N., and Verneris, M. R. (2007) CD56(dim)CD16(+) NK cells downregulate CD16 following target cell induced activation of matrix metalloproteinases. *Leukemia 21*, 356–359; author reply 359.

Chapter 5

Enhanced Migration of Human Dendritic Cells Expressing Inducible CD40

Natalia Lapteva

Abstract

Dendritic cells (DC) are the most potent antigen-presenting cells for priming and activating naïve CD4$^+$ and CD8$^+$ T lymphocytes. This property has led to their use as a cellular vaccine in a number of clinical trials with promising results. However, the clinical efficacy of DC vaccines in patients has been unsatisfactory, probably because of a number of key deficiencies, including limited migration of ex vivo generated DCs to the secondary lymphoid tissues. To enhance human DC-based vaccines, we used the combination of an inducible CD40 receptor (iCD40) along with TLR-4 ligation. The iCD40 receptor permits targeted, reversible activation of CD40. Using iCD40 in combination with lipopolysaccharides (LPS), we enhanced DCs migration in vitro upon escalation of the AP1903 dimerizer drug doses. This result suggests that the use of iCD40-modified and LPS-stimulated DCs is a potent strategy in DC-based cancer immunotherapies.

Key words: Human dendritic cells, migration, chemotaxis.

1. Introduction

Dendritic cells (DCs) are the most potent antigen-presenting cells and therefore they are central in the induction and regulation of adaptive immune responses (1). In the steady state, immature DCs mainly reside in peripheral tissue, where they sample the environment for danger signals. Upon activation with such a signal, DCs become activated (upregulate expression of CD40, CD80, and CD86 co-stimulatory molecules and chemokines receptors, such as CCR7 and CXCR4) and efficiently home to the T-cell zones of lymphoid organs where they present peripheral

P. Yotnda (ed.), *Immunotherapy of Cancer*, Methods in Molecular Biology 651,
DOI 10.1007/978-1-60761-786-0_5, © Springer Science+Business Media, LLC 2010

antigens and activate naïve T lymphocytes. Interestingly, it has been shown that DC migrated to the lymph nodes can transfer the antigens to resident DC and thus spread antigens to a larger pool of cells (2). Also, the increased DC recruitment to the draining lymph nodes induces higher frequency of peripheral antigen-specific T cells (3). Moreover, DCs migrated to the lymph nodes are essential for the proliferation and sustained activation of antigen-specific T cells (4). Therefore, the success of DC-based immunotherapy is highly dependent on efficient trafficking of the DC to T-cell-rich areas in secondary lymphoid tissues.

DC-based cancer vaccines have been in clinical trials in patients with a variety of cancers (1). Despite some encouraging observations in these trials, vaccine-induced antigen-specific T-cell responses have been insufficient to effectively reduce tumor burden or prevent tumor progression in most patients, suggesting that further improvements in the potency of DC-based cancer vaccines are required (5). One of the important aspects of DC-based therapy is efficient cell trafficking to the draining lymph nodes. Several clinical studies have shown that only 0.1–4% of ex vivo generated DCs migrated to the lymph nodes (6, 7). This poor DC recruitment may contribute to the limited clinical responses to DC-based immunotherapies. Here we describe the DC activation system based on targeted temporal control of the CD40 signaling pathway to extend the prostimulatory state of DCs within lymphoid tissues. We have re-engineered CD40 receptor so that the cytoplasmic domain of CD40 was fused to synthetic ligand-binding domains along with a membrane-targeting sequence (8, 9). Activation of the DCs with lipid-permeable, dimerizing drug AP1903 and lipopolysaccharides (LPS) significantly enhanced the dimmer-dependent in vitro migration of DCs toward CCL19.

2. Materials

2.1. Generation of Human Dendritic Cells by Plastic Adherence and Flow Cytometry

1. Leukopaks (Gulf Coast Blood Center, Houston TX)
2. DC medium (Cell Genix GmbH, Antioch, IL)
3. RPMI medium 1640 (Mediatech, Inc, Manassas, VA)
4. D-PBS, 1× (Mediatech, Inc)
5. Lymphoprep Separation Medium (Greiner Bio-One, Inc, Monroe, NC)
6. Human granulocyte-macrophage colony stimulation factor (GM-CSF, R&D Systems, Minneapolis, MN)
7. Human interleukin 4 (IL-4, R&D Systems)

8. 100-mm sterile tissue culture plate (Fisher Scientific, Pittsburgh, PA)

9. T75-cm^2 sterile tissue culture flask (Fisher Scientific)

10. 50-ml sterile tubes (Fisher Scientific)

11. Fetal bovine serum (FBS, InvitroGen, Carlsbad, CA)

12. All anti-human monoclonal antibodies (Ab) used for flow cytometry (HLA-A, B, C, HLA-DR, CD40, CD80, CD83, CD3, CD14, CD16, CD19) are phycoerythrin (PE)-conjugated (BD BioSciences, San Jose, CA)

2.2. Transduction of Human Dendritic Cells with Ad5f35-ihCD40 and Activation with Lipopolysaccharides and AP1903 Dimerizer Drug

1. Ad5f35-ihCD40 (5×10^{12} vp/ml, produced in the Vector core facility of Baylor College of Medicine, Houston, TX)

2. Ad5f35-Luciferase (Ad5f35-Luc) (5×10^{12} vp/ml, produced in the Vector core facility of Baylor College of Medicine)

3. Lipopolysaccharides (LPS), cell culture tested, purified by gel-filtration chromatography, γ-irradiated (Sigma Aldrich Co, St. Louis, MO)

4. AP1903 (Alphora Research, Inc., Ontario, Canada)

5. 48-well flat bottom tissue culture plates (Fisher Scientific)

6. Teflon cell scrapers (Fisher Scientific)

2.3. Chemotaxis Assay

1. Green-CMFDA cell tracker (Invitrogen)

2. Human CCL19 (R&D Systems)

3. 96-well Fluoroblock System with 8-μm pore size (BD BioSciences)

4. FLUOstar OPTIMA (BMG LABTECH GmbH, Offenburg, Germany)

3. Methods

3.1. Generation of Human DCs

DCs were generated from leukopaks obtained from Gulf Coast Blood Center. Leukopaks are bags with approximately 50 ml of human blood cells collected from normal peripheral blood by automated apheresis procedure. Each leukopak contains a mixture of monocytes, lymphocytes, platelets, plasma, and red blood cells. All leukopacks used in this study were derived from healthy donors (*see* **Note 1**).

1. Prewarm D-PBS and lymphoprep to room temperature.

2. Mix 50 ml of leukopak's blood with 150 ml (3 volumes) of D-PBS in a T75-cm^2 culture flask.

3. Layer 40 ml of blood-D-PBS mixture over 10 ml in a 50-ml tube.

4. Spin cells for 30 min at 450 × g at room temperature with the centrifuge's brake set at "Off."

5. Harvest peripheral blood mononuclear cell layer (PBMCs) into two 50-ml tubes, and fill upto 50 ml of D-PBS in each tube.

6. Centrifuge cells at 400 × g for 5 min at room temperature.

7. Loosen the pellets in each tube by finger-flicking. Resuspend cells in each tube in 25 ml of D-PBS and combine cells in one 50-ml tube.

8. Centrifuge cells at 400 × g for 5 min at room temperature.

9. Count the cells and adjust cell concentration to 5×10^6 cells/ml in RPMI 1640 (serum free).

10. Transfer 10 ml of cells into 100-mm tissue culture plates.

11. Incubate cells for 2 h at 37°C in a 5% CO_2 incubator.

12. Wash away the non-adherent cells by rinsing the plates three times with 10 ml/plate room temperature D-PBS (*see* **Note 2**).

13. Replenish the plates with 10 ml of CellGenix DC Medium supplemented with 800 U/ml GM-CSF and 500 U/ml of IL-4 (*see* **Note 3**).

14. Culture cells for 5 or 6 days at 37°C, 5% CO_2 incubator. Cytokine replenishing is not necessary.

3.2. Flow Cytometric Analysis of Immature DCs

DCs are harvested on day 5 of culture and analyzed for expression of DC markers, such as HLA-class I (HLA-A,B,C), HLA-class-II (HLA-DR), CD40, CD80, and CD83. In addition, contamination of the DC sample with CD3+ (T cells), CD19+ (B cells), CD14+ (undifferentiated monocytes and macrophages), and CD16+ (NK cells) is also analyzed (*see* **Note 4**).

1. Resuspend DCs in FACS buffer (D-PBS with 0.5%FBS) at 10^6 cells/ml.

2. Aliquot 50 μl of DCs into FACS tubes and keep them on ice.

3. Add 20 μl of each antibody into each tube. Incubate cells for 30 min at 4°C in the dark.

4. Add and mix 1 ml of FACS buffer to the cells.

5. Centrifuge DCs at room temperature at 400 × g for 5 min.

6. Remove the supernatants and reconstitute cell pellets in 400 μl of FACS buffer.

7. Perform flow cytometric analysis.
An example of typical flow cytometry data on immature DCs harvested on day 5 of culture is shown in **Fig. 5.1**.

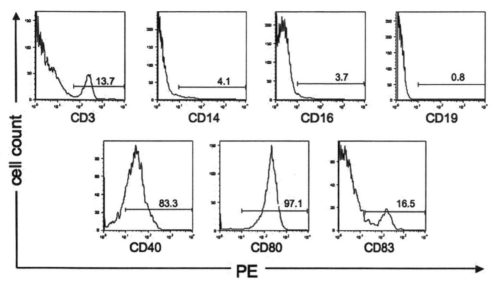

Fig. 5.1. Phenotype of immature DCs cultured for 5 days with GM-CSF and IL-4. Expression of CD40, CD80, and CD83 maturation markers and purity of the cells (CD3+, CD14+, CD16+, and CD19+ contaminating cells) were assessed by flow cytometry.

3.3. Transduction of Human Dendritic Cells with Ad5f35-ihCD40 and Activation with LPS and AP1903 Dimerizer Drug

1. Harvest immature DCs on day 5 or 6 by gentle resuspension (*see* **Note 5**) with a 10-ml serological pipette.

2. To remove remaining adherent cells, add 5 ml of cold D-PBS and incubate plates for 15 min at +4°C.

3. Combine all the cells in 50 ml tubes and centrifuge them at $400 \times g$ for 5 min at room temperature.

4. Discard the supernatants, loosen pellets by finger-flicking, and add 10 ml of CellGenix DC medium.

5. Perform cell count and adjust the cell concentration to 2×10^6 cells/ml in CellGenix DC medium supplemented with 800 U/ml GM-CSF and 500 U/ml of IL-4.

6. Aliquot 250 μl of the cell suspension into each well of 48-well plate and add the 10,000 VP/cell (160 MOI) of Ad5f35-ihCD40 or control adenovirus. Incubate cells with the virus for 2 h at 37°C in a 5% CO_2 incubator.

7. Add 750 μl (containing 800 U/ml GM-CSF and 500 U/ml of IL-4) into each well. Activate DCs with 1 μg/ml LPS and 1, 10, 50, 100, and 300 nM AP1903. Experimental groups are described in **Table 5.1**.

3.4. Chemotaxis Assay

Chemotaxis of DCs is measured in duplicates by migration through a polycarbonate filter with 8-μm pore size in 96-multiwell HTS Fluoroblok plates.

Table 5.1
Experimental conditions

Mock
1 nM AP1903
10 nM AP1903
50 nM AP1903
100 nM AP1903
300 nM AP1903
LPS
Ad5f35-ihCD40
Ad5f35-ihCD40+LPS
Ad5f35-ihCD40+1 nM AP1903
Ad5f35-ihCD40+10 nM AP1903
Ad5f35-ihCD40+50 nM AP1903
Ad5f35-ihCD40+100 nM AP1903
Ad5f35-ihCD40+300 nM AP1903
Ad5f35-ihCD40+1 nM AP1903+LPS
Ad5f35-ihCD40+10 nM AP1903+LPS
Ad5f35-ihCD40+50 nM AP1903+LPS
Ad5f35-ihCD40+100 nM AP1903+LPS
Ad5f35-ihCD40+300 nM AP1903+LPS
Ad5f35-Luc+100 nM AP1903+LPS

1. DCs are harvested after approximately 20 h incubation with activation stimuli.

2. 4 mM CM-FDA staining solution is added and gently resuspended with cells.

3. Incubate DCs for 30 min at 37°C and 5% CO_2. (*see* **Note 6**).

4. Vigorously pipette the cells up and down in the well and then transfer into a sterile 15-ml tube. To remove remaining adherent cells, scrape them using Teflon scraper.

5. Wash DCs three times in 10 ml of 1× D-PBS.

6. Perform cell count and resuspend cells in CellGenix DC medium supplemented with 800 U/ml GM-CSF and 500 U/ml IL-4 at 10^6 cells/ml.

7. Fill the inserts with 50 μl (50,000 cells) of DCs (*see* **Note 7**).

8. Carefully load 250 μl of pre-warmed DC medium containing 100 ng/ml CCL19 or assay medium alone (as a control for spontaneous migration) into the lower chamber. Incubate cells for 1.5–2 h at 37°C and 5% CO_2.

9. Measure the fluorescence of cells migrated through the microporous membrane, using the FLUOstar OPTIMA reader with excitation 485 nm and emission 520 nm. (*see* **Note 8**)

10. The mean fluorescence of spontaneously migrated cells is subtracted from the total number of migrated cells toward CCL19 for each condition. Typical results are presented on **Fig. 5.2**.

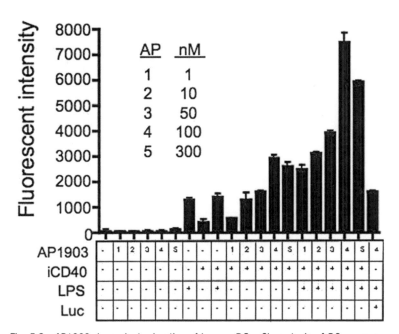

Fig. 5.2. AP1903-dependent migration of human DCs. Chemotaxis of DCs was measured by migration through a polycarbonate filter with 8-μm pore size in 96-multiwell HTS Fluoroblok plates. AP: AP1903, Luc: Ad5f35-Luciferase, iCD40: Ad5f35-ihCD40.

4. Notes

1. All leukopaks are routinely tested in Gulf Coast Blood Center for HIV, hepatitis B and C, HTLV, and syphilis.

2. Cells of healthy donors adhere very well to plastic within 2-h incubation. Therefore, use 10-ml serological pipettes for

washing away non-adherent cells and directly pipette D-PBS on a cell layer.

3. GM-CSF from R&D Systems could be substituted with leukine or sargramostim (GM-CSF) from Bayer Healthcare. 800 U/ml of leukine is used for DC differentiation.

4. The expression of DC markers (CD40, CD80, CD83, HLA-A, HLA-B, HLA-C, and HLA-DR) is measured on DC population gated on side and forward scatter dot plot. The expression of CD3, CD14, CD16, and CD19 is evaluated on all the cells. Typically, the percentage of contaminating monocytes/macrophages, T, B-lymphocytes, and NK cells does not exceed 30% of total cells.

5. Typically, DC yield from one leukopak is approximately 10–20×10^6.

6. Observe cell staining under a fluorescence microscope using FITC filter. Majority of the cells should be green after 30-min incubation with CM-FDA.

7. Handle all inserts under aseptic conditions. Use pre-warmed media to prevent cell shock. Fill the inserts with cells before filling the bottom wells with media. This prevents bubbles from getting trapped underneath the insert. The lower wells can be filled through the sample port using a multi-channel pipette.

8. Fluorescence signal is measured directly on the bottom of the wells.

Acknowledgements

The author would like to thank Professors David Spencer, Kevin Slawin for developing inducible CD40 receptor and for their advice and encouragement, and Mamatha Seethammagari for her technical assistance. The author was supported by an Award from Department of Defense PC060436. The author is also thankful to Ariad Pharmaceuticals for providing AP1903.

References

1. Steinman, R. M., and Banchereau, J. 2007. Taking dendritic cells into medicine. *Nature* *449*, 419–426.
2. Allan, R. S., Waithman, J., Bedoui, S., Jones, C. M., Villadangos, J. A., Zhan, Y., Lew, A. M., Shortman, K., Heath, W. R., and Carbone, F. R. (2006) Migratory dendritic cells transfer antigen to a lymph node-resident dendritic cell population for efficient CTL priming. *Immunity 25*, 153–162.

3. MartIn-Fontecha, A., Sebastiani, S., Hopken, U. E., Uguccioni, M., Lipp, M., Lanzavecchia, A., and Sallusto, F. (2003) Regulation of dendritic cell migration to the draining lymph node: impact on T lymphocyte traffic and priming. *J Exp Med 198*, 615–621.

4. Allenspach, E. J., Lemos, M. P., Porrett, P. M., Turka, L. A., and Laufer, T. M. (2008) Migratory and lymphoid-resident dendritic cells cooperate to efficiently prime naive CD4 T cells. *Immunity 29*, 795–806.

5. Verdijk, P., Aarntzen, E. H., Punt, C. J., de Vries, I. J., and Figdor, C. G. (2008) Maximizing dendritic cell migration in cancer immunotherapy. *Expert Opin Biol Ther 8*, 865–874.

6. De Vries, I. J., Krooshoop, D. J., Scharenborg, N. M., Lesterhuis, W. J., Diepstra, J. H., Van Muijen, G. N., Strijk, S. P., Ruers, T. J., Boerman, O. C., Oyen, W. J., et al. (2003) Effective migration of antigen-pulsed dendritic cells to lymph nodes in melanoma patients is determined by their maturation state. *Cancer Res 63*, 12–17.

7. Quillien, V., Moisan, A., Carsin, A., Lesimple, T., Lefeuvre, C., Adamski, H., Bertho, N., Devillers, A., Leberre, C., and Toujas, L. (2005) Biodistribution of radiolabelled human dendritic cells injected by various routes. *Eur J Nucl Med Mol Imaging 32*, 731–741.

8. Hanks, B. A., Jiang, J., Singh, R. A., Song, W., Barry, M., Huls, M. H., Slawin, K. M., and Spencer, D. M. (2005) Re-engineered CD40 receptor enables potent pharmacological activation of dendritic-cell cancer vaccines in vivo. *Nat Med 11*, 130–137.

9. Lapteva, N., Seethammagari, M. R., Hanks, B. A., Jiang, J., Levitt, J. M., Slawin, K. M., and Spencer, D. M. (2007) Enhanced activation of human dendritic cells by inducible CD40 and Toll-like receptor-4 ligation. *Cancer Res 67*, 10528–10537.

Chapter 6

Differentiation of Human Embryonic Stem Cells into Hematopoietic Cells In Vitro

Eun-Mi Kim and Nicholas Zavazava

Abstract

The ability of embryonic stem cells (ES) cells to form cells and tissues from all three germ layers can be exploited to generate cells that can be used to treat diseases. In particular, successful generation of hematopoietic cells from ES cells could provide safer and less immunogenic cells than bone cells, obviating the need for severe host preconditioning when transplanted across major histocompatibility complex barriers. To generate hematopoietic stem cells, protocols utilizing embryoid body (EB)-induced differentiation of human ES (hES) cells have been applied in the authors' laboratory. While this protocol results in targeted differentiation into hematopoietic cells, much remains to be done to improve these methods and make them more efficient.

Key words: Human embryonic stem cells, embryonic body, differentiation, hematopoiesis, stromal cell lines.

1. Introduction

Pluripotent hES cells can provide new opportunities for developing and establishing new treatments, including the induction of transplantation tolerance, because of their unique characteristics: lack of MHC antigens, poor expression of co-stimulatory molecules, and lack of T cells that can trigger graft-versus-host reaction (1–3). Bone marrow, umbilical cord blood, and mobilized peripheral blood are sources of hematopoietic cells, the application of which is hampered by the need for human leukocyte antigen matching. In contrast, because of their low degree of immunogenicity and high propensity to proliferate, embryonic

P. Yotnda (ed.), *Immunotherapy of Cancer*, Methods in Molecular Biology 651,
DOI 10.1007/978-1-60761-786-0_6, © Springer Science+Business Media, LLC 2010

stem (ES) cells have emerged as a likely and more suitable alternative cell source for generating hematopoietic cells (4–11). For these reasons, ES cell-derived HPCs are an appealing source of hematopoietic therapies.

In recent years, a number of protocols have been successfully developed to coerce hES cells) to differentiate into hematopoietic cells (4, 5, 8, 10, 12–14). They can aggregate into clusters known as embryoid bodies (EBs), characterized by the presence of all the three germ layers (4, 9, 11, 15–18). The EB-induced differentiation of hES cells can generate hematopoietic progenitor cells (HPCs), which can be enhanced by mesoderm inducer bone morphogenetic protein-4 (BMP4) and other hematopoietic cytokines (14). Co-culture of hES cells with stromal cell lines such as S17, OP9, and fetal liver-derived stromal cells has also successfully induced hematopoietic cell differentiation (5, 8, 16, 19–21). We will describe the method that has been successfully applied in our laboratory to obtain hES cells-derived HPCs: uniformed EB-induced differentiation-based derivation of HPCs.

2. Materials

2.1. Generation of Primary Mouse Embryonic Fibroblasts (MEF)

1. E13.5–14.5 pregnant female mice.
2. Dulbecco's phosphate buffered saline (D-PBS) without $CaCl_2$ and $MgCl_2$.
3. MEF medium: combine Dulbecco's modified eagle's medium (DMEM), 10% heat-inactivated fetal bovine serum, 1% penicillin–streptomycin antibiotics, and 1× sodium pyruvate. Sterilize by passing through the filter and store at 4°C.
4. Cryopreservation medium: combine 5 ml of dimethyl sulfoxide (DMSO) and 45 ml of heat-inactivated FBS. Sterilize by passing through the filter and store at 4°C.
5. 0.25% Trypsin-EDTA (ethylenediaminetetraacetic acid).
6. 70-μm cell strainer.
7. Dissecting scissors and forceps.
8. Sterile culture dish.
9. Sterile disposable 10-ml glass pipette.
10. 15- and 50-ml conical centrifuge tubes.
11. 1.5-ml Cryovial.
12. 37°C, 5% CO_2 humidified incubator.

13. Inverted tissue culture microscope with phase contrast microscope ($\times 10$, $\times 20$, and $\times 40$ objectives).

14. Refrigerated centrifuge.

15. Biosafety cabinet with aspirator for tissue culture.

16. 37°C water bath.

17. Gamma irradiator (^{137}Cs).

2.2. Culture of Human Embryonic Stem Cells

1. 0.1% Gelatin: dissolve 0.5 g of the gelatin in 500 ml distilled water. Sterilize by autoclave and store up to 6 months at room temperature.

2. Basic fibroblast growth factor (bFGF, 10 µg/ml): dissolve 10 µg of bFGF in 1 ml D-PBS containing 0.1% bovine serum albumin (BSA) and store at –20°C until use.

3. hES cells medium: Mix 100 ml knockout serum replacement (Invitrogen, cat. no. 10828-028), 2.5 ml GlutaMax (Invitrogen, cat. no. 35050-061), 5 ml non-essential amino acids (100× NEAA, Invitrogen, cat. no. 11140-050), 3.5 µl 2-mercaptoethanol, 5 ml penicillin and streptomycin (100×), and 500 µl of bFGF (10 µg/ml). Fill up to 500 ml with DMEM/F12 (Invitrogen, cat. no. 11330-057), and filter the medium with a bottle-top 0.22 µm filter. Store at 4°C for 2 week.

4. 1 mg/ml Collagenase solution: dissolve 50 mg of Collagenase type IV (Invitrogen, cat. no. 17104-019) in 50 ml DMEM-F12 and filter using a 0.22-µm filter. Store at 4°C for up to 14 days.

5. 0.05% Trypsin-EDTA.

6. 6-well tissue culture plates.

7. 5- and 10-ml sterile glass serological pipettes.

8. 15- and 50-ml conical centrifuge tubes.

9. 0.22-µm bottle-top filter (500 ml).

2.3. In Vitro Differentiation of ES Cells into HPCs

1. EB medium: mix 100 ml Knockout serum replacement, 2.5 ml GlutaMax, 5 ml non-essential amino acids, 3.5 µl 2-mercaptoethanol, 5 ml penicillin–streptomycin (100×). Fill up to 500 ml with DMEM/F12. Filter the medium with a 0.22-µm bottle-top filter and store at 4°C for 1 month.

2. Differentiation medium: Mix 50 ng/ml bone morphogenetic protein 4 (BMP-4), 300 ng/ml stem cell factor (SCF), 10 ng/ml IL-3, 10 ng/ml IL-6, 50 ng/ml G-CSF, and 300 ng/ml Flt3 ligand in EB medium.

3. Recombinant human stem cell factor (R&D, cat. no. 255-SC), Flt3 ligand (R&D, cat. no. 308-FK), BMP-4 (R&D,

cat. no. 314-BP), IL-3 (R&D, cat. no. 203-IL), and IL-6 (R&D, cat. no. 206-IL): reconstitute lyophilized powders at 10 μg/ml in sterile DPBS containing 0.1% BSA and store in 50-μl aliquots at −80°C (store thawed aliquots for 1–2 weeks at 4°C).

4. Recombinant human G-CSF (Amgen, cat. no. 3105100): Store in 50-μl aliquots at −80°C. Store thawed aliquots no longer than 3 months at −20°C and thawed aliquots for 1–2 weeks at 4°C.

5. AggreWell™ 400 plates (STEMCELL Technologies, cat. no. 27845).

6. Y-27632 ROCK inhibitor (Calbiochem, cat. no. 688000).

7. TrypLE™ Express (Invitrogen, cat. no. 12604).

8. 6-well ultra-low adherence plate (STEMCELL Technologies, cat. no. 27145).

9. 40-μm cell strainer.

10. MACS buffer (Miltenyi Biotec, cat. no. 130-091-221).

11. CD34 MultiSort Microbeads (Miltenyi Biotec, cat. no. 130-056-701).

3. Methods

3.1. Generation of Primary Mouse Embryonic Fibroblasts

3.1.1. Isolation of Primary Mouse Embryonic Fibroblast

1. Sacrifice an E13.5-14.5 pregnant female mouse by carbon-dioxide asphyxiation.

2. Swab it with 70% ethanol, lay it on its back, and make a fine incision to expose the abdominal cavity carefully.

3. Locate the uterine horns and carefully dissect them out into a sterile 10-cm sterile tissue culture dish containing 1× PBS. Wash the uterine horns carefully and transfer them into a second sterile tissue culture dish containing 1× PBS: Use only serological pipettes.

4. Dissect out the uterine horns and remove all of the embryos along with the embryonic sacs. Gently remove the embryos from the embryonic sacs and transfer all of the embryos into another sterile tissue culture dish containing 1× PBS and wash three times with 10 ml PBS.

5. Decapitate each embryo and remove all of its limbs and perform evisceration under a dissecting microscope to remove various internal organs.

6. Transfer the remainder of the embryo into a sterile tissue culture dish and finely mince it using sharp surgical blade. Add 0.25% Trypsin-EDTA to completely cover the minced tissue.

7. Incubate the contents at 37°C for 15 min 2–3 times and pass the cell suspension through a 40-μm cell strainer to remove the undigested tissue chunks. Add DMEM containing 10% FBS to neutralize trypsin activity.

8. Centrifuge at 300 × g for 10 min at 4°C. Discard the supernatant and resuspend the cell pellet in 50 ml of DMEM supplemented with 10% FBS and 1% penicillin–streptomycin.

9. Plate the cells into the same number of 100-mm dishes as the number of fetuses used and culture until confluent.

3.1.2. Harvest Mouse Embryonic Fibroblast (MEFs) and Freeze

1. Wash the mouse embryonic fibroblast (MEF) cells in each dish with 5 ml PBS.

2. Add 3 ml 0.25% Trypsin-EDTA solution to the dishes and incubate cells for 3 min.

3. Add 5 ml MEF culture medium to each dish and mix well with Trypsin-EDTA solution to neutralize.

4. Transfer the cells to a 50-ml conical tube and centrifuge the suspension at 300 × g for 5 min.

5. Aspirate the supernatant and resuspend the cell pellet with 1 ml cryopreservation medium.

6. Add 1 ml of cell suspension to 1.5-ml cryovial.

7. Immediately freeze the cells in –80°C freezer.

3.1.3. Mouse Embryonic Fibroblasts Culture and Propagation

1. Thaw one vial of MEFs quickly in 37°C water bath and transfer the thawed cell suspension to a 50-ml conical tube containing 10 ml of MEF medium.

2. Centrifuge the cells at 300 × g for 5 min and remove the supernatant by aspiration.

3. Resuspend the cell pellet in 50 ml of MEF medium and plate into five 100-mm culture dishes not coated with gelatin.

4. Culture the cells in a 37°C, 5% CO_2 humidified incubator for 2–3 days. Monitor cell density daily.

5. When the cells reach about 80% confluence, wash each dish with 5 ml PBS and trypsinize the cells for 3 min at 37°C with 2 ml of Trypsin-EDTA solution.

6. Harvest and transfer the cells to a 50-ml conical tube containing 10 ml of MEF medium. Centrifuge at $300 \times g$ for 5 min and remove the supernatant by aspiration.

7. Resuspend the cell pellet in 50 ml of MEF medium and split the cells into twenty-five 100-mm culture dishes containing 8 ml of MEF medium.

8. Repeat steps 4–6.

9. Resuspend cell pellet in 20 ml of MEF medium and count the cells then transfer calculated amount of cells to a 15-ml conical tube. (*see* **Note 2**).

10. Irradiate the cells with 3000 rads of gamma irradiation, then centrifuge at $300 \times g$ for 5 min, and remove the supernatant by aspiration.

11. Resuspend the cell pellet at 2×10^6 cells/ml with freezing medium and aliquot cells into cryovials, then keep at -80°C freezer.

3.2. Culture of Human Embryonic Stem Cells (hES Cells)

3.2.1. Gelatin Coating of Tissue Culture Plate

1. Add 2 ml of 0.1% gelatin solution to each well of the 6-well plate.

2. Leave the 6-well plate at room temperature for 30 min.

3. Remove the gelatin solution and wash the plate with PBS.

3.2.2. Preparation of MEFs Feeder Plate

1. Prepare 0.1% gelatin-coated 6-well plate.

2. Thaw one vial (2×10^6 cells) of irradiated MEFs by swirling in 37°C water bath (*see* **Note 3**).

3. Transfer the MEFs into 15-ml conical tube containing 4 ml prewarmed MEF medium.

4. Centrifuge the cells at $300 \times g$ for 5 min and remove the supernatant.

5. Resuspend the MEFs in 12 ml MEF medium and add 1 ml of MEF suspension to each well of the 6-well plate containing 1 ml fresh MEF medium per well.

6. Incubate the cells in a 37°C, 5% CO_2 humidified incubator for 24 h.

3.2.3. Maintenance of Human Embryonic Stem Cells

1. Thaw one vial of H13 hES cells quickly in 37°C water bath and transfer the thawed cells to a 15-ml conical tube containing hES cell medium.

2. Centrifuge the cells at $200 \times g$ for 5 min and remove the supernatant by aspiration.

3. Resuspend the hES cells in 6 ml of hES cell medium.

4. Aspirate the medium from a MEFs feeder plate and add 1 ml hES medium to each well of the 6 well plate containing MEF cells.

5. Add 1 ml of hES cells to each well of the MEFs feeder plate.

6. Incubate the cells in a 37°C, 5% CO_2 humidified incubator.

7. Refresh the hES cell culture medium daily.

8. After 5–7 days, aspirate the hES cell culture medium from hES cells plate.

9. Add 1 ml Collagenase solution (1 mg/ml) to each well and incubate for 5 min at 37°C (*see* **Note 4**).

10. When the cells have began to peel up, aspirate the Collagenase solution with a Pasteur pipette, without disturbing the attached cell layer.

11. Add 2 ml of hES cell culture medium to each well.

12. Hold a 5-ml pipette perpendicular to the surface of plate and gently scrape the surface of the plate while pipetting up and down (be careful not to create bubbles).

13. Transfer the hES cells into the 15-ml conical tube and suspend the cells gently to separate cell colonies.

14. Centrifuge the hES cells at 200 × g for 5 min and aspirate the MEF culture medium from a 6-well feeder plate containing the irradiated MEFs (1×10^6 cells/plate).

15. Add 1 ml of hES cells culture medium to each well.

16. Aspirate the supernatant from the hES cells pellet and resuspend the pellet with 6 ml of hES cells culture medium.

17. Add 1 ml of the cell suspension drop-wise to each well to ensure even distribution.

18. Incubate the cells overnight in a 37°C, 5% CO_2 humidified incubator to allow colonies to attach.

19. Refresh the hES cell culture medium daily and keep undifferentiated hES cells (**Fig. 6.1**).

3.3. In Vitro Differentiation of hES Cells into HPCs (Hematopoietic Progenitor Cells)

3.3.1. Formation of EBs

1. Culture the undifferentiated hES cells in 6-well plates until 70–80% confluence is reached.

2. Aspirate the medium and rinse the cells once with 2 ml of PBS.

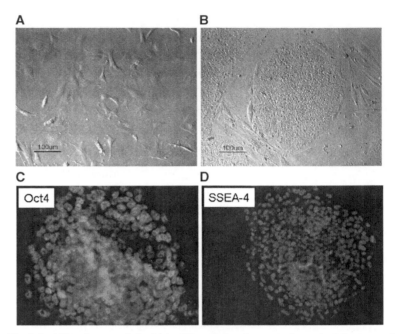

Fig. 6.1. hES cells expanded prior to differentiation form colonies and retain stem cell marker expression. (**A**) Mouse embryonic fibroblasts. (**B**) Phase contrast image of hES cells (H13). (**C**), (**D**) Immunofluorescent image of hES cells stained for Oct4 and SSEA-4 indicate that they retain an undifferentiated phenotype.

3. Add 0.75 ml of prewarmed 0.05% Trypsin-EDTA to each well and incubate at 37°C for 2 min.

4. Gently pipette the cell suspension 2–3 times with a serological pipette.

5. Transfer the cells to a 15-ml conical tube.

6. Centrifuge the cells at $300 \times g$ for 5 min at room temperature. Aspirate the supernatant and resuspend the pellet in 2 ml of EB medium.

7. Count viable cells using trypan blue.

8. Prepare the AggreWell^{TM} 400 plate (**Fig. 6.2A**) (*see* **Note 5**).

9. Rinse each well to be used with 1 ml of DMEM/F12 and aspirate the medium.

10. Add 1 ml of EB formation medium per well of an AggreWell^{TM} 400 plate.

11. Centrifuge the AggreWell^{TM} 400 plate at $3000 \times g$ for 2 min in a swinging bucket rotor.

12. Add 1.2×10^6 cells to each well of AggreWell^{TM} 400 plate to a final volume of 2 ml of EB medium.

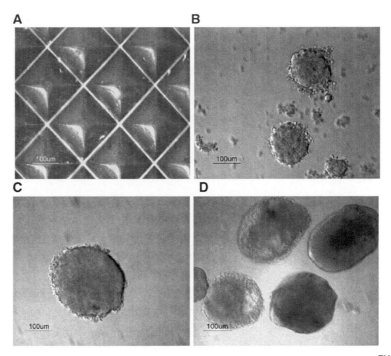

Fig. 6.2. Generation of uniformed embryoid bodies (EBs). (**A**) Picture of AggreWell™ 400 plates contains microwells to make uniform cell aggregates. (**B**) EBs formed using AggreWell™ 400 plates have a uniform shape on day 1. (**C, D**) Morphology of EBs on day 1 and 8, respectively.

13. Add Y-27632 ROCK inhibitor to a final concentration of 10 μM to enhance cell survival during EB formation.

14. Centrifuge the AggreWell™ 400 plate at $100 \times g$ for 3 min to capture the cells in the microwells.

15. Incubate the cells in a 37°C, 5% CO_2 humidified incubator for 24 h.

3.3.2. EB-Derived Hematopoietic Differentiation

1. Harvest the EBs by gently pipetting up and down three times.

2. Pass the EBs suspension through an inverted 40-μm cell strainer on top of a 50-ml conical tube to remove single cells. The aggregates will remain on top of the inverted cell strainer.

3. Turn the cell strainer right-side up over a fresh 50-ml conical tube and collect the aggregates by washing with 5 ml of EB medium.

4. Allow the EBs to settle to the bottom of a 50-ml conical tube by leaving them undisturbed for 5 min at room temperature.

5. Carefully remove the medium and replace with 4 ml of EB medium supplemented with SCF, Flt3L, IL-3, IL-6, G-CSF, and BMP-4.

6. Transfer the EBs to one well of the low attachment 6-well plates and incubate in a 37°C, 5% CO_2 humidified incubator (**Fig. 6.2B–D**).

7. Change the EB medium containing SCF, Flt3L, IL-3, IL-6, G-CSF, and BMP-4 every 4–5 days.

8. After 15 days to 18 days, transfer the EBs to a 15-ml conical tube.

9. Centrifuge the EBs at 200 × g for 3 min and aspirate the supernatant.

10. Wash the EBs with PBS to remove differentiation medium and centrifuge the EBs at 200 × g for 3 min and aspirate the supernatant.

11. Add 2 ml of TrypLE™ Express and place tube for 15 min in a 37°C water bath.

12. After incubation in TrypLE™ Express, gently dissociate the cells by passing the EBs three times through a 23-G needle attached to a 1-ml syringe. As the EBs breaks apart and dissociate into single cells, the solution becomes cloudy.

13. Add 5 ml of differentiation medium without cytokines to tube to dilute the TrypLE™ Express.

14. Centrifuge the cells at 400 × g for 5 min and aspirate the supernatant.

15. Add 5 ml PBS and suspend the cells and filter through a sterile 40-μm cell strainer.

16. Centrifuge the cells for 5 min at 400 × g and aspirate the supernatant and re-suspend the cells with PBS.

17. Count viable cells by trypan blue exclusion using a hemacytometer and resuspend in the buffer or medium for analysis (FACS anaysis, CFU assay, in vivo transplantation).

3.3.3. Isolation of CD34+ HPCs

1. Harvest the differentiated cells and transfer them to a 15 ml conical tube.

2. Centrifuge the cells at 400 × g for 5 min.

3. Aspirate the supernatant and resuspend the cells in 300 μl of MACS buffer.

4. Add 100 μl of FcR blocking reagent and 100 μl of CD34 MultiSort Microbeads.

5. Mix well and incubate the cells for 30 min at 4°C.

6. Wash the cells by adding 1 ml MACS buffer and centrifuge the cells at $300 \times g$ for 2 min. Discard the supernatant and resuspend the cell pellet in 500 µl MACS buffer.

7. Assemble the MS column and prepare column by rinsing with 500 µl MACS buffer.

8. Apply the cell suspension onto the column and wash the column with 2 ml MACS buffer.

9. Remove the column from MACS and place it on a 15 ml tube and add 3 ml MACS buffer into the column.

10. Flush out the magnetically labeled cells by firmly pushing the plunger into the column and centrifuge at $400 \times g$ for 5 min.

11. Aspirate the supernatant and resuspend the cells with PBS.

12. Count viable cells by trypan blue exclusion and resuspend the cells in buffer or medium for analysis (FACS analysis for purity, in vivo transplantation).

4. Notes

1. All procedures require sterilization facilities and a standard cell culture workplace.

2. To ensure complete inactivation of the MEF cells, do not exceed a density greater that 2×10^6 cells/plate.

3. The thawing procedure must be performed as quickly as possible to ensure optimal cells recovery.

4. Do not use old Collagenase solution and do not incubate the cells in Collagenase solution over 15 min.

5. AggreWell^{TM} 400 plates contain microwells, which can be used to aggregate hES cells. EBs generated using AggreWell^{TM} 400 plate are consistent in size and shape.

Acknowledgements

This study was made possible by aVA Merit Review Award and Grant Number NIH/NHLBI #R01 HLO73015 to N.Z.

References

1. Amit, M., Carpenter, M. K., Inokuma, M. S., Chiu, C. P., Harris, C. P., Waknitz, M. A., Itskovitz-Eldor, J., and Thomson, J. A. (2000) Clonally derived human embryonic stem cell lines maintain pluripotency and proliferative potential for prolonged periods of culture. *Dev Biol 227*, 271–278.

2. Basu, S., and Broxmeyer, H. E. (2005) Transforming growth factor-{beta} modulates responses of CD34+ cord blood cells to stromal cell-derived factor-1/CXCL12. *Blood 106*, 485–493.

3. Ledran, M. H., Krassowska, A., Armstrong, L., Dimmick, I., Renstrom, J., Lang, R., Yung, S., Santibanez-Coref, M., Dzierzak, E., Stojkovic, M. (2008) Efficient hematopoietic differentiation of human embryonic stem cells on stromal cells derived from hematopoietic niches. *Cell Stem Cell 3*, 85–98.

4. Chadwick, K., Wang, L., Li, L., Menendez, P., Murdoch, B., Rouleau, A., and Bhatia, M. (2003) Cytokines and BMP-4 promote hematopoietic differentiation of human embryonic stem cells. *Blood 102*, 906–915.

5. Kaufman, D. S., Hanson, E. T., Lewis, R. L., Auerbach, R., and Thomson, J. A. (2001) Hematopoietic colony-forming cells derived from human embryonic stem cells. *Proc Natl Acad Sci USA 98*, 10716–10721.

6. Lu, S. J., Li, F., Vida, L., and Honig, G. R. (2004) CD34+ CD38- hematopoietic precursors derived from human embryonic stem cells exhibit an embryonic gene expression pattern. *Blood 103*, 4134–4141.

7. Perlingeiro, R. C., Kyba, M., and Daley, G. Q. (2001) Clonal analysis of differentiating embryonic stem cells reveals a hematopoietic progenitor with primitive erythroid and adult lymphoid-myeloid potential. *Development 128*, 4597–4604.

8. Vodyanik, M. A., Bork, J. A., Thomson, J. A., and Slukvin, I. I. (2005) Human embryonic stem cell-derived CD34+ cells: Efficient production in the coculture with OP9 stromal cells and analysis of lymphohematopoietic potential. *Blood 105*, 617–626.

9. Wang, L., Li, L., Shojaei, F., Levac, K., Cerdan, C., Menendez, P., Martin, T., Rouleau, A., and Bhatia, M. (2004) Endothelial and hematopoietic cell fate of human embryonic stem cells originates from primitive endothelium with hemangioblastic properties. *Immunity 21*, 31–41.

10. Zambidis, E. T., Peault, B., Park, T. S., Bunz, F., and Civin, C. I. (2005) Hematopoietic differentiation of human embryonic stem cells progresses through sequential hematoendothelial, primitive, and definitive stages resembling human yolk sac development. *Blood 106*, 860–870.

11. Zhan, X., Dravid, G., Ye, Z., Hammond, H., Shamblott, M., Gearhart, J., and Cheng, L. (2004) Functional antigen-presenting leucocytes derived from human embryonic stem cells in vitro. *Lancet 364*, 163–171.

12. Kennedy, M., D'Souza,S.L., Lynch-Kattman, M., Schwantz, S., and Keller, G. (2007) Development of the hemangioblast defines the onset of hematopoiesis in human ES cell differentiation cultures. *Blood 109*, 2679–2687.

13. Ng, E. S., Davis, R. P., Azzola, L., Stanley, E. G., and Elefanty, A. G. (2005) Forced aggregation of defined numbers of human embryonic stem cells into embryoid bodies fosters robust, reproducible hematopoietic differentiation. *Blood 106*, 1601–1603.

14. Pick, M., Azzola, L., Mossman, A., Stanley, E. G., and Elefanty, A. G. (2007) Differentiation of human embryonic stem cells in serum-free medium reveals distinct roles for bone morphogenetic protein 4, vascular endothelial growth factor, stem cell factor, and fibroblast growth factor 2 in hematopoiesis. *Stem Cells 25*, 2206–2214.

15. Cerdan, C., Rouleau, A., and Bhatia, M. (2004) VEGF-A165 augments erythropoietic development from human embryonic stem cells. *Blood 103*, 2504–2512.

16. Tian, X., Morris, J. K., Linehan, J. L., and Kaufman, D. S. (2004) Cytokine requirements differ for stroma and embryoid body-mediated hematopoiesis from human embryonic stem cells. *Exp Hematol 32*, 1000–1009.

17. Bauwens, C. L., Peerani, R., Niebruegge, S., Woodhouse, K. A., Kumacheva, E., Husain, M., and Zandstra, P. W. (2008) Control of human embryonic stem cell colony and aggregate size heterogeneity influences differentiation trajectories. *Stem Cells 26*, 2300–2310.

18. Ungrin, M. D., Joshi, C., Nica, A., Bauwens, C., and Zandstra, P. W. (2008) Reproducible, ultra high-throughput formation of multicellular organization from single cell suspension-derived human embryonic stem cell aggregates. *PLoS ONE. 3*, e1565.

19. Narayan, A. D., Chase, J. L., Lewis, R. L., Tian, X., Kaufman, D. S., Thomson, J. A., and Zanjani, E. D. (2006) Human embry-

onic stem cell-derived hematopoietic cells are capable of engrafting primary as well as secondary fetal sheep recipients. *Blood 107*, 2180–2183.

20. Qiu, C., Hanson, E., Olivier, E., Inada, M., Kaufman, D. S., Gupta, S., and Bouhassira, E. E. (2005) Differentiation of human embryonic stem cells into hematopoietic cells by coculture with human fetal liver cells recapitulates the globin switch that occurs early in development. *Exp. Hematol. 33*, 1450–1458.

21. Slukvin, I., Vodyanik, M. A., Thomson, J. A., Gumenyuk, M. E., and Choi, K. D. (2006) Directed differentiation of human embryonic stem cells into functional dendritic cells through the myeloid pathway. *J Immunol 176*, 2924–2932.

Chapter 7

Gene Therapy to Improve Migration of T Cells to the Tumor Site

Antonio Di Stasi, Biagio De Angelis, and Barbara Savoldo

Abstract

One requirement for anti-tumor T cells to be effective is their successful traffic to tumor sites. Trafficking of T cells to lymphoid organs and peripheral tissues is a multistage process. Soluble and tissue-bonded chemokines interacting with chemokine receptors expressed by T lymphocytes certainly play a pivotal role in determining migration under physiologic conditions and during inflammation. Therefore a match between the chemokines the tumor produces and the chemokine receptors the effector T cells express is required. Since chemokine produced by the targeted tumor may not match the subset of chemokine receptors expressed by T cells, gene therapy can be used to force the expression of the specific chemokine receptor by effector T cells so that the anti-tumor activity of adoptively transferred anti-tumor T cells is maximized.

Key words: Chemokine, chemokine receptor, T cells, migration assay.

1. Introduction

1.1. Chemokines and Migration

Chemokines are small proteins (8–10 kDa) with chemoattractant properties (1). They are divided into four groups (C, CC, CXC, and CX3C), according to the number and the spacing of the first two cysteine residues in the amino-terminal part of the protein. Their effects are exerted through the binding of seven-transmembrane domain G protein-coupled receptors (7TM-GPCR). Chemokines play critical role in regulating homeostatic trafficking and inflammatory responses of hematopoietic stem cells, lymphocytes, and dendritic cells (2). In addition, chemokines are implicated in promoting autocrine or paracrine

P. Yotnda (ed.), *Immunotherapy of Cancer*, Methods in Molecular Biology 651,
DOI 10.1007/978-1-60761-786-0_7, © Springer Science+Business Media, LLC 2010

growth of cancer cells, in regulating angiogenesis, cancer cell invasion, and metastasis, and in supporting immune cells infiltration into tumors (3).

1.1.1. Migration of Immune Cells from the Circulation

Cells circulating in the blood flow exit the vasculature at postcapillary venules, after an initially loose attach (tether) and roll on endothelial cells (recruitment stage, step 1). This first step is mediated through the interaction of homing receptors present on the surface of T cells (mostly selectins but also some integrins) with their respective ligands expressed on endothelial cells, and allows cells to be exposed to chemical signals (step 2, up-regulation of adhesive capabilities) consisting of chemokines, cytokines, inflammatory lipid mediators, complement proteins such as C3a and C5a, and microbial products. This interaction results in the activation-dependent up-regulation of integrin adhesive capabilities, with arrest (step 3, firm arrest) and then exit of the circulating cell from the vasculature into tissue(s) (step 4, transmigration) (4).

1.1.2. Migration of Immune Cells to Tumors

Tumors develop when transformed cells evade the surveillance of the immune system (5). Although the majority of tumors contain immune cells, their presence is not sufficient to control cancer cells growth and/or spread (6). Predominant cell types at tumor sites are macrophages and lymphocytes. In some cancers the presence of natural killer cells, eosinophils, granulocytes, and B cells has been reported (7). Chemokines are critical players in causing infiltration by immune cells. Their role can be dual, as they can favor the infiltration of effector T cells or induce migration of cells that create a favorable environment for the tumor. Chemokines that promote recruitment of Th1 cells are small inducible cytokine A4 (MIP-1-beta), interferon inducible protein 10 (IP-10), Rantes, MIP-1 alfa, and MCP-1 (8–11). However, many chemokines can be produced by the tumor itself to escape immune surveillance (12). For instance, the chemokine CCL2 attracts type II (or M2) polarized macrophages (tumor-associated macrophages, TAM) with primarily pro-tumor functions, as they produce factors promoting angiogenesis and impairing NF-kB inflammatory pathways, and inhibitory cytokines, such as IL-10 and PGE-2 (13, 14). In addition, TAMs produce other chemokines such as CCL18 (15), which recruit naïve T cells that become anergic because of the presence of M2 and immature dendritic cells (DC), and CCL17 and CCL22, which attract CCR4+ expressed on Th2 and regulatory T cells (Treg cells), which provide another immunoevasion strategy (16). CCL17 and CCL22 can be produced by the tumor itself (for example, by Reed-Sternberg cells in Hodgkin lymphoma) to attract CCR4+ Th2, Treg cells as well as monocytes (17).

1.2. Significance of Studying Migration and Chemoattraction

The development of in vitro and in vivo assays to study cell migration can help in better understanding the physiological mechanisms involved in cells migration and define the components implicated in the process. For oncological applications, characterizing the interactions between chemokines and chemokine receptors offers the opportunity to improve the homing of effector T cells to the tumor side, by chemokine receptor genetic modification. An example of this application is presented in this chapter where Hodgkin lymphoma (HL) is used as a model. Indeed, this tumor generates a chemokine milieu that significantly influences which T-cell subtypes traffic to and accumulate in the tumor (17, 18). For instance, Reed-Stemberg cells produce the chemokines TARC/CCL17 and MDC/CCL22 that attract Th2 cells and Tregs, which express CCR4, the receptor for these chemokines (17, 19–22). In contrast, CD8+ effector T cells, which lack CCR4 expression, are rarely detected within HL tumors, a result likely attributable to an incompatible match between the chemokines secreted by the tumor cells and the chemokine receptors expressed by the effector T cells. The abundance of Tregs (and Th2 cells) in tumors including HL can create a hostile immune microenvironment by impairing the anti-tumor activity of the few cytotoxic-effector T lymphocytes able to reach the tumor site (23). Thus, increasing the number of cytototxic T cells that efficiently reach the tumor site should enhance anti-tumor responses. Here we describe how improved migration of T cells at the tumor site can be studied using in vitro and in vivo assays.

1.3. In Vitro Evaluation of Migration: Transwell Migration Assay

Available techniques to examine in vitro migration have been reviewed by Wilkinson et al. (24). Here we describe an in vitro transwell migration assay protocol based on radioactive labeling with ^{51}Cr(25) to evaluate migration of T cells genetically modified to overexpress CCR4, the specific chemokine receptor for TARC.

1.3.1. Filter-Based Assay

Filter assays have been widely used by various authors since they are of easy accessibility and execution (26). However, because the cells cannot be observed in real time, any evidence of chemotaxis is indirect. The single-well Boyden chamber was first introduced in 1962, but several modified versions have since been developed. In Boyden's initial experiments, a 150-μm thick, cellulose ester membrane containing pores of 3-μm diameter was used to separate two compartments (upper and lower) of a chamber. A solution containing a potential chemoattractant was placed in the lower compartment, and a leukocyte suspension was placed in the upper compartment of the chamber, on top of the filter membrane. Migration was measured by counting the leukocytes that had moved through the filter pores to the underside of the membrane in response to presentation of the chemoattractant for 1–4 h at 37°C. This system required large volumes of chemoattractants and numbers of cells.

Polycarbonate filters are more commonly used today (27). Unlike the cellulose, ester polycarbonate filters are thinner (10 μm). The pores are holes punched by neutron bombardment and the migration is dependent on a 2-D surface, whereas in cellulose filters, the cells are moving through a 3-D matrix. Despite this, the polycarbonate filter assays are more popular because they are easy to run and automatized multi-well microplates are now available, increasing the throughput of this procedure (28). By precoating the filter with either monolayer of endothelial cells (29), or extracellular matrix protein, or migration across an endothelium into a fibrillar matrix, is possible to recreate more physiological conditions.

1.3.2. Estimation of Chemotaxis

To indirectly quantify the number of migrated cells through microscope evaluation, cells can be labeled with fluorescent dyes, such as BCECF-AM and calcein AM (30, 31). Migrated cells can be more accurately quantified by simple counting or using analytic techniques, such as radioactive labeling with ^{51}Cr (25), propidium-iodide-based laser scanning cytometry (32), fluorescent-beads-based flow cytometric cell counting (33), or firefly luciferase in a high-throughput assay (34).

1.4. In Vivo Evaluation of Migration

Some of the available techniques to examine cell trafficking are based on cell labeling with tracing dyes (fluorescent dyes such as CFSE (carboxyfluorescein diacetate), bromodeoxyuridine, or radioisotopes). The major drawbacks of these techniques are the cell toxicity mediated by the dye, and the labeling loss through dilution during cell division (35, 36). To overcome such limitations, reporter genes, such as green fluorescent proteins (GFP), have been introduced (37). These optical markers allow examination of labeled cells by fluorescence microscopy and flow cytometry. However for many of these techniques, tissue/cell isolation is required, with no temporal information about dynamic cellular processes. Optical imaging techniques can overcome this problem as mammalian tissues, while relatively opaque, permit transmission of light in the visible and near infrared region of the spectrum. The bioluminescence imaging (BI) (36) is an optical imaging modality that detect externally light emitted from internal biological sources using a light-tight chamber equipped with a cooled sensitive charge-coupled device (CCD) camera (for higher sensitivity) and appropriate lenses (38). Here we describe the use of BI to evaluate migration in vivo of T cells genetically modified to overexpress CCR4, to the site of a tumor producing TARC.

Other validated methods to study in vivo migration of cells have been reviewed by Mandl et al. (36).

1.4.1. Bioluminescence Imaging

Reporter genes that encode bioluminescent enzymes (e.g., Firefly luciferase and Renilla luciferase) have been used as internal biological light sources. Since using two different substrates, they can be used together to monitor two populations simultaneously (i.e., effector and tumor cells) (39). The most frequently used enzyme is Firefly luciferase (*Photinus*). This enzyme produces light by catalyzing the oxidation of its small molecule substrate luciferin D (luciferin (D-(−)-2-(60-hydroxy-20-benzo-thiazolyl) thiazone-4-carbozylic acid) in an ATP-dependent process, with the final release of oxyluciferin, AMP, and light. The reaction is very energetically efficient: nearly all of the energy input into the reaction is transformed into light. In the last few decades, many luciferase genes have been isolated and used to build DNA vectors (40). The advantages of genome integration of such reporter genes are the possibility to carry on long-term studies and the development of animal models of neoplastic diseases. A popular device to measure bioluminescence is the IVIS® Imaging System. Some of the characteristic of the IVIS system are tridimensional spatial localization and co-registration with other imaging modes (computerized tomography (CT), MRI, bioluminescence, and fluorescent data simultaneously collected), ability to detect as few as 50 cells in vivo (one cell in vitro), and combination of epi- and trans-illumination for both superficial and deep tissue visualization. A recent report described the molecular optimization of firefly luciferase retroviral system to detect fewer than ten mouse T cells in an immunocompetent mouse model of cancer using this device (41).

2. Materials

2.1. Cell Lines Culture

1. There are several HL-derived cell lines available that produce the chemokine TARC. Examples are HDLM-2 and L-428 (German Collection of Cell Cultures, DMSZ, Braunschweig, Germany). As negative control, an anaplastic large cell lymphoma (ALCL)-derived cell line, Karpas-299 (German Collection of Cell Cultures, DMSZ), that does not produce TARC can be used. For experimental purposes, this cell line has also been genetically engineered to stably produce TARC by retroviral vector transduction (42).

2. T25/T75 tissue culture-treated flasks (Corning Life Sciences, Lowell, MA).

3. RPMI-1640 medium (Hyclone, Logan, Utah) containing 10% fetal bovine serum (FBS, Hyclone) and 2 mM L-glutamine (GIBCO-BRL, Gaithersburg, MD). Store at 4°C. Warm at 37°C before use.

4. Serum-free medium: AIM-V (GIBCO-BRL, Gaithersburg, MD). Store at 4°C. Warm at 37°C before use.

2.2. Genetically Modified Activated T Cells

1. Peripheral blood mononuclear cells (PBMCs).

2. OKT3 (ortho-Biotech) 1 mg/ml (Bridgewater, NJ). Store at 4°C.

3. Purified Mouse Anti-Human CD28 1 mg/ml (BD Pharmingen, San Diego, CA). Store at 4°C.

4. Sterile water (Baxter Healthcare Corporation).

5. Recombinant human interleukin-2 (IL-2) (Chiron, Emeryville, CA). Reconstitute in medium at 200 IU/μl. Store at –80°C in aliquots that can be used 5 or 6 times.

6. 24-well non-tissue culture-treated plates (BD Biosciences, San Jose, CA).

7. 24-well tissue culture plate (BD Biosciences).

8. Recombinant fibronectin fragment (FN CH-296; Retronectin; Takara Shuzo, Otsu, Japan). Reconstitute in water at 1 mg/ml and store aliquots at –20°C.

9. SFG-CCR4 retroviral supernatant (Vector Production Facility, Baylor College, Houston, TX). Store at –80°C in appropriate aliquots (*see* **Note 1**).

10. T cells medium: 45% RPMI (Hyclone, Logan UT), 45% Click's (Irvine, Scientific, Santa Ana, CA), 10% FBS, and 2 mM Glutamine (Gibco-BRL, Gaithersburg MD). Store at 4°C. Warm at 37°C before use.

11. Cell dissociation solution (Sigma-Aldrich, St Louis, MO). Store at 4°C.

12. IgG1-PE, IgG1-PerCP, CCR4-PE, CD8-PerCP, CD4-APC antibodies (BD Bioscience, San Jose, CA).

2.3. Transswell Migration Assay

1. 0.5-μm pore 24-well transwell plates (Corning Life Sciences, Lowell, MA).

2. AIM V medium (Gibco-BRL). Store at 4°C. Warm at 37°C before use.

3. Anti-human CCL17/TARC Antibody (R&D system, Minneapolis, MN). Reconstitute in DPBS (Gibco-BRL) at a concentration of 0.1 mg/ml. Store aliquots at –20°C to –70°C for 6 months. Avoid repeated freeze–thaw cycles.

4. Mouse anti-human IgG1 (R&D system). Reconstitute in DPBS (Gibco-BRL) at a concentration of 0.1 mg/ml. Store aliquots at −20°C. Avoid repeated freeze–thaw cycles.

2.4. Effector Cells Radiolabeling

1. ^{51}Cr (100 μcurie) (MP Biomedical, Solon, OH).

2. 1%-Triton X solution (Sigma).

3. Gamma counter Packard cobra quantum (Packard Instrument Company, Downers Grove, IL).

2.5. In Vivo Imaging

1. SFG-eGFP-FFluciferase retroviral supernatant (Vector Production Facility, Baylor College, Houston, TX). Store at −80°C in appropriate aliquots

2. Matrigel (BD Biosciences, San Jose, CA). Store at −20°C. Thaw on ice and keep it on ice when in use.

3. CB17/SCID mice (Harlan-Sprague, Indianapolis, IN).

4. IVIS® Imaging System 100 Series equipment (Caliper Life Sciences, Hopkinton, MA).

5. rhIL-2 (Teceleukin, Fisher Bioservices, Rockville, MD). Reconstitute at 200 IU/μl and store at −80°C.

6. D-luciferin, firefly, potassium salt, 1.0 g/vial (Caliper Life Sciences, Hopkinton, MA). Reconstitute D-luciferin in PBS w/o Mg^{2+} and Ca^{2+} at a concentration of 15 mg/ml, filter sterilize through a 0.2–μm filter and store at −20°C.

3. Methods

3.1. Generation and Transduction of Activated T Cells

1. On day 0, coat the appropriate amount of wells of a 24-well non-tissue culture treated plate with 0.5 ml of water containing 1 μg/ml of OKT3 and 1 μg/ml of anti-CD28 and incubate for 3–4 h at 37°C.

2. Aspirate the antibody/solution and wash with 2 ml of complete medium.

3. Resuspend PBMC at 0.5×10^6 ml^{-1} in T-cell medium, add 2 ml/well, and incubate at 37°C, 5% CO_2.

4. On day 1, remove 1 ml of medium and replace with fresh T-cell medium containing rhIL-2 (100 U/ml).

5. On day 1, also, coat the required number of wells of a non-tissue culture-treated 24-well plate, with retronectin at a concentration of 7 μg/ml/well. Incubate at 4°C for 16–24 h.

6. On day 2 remove the retronectin-coated plate from 4°C, aspirate retronectin, and wash with medium.

7. Add 0.5 ml of SFG-CCR4 retroviral supernatant and incubate for 20 min in the biosafety cabinet. Aspirate and add another 0.5 ml of retroviral sup for 20 min.

8. Aspirate, add 1.5 ml of retroviral sup and add 0.5 ml of T cells resuspended at the concentration of 1×10^6 ml^{-1} in complete medium containing rhIL-2 (100 IU/ml) (*see* **Note 2**).

9. Spin plate at 1000 g for 20 min and incubate at 37°C for at least 48 h.

10. Two days after transduction, remove 1 ml of medium/sup from each well.

11. Add 1 ml of eGFP-FFLuc supernatant to each well and IL-2 (100 U/ml).

12. Spin plate at 1000 g for 20 min and incubate at 37°C for 48 h.

13. After 48 h of incubation, collect cells from each well and remove eventual adherent cells by using cell dissociation medium.

14. Count cells (both transduced and NT), resuspend them at the concentration of 0.5×10^6 ml^{-1} in complete medium containing rhIL-2 (50 U/ ml), and aliquot 2 ml/well.

15. Feed cells every 3–4 days with medium containing rhIL-2 (50 U/ml). Once a week, collect cells, count them, and replate them as described in **Section 3.1**, Step 11 until the number of cells is sufficient to perform the assays described below (**Sections 3.2** and **3.3**) is achieved.

3.2.
Immunophenotype

Assess transduction efficiency of T cells by FACS analysis.

1. Collect 1×10^6 of T cells and wash with PBS containing 1% FBS.

2. Aliquot 1×10^5 T cells/tube.

3. Add 5 μl (or as recommended by the manufacturer) of appropriate antibodies combination to each tube:
control: isotype PE and isotype PerCP;
test tube: CCR4-PE and CD3-PerCP (or CD4-PerCP or CD8-PerCP).

4. Incubate in the dark for 20 min (*see* **Note 3**).

5. Wash cells with PBS/1% FBS.

6. Analyze using FACScan (Becton Dickinson) equipped with the filter set for triple fluorescence signals and cell quest software (*see* **Note 4**).

The results of a representative transduction experiment are shown in **Fig. 7.1**.

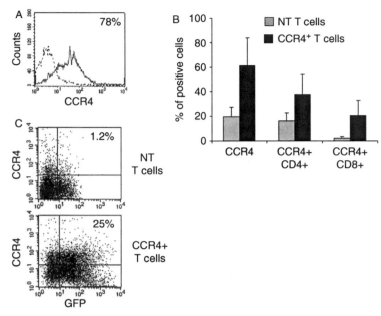

Fig. 7.1. Panel A shows phenotypic analysis of T cells generated from one healthy donor and transduced with CCR4 retroviral vector. The histogram shows the expression of CCR4 in control (Non-Transduced, NT; *dotted line*) T cells and in CCR4$^+$ T lymphocytes (*solid line*). Surface expression of CCR4 was evaluated by FACS analysis. Panel B shows the expression of CCR4, evaluated on CD4$^+$ and CD8$^+$ T cells, of NT T cells (gray bars) and CCR4$^+$ T cells (*black bars*). Bars represent the average ± standard deviation of T cells from 4 experiments. Panel C shows the expression of FF-lucifarese of NT (*upper plot*) and CCR4$^+$ (*lower plot*) T cells evaluated by FACS based on GFP expression.

3.3. Transwell Migration Assay

3.3.1. Preparation of Supernatant and of Effector T Lymphocytes

1. Cell lines producing the chemokine of interest are kept in culture in complete medium in T75 flasks. Cells should be fed at least twice weekly, by removing half of the medium and replacing it with fresh medium.

2. To perform the assay, culture the cell lines HDLM-2, L-428, Karpas, and Karpas/TARC for 16 h in serum-free medium (i.e., AIM V, to reduce the chemoattractant effect of protein contained in the medium) at a concentration of 10^6 ml^{-1} in T25 tissue culture-treated flasks (*see* **Note 5**).

3. Collect, count, and wash effector T cells in complete medium. Label at least 2–3 × 10^6 cells (*see* **Note 6**).

4. Resuspend pelleted T cells by finger-flicking and perform radiolabeling by adding 100 μCi of ^{51}Cr in a radioactive safety cabinet. Labeled cells are then incubated for 1 h at 37°C, gently resuspending cells by finger-flicking every 15 min (*see* **Note 7**).

3.3.2. Lower Chamber Preparation

1. Set up the same experimental condition for each set of effector cells, i.e., in this case NT – T cells and SFG-CCR4$^+$ transduced T cells (*see* **Note 8**).

2. Collect the supernatant, containing the chemokine of interest, from the T25 flasks in a conical tube and spin at 400 g for 5 min to remove residual cells.

3. Load the lower chamber with 500 μl of supernatant and incubate at 37°C while preparing effector cells. For example, for this particular setting add the following:
   a. HDLM-2 supernatant to two wells (one well for NT and one well for CCR4$^+$);
   b. L-428 supernatant to two wells (one well for NT and one well for CCR4$^+$);
   c. Karpas-299 supernatant to two wells (one well for NT and one well for CCR4$^+$),
   d. Karpas-299/TARC supernatant to six wells (one well for NT, one well for NT + isotype Ab, one well for NT + anti-TACR Ab; one well for CCR4$^+$, one well for CCR4$^+$ T cells + Isotype Ab, one well for CCR4$^+$ T cells + anti-TACR Ab) (*see* **Note 9**).

4. Place 500 μl of the serum-free medium in one well as negative control (to measure random migration).

5. Place 400 μl of the serum-free medium in one well where later T cells will be added (*see* **Section 3.3.3**, Step 3) (to measure maximal migration).

3.3.3. Upper Chamber Preparation

1. Wash ^{51}Cr-labeled T lymphocytes by centrifugation at 400 g for 5 min using 5 ml of complete medium; count cells after the third wash, and then resuspend them at the concentration of 1×10^6 ml^{-1} in AIM-V medium.

2. Add 100 μl of T cells into appropriate transwell inserts (upper compartment of the plate).

3. Add 100 μl of cells to the lower compartment of well containing the 400 μl of medium (*see* **Section 3.3.2**, Step 5, maximal migration).

4. Incubate the plates for 4–5 h at 37°C, 5% CO_2 (*see* **Note 10**).

3.3.4. Collection of Migrated Cells

1. After the incubation time, carefully remove the transwell inserts.

2. Add 100 μL of 1% Triton X solution to lyse cells to release the ^{51}Cr from migrated cells.

3. Collect the content of the lower chamber (migrated cells) and read using a gamma counter.

*3.3.5. Measurements
and Analysis of the
Results (see Note 11)*

1. Measure ^{51}Cr release for each specimen.

2. The chemotactic index is calculated by dividing the number of migrated cells by the random migration in the presence of medium only.

3. The percent of migration is calculated as follows: [cpm from experimental supernatant (cells migrated in the lower chamber) – cpm in the presence of medium only (random migration)]/[cpm of maximal migration – cpm of random migration] x 100.

The results of a representative migration experiment are shown in **Fig. 7.2**.

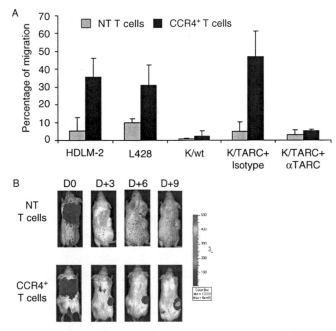

Fig. 7.2. Panel A shows the migration of NT (*gray bars*) and CCR4$^+$ (*black bars*) T cells toward TARC gradients, using the transwell migration assay in one representative donor (average ± standard deviation). T-cell migration was evaluated using culture supernatants collect from the two HL-derived cell lines (HDLM-2 and L428) that physiologically produce high amount of TARC, and from the Karpas-299 cell line genetically modified to produce TARC (K/TARC). Unmodified Karpas-299 (K/wt) was used as a control. The panel shows that migration toward TARC is significantly improved if T cells are genetically modified to overexpress CCR4 and that this improved migration of CCR4$^+$ T cells (*black bars*) is TARC-mediated as inhibited by addition of anti-TARC antibodies but not by the addition of isotype control. Panel B shows the bioluminescence signal from NT and CCR4$^+$ T cells in a SCID mouse engrafted with TARC$^-$ tumor (K/wt) on the left side and the TARC$^+$ tumor (K/TARC) on the right side. While no significant expansion of the bioluminescent signal was observed to either site of tumor in mice receiving NT T cells (*upper pictures*), increase of bioluminescence was observed in mice receiving CCR4$^+$ T cells (*lower pictures*) only at the site of tumor-producing TARC.

3.4. In Vivo Migration

3.4.1. In Vivo Tumor Model

1. Sublethally irradiate (230 cGy) 6- to 8-week-old CB17/SCID mice to oblate NK cells.

2. Inject subcutaneously (s.c.) 5×10^6 tumor cells resuspended in 200 µL of matrigel. Karpas-299 (tumor cell that does not produce TARC) can be injected on the left flank, while Karpas-299 genetically modified to express TARC can be injected on the right flank of the same animal (*see* **Note 12** and **Note 13**).

3. When tumor is palpable (0.5 cm; 5–7 days later), inject intravenously via tail vein 10×10^6 FFluciferase⁺ T cells (control group) or CCR4⁺FFluciferase⁺ T cells (experimental group) (*see* **Note 14**).

4. Inject intraperitoneally (i.p.) IL-2 (500 U/mouse) three times a week to sustain T cells' expansion.

3.4.2. In Vivo Imaging Assessment System

1. Anesthetize mice in a clear Plexiglas chamber filled with 2.5% Isoflurane/air mixture (*see* **Notes 15** and **16**).

2. Inject D-luciferin intraperitoneally at a concentration of 150 mg/kg body weight (10 µl/g of body weight, i.e., for mouse 100µL of the 15 mg/ml solution to deliver 1.5 mg of D-luciferin) (*see* **Notes 17** and **18**).

3. Allow 10 min for D-luciferin distribution (*see* **Note 19**).

4. Place mice fully anesthetized in the light-tight chamber (ensure isoflurane/air deliver through the nose cones attached to the manifold).

5. Close the door of the chamber and begin acquisition using the living image program on the computer screen.

6. Expose mice for appropriate time (ranging from 5 min to <10 seconds, depending on the strength of signal). The mice position may be dorsal or ventral depending on the experiment. When the mice are turned from dorsal to ventral (or vice versa) attention must be paid to any sign of distress.

7. Select appropriate parameters, according to experimental conditions, including filters (f/stop), binning, photography (low f number and high diameter lens gives higher sensitivity and uniform light collection), and field of view (*see* **Note 20**).

8. After imaging is complete, mice are returned to their cages where they should wake up quickly. However, in this phase mice should be monitored for any possible sign of distress (rare).

9. Using the appropriate program analysis, draw a constant region of interest (ROI) over the tumor regions and measure the intensity of the signal as total photon/sec/cm^2/sr (p/s/cm^2/sr). The image data can be exported directly on an excel worksheet for further analysis (*see* **Notes 20** and **21**).

Results of a representative migration experiment are shown in **Fig. 7.2**.

4. Notes

1. Do not refreeze unused viral supernatant.

2. Keep some T cells as Non-Transduced (NT, control). These cells will need to be plated at the same concentration in complete medium containing IL-2 (100 U/ml) in a 24-well tissue culture-treated plate.

3. Room temperature is recommended when testing for CCR4 chemokine receptor.

4. Assess for GFP using the FL-1 channel.

5. The production of chemokines can be tested for each cell line to determine the types and amount of chemokine produced. Supernatant should be tested using commercially available ELISA kits (R&D System or Peprotech).

6. To estimate the required number of cells, consider that about 1×10^5 will be needed for each well of the transwell plate. However, cells will be lost during cell washes so it is recommended to start from $\sim 5 \times 10^5$ T cells for every 1×10^5 required.

7. Wear appropriate radio-protection equipment and monitor the work area using a survey meter; label and dispose of radioactive waste according to approved guidelines; personnel monitoring with thermoluminescence dosimetry is recommended.

8. It is recommended that experiments are set in duplicate or triplicate for each condition.

9. For the wells containing supernatant and antibodies (isotype antibody or chemoattractant blocking antibody) incubate for at least 20 min prior the loading of the effector T cells in the upper transwell compartment.

10. A time-course evaluation before setting up experiment is required to evaluate the optimal period of incubation for a particular set of experimental conditions.

11. A different option to this protocol is to quantitate the migrated cells by direct counting. In this case, you will not need to label cells with ^{51}Cr. In addition, it is recommended to plate at least 1×10^6 cells in the upper compartment. Then follow the alternative step in **Section 3.3.4** Migrated cells collection: after incubation, carefully remove the transwell inserts and collect the content of the lower chamber making sure to collect all the migrated cells; count viable cells after dilution with trypan blue. The percent of migration is calculated as above (**Section 3.3.5**, Step 3) using the cell number as the parameter.

12. Using this approach each mouse acts as a "self-control" for unmodified and CCR4$^+$ T cells.

13. Ensure that the two cell lines have comparable in vivo growth.

14. Collect T cells and wash them with DPBS; then count and resuspend them in DPBS in 200 μl final volume.

15. In vivo imaging assessment can be performed starting from the day of lymphocyte injection and subsequently three times a week.

16. A clear chamber allows unimpeded visual monitoring of the animals, e.g., to easily determine if the animals are breathing.

17. A D-luciferin kinetic study should be performed for each animal model to determine peak signal time. Preferred site for injection is the animal's lower left abdominal quadrant. Mice can be manually restrained, dorsal recumbency (abdomen side up), with cranial (head) end of animal pointed down. Needle should be bevel-side up and slightly angled when entering the abdominal cavity. Penetrate just through abdominal wall (about 4–5 mm). The tip of the needle should just penetrate the abdominal wall of the animal's left lower abdominal quadrant.

18. Recommended needle size is 25 gauge (usually used with 1-cc syringe).

19. Ten minutes post-substrate administration, the D-luciferin has been shown to distribute in saturation levels broadly to tissues throughout the body and can cross the blood–brain barrier and placental barrier (38).

20. Refer to IVIS manual and software for further information.

21. When using photon/sec/cm^2/sr, measured signals are automatically corrected for these variables; autofluorescent background is automatically subtracted as well.

References

1. Mackay, C. R. (2001) Chemokines: Immunology's high impact factors. *Nat Immunol 2*, 95–101.
2. Mantovani, A., Allavena, P., Sozzani, S., Vecchi, A., Locati, M., and Sica, A. (2004) Chemokines in the recruitment and shaping of the leukocyte infiltrate of tumors. *Semin Cancer Biol 14*, 155–160.
3. Balkwill, F. (2004) Cancer and the chemokine network. *Nat Rev Cancer 4*, 540–550.
4. Sackstein, R. (2005) The lymphocyte homing receptors: gatekeepers of the multistep paradigm. *Curr Opin Hematol 12*, 444–450.
5. Liotta, L. A. and Kohn, E. C. (2001) The microenvironment of the tumour-host interface. *Nature 411*, 375–379.
6. Dunn, G. P., Old, L. J., and Schreiber, R. D. (2004) The immunobiology of cancer immunosurveillance and immunoediting. *Immunity 21*, 137–148.
7. Vicari, A. P. and Caux, C. (2002) Chemokines in cancer. *Cytokine Growth Factor Rev 13*, 143–154.
8. Moran, C. J., Arenberg, D. A., Huang, C. C., Giordano, T. J., Thomas, D. G., Misek, D. E., Chen, G., Iannettoni, M. D., Orringer, M. B., Hanash, S., and Beer, D. G. (2002) RANTES expression is a predictor of survival in stage I lung adenocarcinoma. *Clin Cancer Res 8*, 3803–3812.
9. Tang, K. F., Tan, S. Y., Chan, S. H., Chong, S. M., Loh, K. S., Tan, L. K., and Hu, H. (2001) A distinct expression of CC chemokines by macrophages in nasopharyngeal carcinoma: implication for the intense tumor infiltration by T lymphocytes and macrophages. *Hum Pathol 32*, 42–49.
10. Negus, R. P., Stamp, G. W., Hadley, J., and Balkwill, F. R. (1997) Quantitative assessment of the leukocyte infiltrate in ovarian cancer and its relationship to the expression of C-C chemokines. *Am J Pathol 150*, 1723–1734.
11. Monti, P., Leone, B. E., Marchesi, F., Balzano, G., Zerbi, A., Scaltrini, F., Pasquali, C., Calori, G., Pessi, F., Sperti, C., Di, C. V, Allavena, P., and Piemonti, L. (2003) The CC chemokine MCP-1/CCL2 in pancreatic cancer progression: regulation of expression and potential mechanisms of antimalignant activity. *Cancer Res 63*, 7451–7461.
12. Gabrilovich, D. (2004) Mechanisms and functional significance of tumour-induced dendritic-cell defects. *Nat Rev Immunol 4*, 941–952.
13. Elgert, K. D., Alleva, D. G., and Mullins, D. W. (1998) Tumor-induced immune dysfunction: the macrophage connection. *J Leukoc Biol 64*, 275–290.
14. Mantovani, A., Sozzani, S., Locati, M., Allavena, P., and Sica, A. (2002) Macrophage polarization: tumor-associated macrophages as a paradigm for polarized M2 mononuclear phagocytes. *Trends Immunol 23*, 549–555.
15. Adema, G. J., Hartgers, F., Verstraten, R., de, V. E., Marland, G., Menon, S., Foster, J., Xu, Y., Nooyen, P., McClanahan, T., Bacon, K. B., and Figdor, C. G. (1997) A dendritic-cell-derived C-C chemokine that preferentially attracts naive T cells. *Nature 387*, 713–717.
16. Balkwill, F. (2004) Cancer and the chemokine network. *Nat Rev Cancer 4*, 540–550.
17. van den, B. A., Visser, L., and Poppema, S. (1999) High expression of the CC chemokine TARC in Reed-Sternberg cells. A possible explanation for the characteristic T-cell infiltratein Hodgkin's lymphoma. *Am J Pathol 154*, 1685–1691.
18. Maggio, E. M., van den, B. A., Visser, L., Diepstra, A., Kluiver, J., Emmens, R., and Poppema, S. (2002) Common and differential chemokine expression patterns in rs cells of NLP, EBV positive and negative classical Hodgkin lymphomas. *Int J Cancer 99*, 665–672.
19. Ishida, T., Ishii, T., Inagaki, A., Yano, H., Komatsu, H., Iida, S., Inagaki, H., and Ueda, R. (2006) Specific recruitment of CC chemokine receptor 4-positive regulatory T cells in Hodgkin lymphoma fosters immune privilege. *Cancer Res 66*, 5716–5722.
20. Iellem, A., Mariani, M., Lang, R., Recalde, H., Panina-Bordignon, P., Sinigaglia, F., and D'Ambrosio, D. (2001) Unique chemotactic response profile and specific expression of chemokine receptors CCR4 and CCR8 by CD4(+)CD25(+) regulatory T cells. *J Exp Med 194*, 847–853.
21. D'Ambrosio, D., Iellem, A., Bonecchi, R., Mazzeo, D., Sozzani, S., Mantovani, A., and Sinigaglia, F. (1998) Selective up-regulation of chemokine receptors CCR4 and CCR8 upon activation of polarized human type 2 Th cells. *J Immunol 161*, 5111–5115.
22. Marshall, N. A., Christie, L. E., Munro, L. R., Culligan, D. J., Johnston, P. W., Barker, R. N., and Vickers, M. A. (2004) Immunosuppressive regulatory T cells are abundant in the reactive lymphocytes of Hodgkin lymphoma. *Blood 103*, 1755–1762.

23. Curiel, T. J., Coukos, G., Zou, L., Alvarez, X., Cheng, P., Mottram, P., Evdemon-Hogan, M., Conejo-Garcia, J. R., Zhang, L., Burow, M., Zhu, Y., Wei, S., Kryczek, I., Daniel, B., Gordon, A., Myers, L., Lackner, A., Disis, M. L., Knutson, K. L., Chen, L., and Zou, W. (2004) Specific recruitment of regulatory T cells in ovarian carcinoma fosters immune privilege and predicts reduced survival. *Nat Med 10*, 942–949.

24. Wilkinson, P. C. (1998) Assays of leukocyte locomotion and chemotaxis. *J Immunol Methods 216*, 139–153.

25. Capsoni, F., Minonzio, F., Ongari, A. M., and Zanussi, C. (1989) A new simplified single-filter assay for 'in vitro' evaluation of chemotaxis of 51Cr-labeled polymorphonuclear leukocytes. *J Immunol Methods 120*, 125–131.

26. Wilkinson, P. C. (1998) Assays of leukocyte locomotion and chemotaxis. *J Immunol Methods 216*, 139–153.

27. Horwitz, D. A. and Garrett, M. A. (1971) Use of leukocyte chemotaxis in vitro to assay mediators generated by immune reactions. I. Quantitation of mononuclear and polymorphonuclear leukocyte chemotaxis with polycarbonate (nuclepore) filters. *J Immunol 106*, 649–655.

28. Falk, W., Goodwin, R. H., Jr., and Leonard, E. J. (1980) A 48-well micro chemotaxis assembly for rapid and accurate measurement of leukocyte migration, *J Immunol Methods 33*, 239–247.

29. Roth, S. J., Carr, M. W., Rose, S. S., and Springer, T. A. (1995) Characterization of transendothelial chemotaxis of T lymphocytes. *J Immunol Methods 188*, 97–116.

30. De Clerck, L. S., Bridts, C. H., Mertens, A. M., Moens, M. M., and Stevens, W. J. (1994) Use of fluorescent dyes in the determination of adherence of human leucocytes to endothelial cells and the effect of fluorochromes on cellular function. *J Immunol Methods 172*, 115–124.

31. Frevert, C. W., Wong, V. A., Goodman, R. B., Goodwin, R., and Martin, T. R. (1998) Rapid fluorescence-based measurement of neutrophil migration in vitro. *J Immunol Methods 213*, 41–52.

32. Butt, O. I., Krishnan, P., Kulkarni, S. S., Moldovan, L., and Moldovan, N. I. (2005) Quantification and functional analysis of chemotaxis by laser scanning cytometry. *Cytometry A 64*, 10–15.

33. Molema, G., Mesander, G., Kroesen, B. J., Helfrich, W., Meijer, D. K., and de Leij, L. F. (1998) Analysis of in vitro lymphocyte adhesion and transendothelial migration by fluorescent-beads-based flow cytometric cell counting. *Cytometry 32*, 37–43.

34. Vishwanath, R. P., Brown, C. E., Wagner, J. R., Meechoovet, H. B., Naranjo, A., Wright, C. L., Olivares, S., Qian, D., Cooper, L. J., and Jensen, M. C. (2005) A quantitative high-throughput chemotaxis assay using bioluminescent reporter cells. *J Immunol. Methods 302*, 78–89.

35. Lyons, A. B. (2000) Analysing cell division in vivo and in vitro using flow cytometric measurement of CFSE dye dilution. *J Immunol Methods 243*, 147–154.

36. Mandl, S., Schimmelpfennig, C., Edinger, M., Negrin, R. S., and Contag, C. H. (2002) Understanding immune cell trafficking patterns via in vivo bioluminescence imaging. *J Cell Biochem. Suppl 39*, 239–248.

37. Okabe, M., Ikawa, M., Kominami, K., Nakanishi, T., and Nishimune, Y. (1997) 'Green mice' as a source of ubiquitous green cells. *FEBS Lett 407*, 313–319.

38. Edinger, M., Hoffmann, P., Contag, C. H., and Negrin, R. S. (2003) Evaluation of effector cell fate and function by in vivo bioluminescence imaging. *Methods 31*, 172–179.

39. Bhaumik, S. and Gambhir, S. S. (2002) Optical imaging of Renilla luciferase reporter gene expression in living mice. *Proc Natl Acad Sci. US A 99*, 377–382.

40. Greer, L. F., III and Szalay, A. A. (2002) Imaging of light emission from the expression of luciferases in living cells and organisms: A review. *Luminescence 17*, 43–74.

41. Rabinovich, B. A., Ye, Y., Etto, T., Chen, J. Q., Levitsky, H. I., Overwijk, W. W., Cooper, L. J., Gelovani, J., and Hwu, P. (2008) Visualizing fewer than 10 mouse T cells with an enhanced firefly luciferase in immunocompetent mouse models of cancer. *Proc Natl Acad Sci USA 105*, 14342–14346.

42. Di Stasi, A., De Angelis, B., Rooney, C. M., Zhang, L., Mahendravada, A., Foster, A. E., Heslop, H. E., Brenner, M. K., Dotti, G., and Savoldo, B. (2009) T lymphocytes coexpressing CCR4 and a chimeric antigen receptor targeting CD30 have improved homing and antitumor activity in a Hodgkin tumor model. *Blood 113*, 6392–6402.

Chapter 8

Gene Therapy to Improve Function of T Cells for Adoptive Immunotherapy

Concetta Quintarelli, Barbara Savoldo, and Gianpietro Dotti

Abstract

Adoptive immunotherapy with cytotoxic T cells has shown promising clinical results in patients with metastatic melanoma and post-transplant-associated viral infections. However, the antitumor effect of adoptively transferred tumor-specific cytotoxic T lymphocytes (CTLs) is impaired by the limited capacity of these cells to expand within the tumor microenvironment. Administration of interleukin 2 (IL-2) has been used to overcome this limitation, but the systemic toxicity and the expansion of unwanted cells, including regulatory T cells, limit the clinical value of this strategy. To discover whether transgenic expression of lymphokines by the CTLs themselves might overcome these limitations, we evaluated the effects of transgenic expression of IL-2 and IL-15 in our model of Epstein-Barr Virus-specific CTLs (EBV-CTLs). We found that transgenic expression of IL-2 or IL-15 increased the expansion of EBV-CTLs in vitro and that these gene-modified EBV-CTL had enhanced antitumor activity, while maintaining their antigen-specificity. Although the proliferation of these cytokine gene transduced CTLs remained strictly antigen dependent, clinical application of this approach likely requires the inclusion of a suicide gene to deal with the potential development of T-cell mutants with autonomous growth. We found that the incorporation of an inducible caspase-9 suicide gene allowed efficient elimination of transgenic CTLs after exposure to a chemical inducer of dimerization, thereby increasing the safety and feasibility of the approach.

Key words: Cytotoxic T cells, EBV, IL-2, IL-15, suicide gene, retroviral vector, T-cell proliferation.

1. Introduction

Adoptive immunotherapy is a promising approach for the treatment of infectious diseases and cancer. Several immunotherapeutic lines of research are currently focusing on the treatment of viral infections, such as cytomegalovirus (CMV), Epstein-Barr virus (EBV), and HIV, as well as a variety of malignancies,

P. Yotnda (ed.), *Immunotherapy of Cancer*, Methods in Molecular Biology 651,
DOI 10.1007/978-1-60761-786-0_8, © Springer Science+Business Media, LLC 2010

including melanoma, Hodgkin lymphoma, nasopharyngeal carcinoma, and several other EBV-associated lymphoproliferative disorders. Adoptive T-cell transfer involves the ex vivo generation and expansion of antigen-specific autologous T cells over a short period of time, from low precursor frequencies to clinically relevant cell numbers, followed by re-infusion into patients. Although a variety of different approaches have been developed, improvements are required to generate antigen-specific cytotoxic T lymphocytes (CTLs) that efficiently persist in vivo. Indeed, the antitumor activity of adoptively transferred CTLs is hampered by the limited capacity of these cells to significantly expand within the tumor microenvironment. Several studies of cancer immunotherapy have focused on the development of strategies to overcome this restriction by controlling the distribution of immune cells at the tumor site through the characterization of various chemokines and receptors modulating the immune system.

Recently, attention has been addressed to two positive growth factors for T cells, IL2 and IL15, to improve T-cell persistence in the tumor environment. Both cytokines are critically involved both in innate and adaptive immune responses (1). Their receptors share two subunits (β and γ) that mediate a set of signal transduction events after ligand binding, but have their own, "private" α-chains, which presumably ensure the binding of the appropriate cytokine and the specificity of the immune response (2, 3). Through the combination of these various subunits, several forms of receptor complexes exist at the cell surface. Biological effects of IL-2 are achieved mainly when this cytokine binds to the trimetric-, high-affine IL-2R complex (IL-2R$\alpha\beta\gamma$). The IL-15R$\alpha\beta\gamma$ complex has a similar high affinity but for IL-15. When this receptor constellation is utilized, IL-2 and IL-15 activate similar janus kinase/signal transducer and activator of transcription (JAK/STAT)-dependent signaling pathways (4). Thus, IL-2 and IL-15 are redundant in stimulating T-cell proliferation in vitro. However, each may have distinct functions and regulate distinct aspects of T-cell activation. Studies have shown that IL-15 is a critical growth factor in initiating T-cell divisions in vivo, whereas IL-2 limits continued T-cell expansion via downregulation of the γ-c expression, with consequent decreased Bcl-2 expression and increased susceptibility to apoptotic cell death. Although the role of IL-2 in the generation and maintenance of antigen-specific T-cell responses in vivo remains unclear, with data supporting both positive and negative effects, IL-2 is currently used to enhance T-cell responses to viral and tumor antigens in patients, including those with HIV or metastatic cancer.

Since adoptively transferred antigen-specific CTLs are highly dependent on exogenous cytokines for their continued growth and survival, systemic administration of IL-2 has been used to enhance their in vivo expansion and persistence. However, high-dose IL-2 therapy is limited by its toxicity resulting from vascular leakage and the serious side effects associated with the prolonged administration of IL-2 limit the amount and duration of this cytokine administration (5–8). Further, the effects of systemically administered cytokines may be non-selective, with potential expansion of unwanted cell subsets, such as regulatory T cells, that constitutively express the IL-2 receptor and adversely affect the function of antitumor CTLs (9).

To overcome these effects, CTLs can be genetically manipulated, using retroviral vectors, to produce their own growth cytokines such as IL-2 and IL-15. In this way CTLs are rendered less helper-cell dependent and better able to sustain their proliferation and activation after antigenic stimulation (10). Because for clinical applications, constitutive expression of transgenic cytokines would likely raise concerns about autonomous and uncontrolled growth of CTLs, the presence of a suicide gene inducible caspase-9 (iCasp-9) protein is required. This proapoptotic gene product is activated after exposure to CID (AP20187), an analog of FK506, that has been safely tested in a phase I study (11). A third gene based on a truncated form of the CD34 molecule (ΔCD34) is also necessary in the construct to allow efficient evaluation and selection of transduced cells.

In this chapter, we describe an in vitro protocol to transduce with retroviral vectors EBV-CTLs and test the expression and functionality of each transgene, while ensuring that these transduced CTL retain their characteristics. All these steps are required to guarantee that this gene manipulation is effective and safe.

2. Materials

2.1. Genetic Modification of EBV-CTLs

1. CTL medium: RPMI 1640 45% (Hyclone, Ogden, UT), Click medium (Irvine Scientific, Santa Ana, CA) 45%, supplemented with 10% fetal bovine serum (FBS, HyClone), 2 mM L-glutamine and penicillin-streptomycin (Gibco/BRL, Bethesda, MD).

2. EBV-LCLs are maintained in RPMI medium, supplemented with 10% fetal bovine serum, 2 mM L-glutamine, 100 IU/ml penicillin, and 100 μg/ml streptomycin in T75 tissue culture flasks.

3. Peripheral blood mononuclear cells (PBMCs) from EBV-seropositive donors.

4. Recombinant human interleukin-2 (IL-2) (Chiron, Emeryville, CA). Reconstitute in medium at 200 U/μl. Store at −80°C in aliquots that can be used 5–6 times.

5. 24-well non-tissue culture-treated plates (BD Biosciences, San Jose, CA).

6. 24-well tissue culture plates (BD Biosciences, San Jose, CA).

7. Recombinant fibronectin fragment (FN CH-296; Retronectin; Takara Shuzo, Otsu, Japan). Reconstitute in water at 1 mg/ml and store aliquots at –20°C.

8. ΔCD34, iC.ΔCD34-IL2, or iC.ΔCD34–IL15 retroviral supernatant (Vector Production Facility, Baylor College, Houston, TX). Store at –80°C.

9. Recombinant human IL-15 (R&D Systems, Minneapolis, MN). Reconstitute in medium at 5 ng/μl and store aliquots at –80°C.

10. Enzyme-Free Cell Dissociation Solution cell (Invitrogen).

11. Trypan blue (Sigma).

12. Cytokine-specific *ELISA* kits containing Microplate-96 wells, Ab-Conjugate, Standard, Assay Diluent, Calibrator Diluent, Wash Buffer Concentrate, Color Reagent A, Color Reagent B, Stop Solution, Plate Covers (R&D System).

13. Plate washer (Bioscan, Inc).

14. Microplate Reader (Bioscan, Inc).

15. Chemical inducer of dimerization (CID) (AP20187; ARIAD Pharmaceuticals, Cambridge, MA), kindly provided by Dr. Spencer (Baylor College of Medicine). CID is resuspended in Ethanol at the final concentration of 2 μM and stored at –20°C. For culture experiments resuspend CID at the final concentration of 50 nM in complete RPMI.

2.2. Immunophenotype

1. Monoclonal antibodies conjugated with different fluorocromes: CD34 APC; CD8 FITC, CD3 PerCP (all from BD Bioscience).

2. 5-ml polystirene tubes (Falcon).

3. FACS Wash buffer: PBS+1% FBS.

4. FACScan (Becton Dickinson) equipped with the filter set for triple fluorescence signals and cell quest software.

5. PE-conjugated MHC Class I tetramers, synthesized in the Baylor College of Medicine Immunologic facility.

6. IOTest ßMark kit (Immunotech, Emeryville, CA), a multiparametric analysis tool designed for quantitative determination of the TCR Vβ repertoire of T lymphocytes by flow cytometry.

7. AnnexinV-FITC, 7-Amino-Actinomycin (7-AAD), and $1\times$ Annexin V Binding Buffer (BD Pharmingen).

2.3. Cytotoxicity Assay

1. ^{51}Cr (100 μcurie) (MP Biomedical, Solon, OH).

2. 96-well plate, V-bottom (Costar).

3. Triton-X (Sigma).

4. Gamma counter Packard cobra quantum (Packard Instrument Company, Downers Grove, IL).

5. Target cells are: autologous LCL; HLA-mismatched LCL; K562. These cells are maintained in culture in T75 flasks in complete medium at 37°C, 5%CO_2.

2.4. Elispot Assay

1. IFN gamma Coating Antibody [Catcher-mAB(1-DIK)] and IFN gamma Detection Antibody [Detector-mAB (7-B6-1-Biotin)] (MABTECH Inc., Mariemont, OH).

2. Streptavidin-AP Concentrate (Thermo Fisher Scientific Inc, Rockford, IL).

3. Millipore MultiScreen$_{HTS}$-IP Filter Plates (Millipore).

4. Elispot medium: RPMI 1640 (Hyclone) supplemented with 5% human AB serum (BioWhittaker), 2 mM L-glutamine and filtered using 0.45-μ filter.

5. PBS (Sigma) containing 0.05% of Tween-20 (Sigma).

6. Avidin-Peroxidase-Complex (ABC kit, Vectastan, Burlingame, CA): add 1 drop of Solution A and 1 drop of Solution B to 10 ml PBS/0.1% Tween-20.

7. AEC substrate: dissolve 1 AEC tablet (Sigma) in 2.5 ml dimethylformamide (Sigma); then add 47.5 ml of a solution consisting of 4.6 ml of 0.1 N of Acetic Acid (Sigma), 11 ml of 0.1 M sodium acetate (Sigma) and 46.9 ml of water (Baxter), add 25 μl 30% hydrogen peroxide (Sigma), and filter using 0.45-μ filter.

8. Zellnet Consulting (Fort Lee, NJ) provides Elispot evaluation service.

3. Methods

3.1. Genetic Modification of EBV-CTLs

1. Thaw PBMC, count, and resuspend at 2×10^6/ml in complete medium. Plate 1 ml/well in a 24-well plate and add 1 ml of irradiated autologous EBV-LCL (40 Gy) resuspended at 5×10^4 cell/ml in complete medium (40:1 effector:target ratio).

2. After 10–12 days, collect CTL, count, and resuspend at 1×10^6/ml in complete medium. Plate 1 ml/well in a 24-well plate and add 1 ml of irradiated autologous EBV-LCL (40 Gy) resuspended at 2.5×10^5 cell/ml in complete medium (4:1 effector:target ratio).

3. After 3–4 days remove 1 ml of medium and replace with complete medium containing IL-2 (50 U/ml).

4. After 3 days, collect CTLs, count, and resuspend them at 1×10^6 cells/ml and aliquot 1 ml/well in 24-well tissue culture plate; add 1 ml of irradiated autologous EBV-LCL (40 Gy) resuspended at 2.5×10^5 cell/ml in complete medium containing IL-2 (50 U/ml).

5. On day 3, coat the required number of wells of a non-tissue culture-treated 24-well plate, with RetroNectin at a concentration of 7 μg/ml/well and incubate at 4°C for 16–24 h.

6. On day 4 remove the retronectin-coated plate from 4°C, aspirate retronectin, and wash wells with 1 ml of complete medium.

7. Add 0.5 ml/well of appropriate retroviral supernatant and incubate for 20 min in the biosafety cabinet. Aspirate and add another 0.5 ml of retroviral supernatant for 20 min.

8. Aspirate, add 1.5 ml of retroviral supernatant, and 0.5 ml of T cells resuspended at the concentration of 1×10^6/ml in complete medium containing rhIL-2 (100 IU/ml) (*see* **Note 1**).

9. Spin plate at $1000 \times g$ for 20 min and incubate at 37°C for at least 48 h.

10. After 48 h of incubation collect cells from each well and remove eventual adherent cells by using cell dissociation medium and restimulate weekly with irradiated (40 Gy) autologous LCL (4:1 Effector:Traget ratio), with or without the addition of exogenous rhIL-2 (50 U/ml) or rhIL-15 (5 ng/ml).

11. Assess transduction efficiency of CTL by FACS analysis, using CD34 APC antibody (*see* **Section 3.3**).

3.2. Testing Functionality of the Transgenes

3.2.1. Expansion of Gene-Modified EBV-CTLs

1. Collect and count CTLs using Trypan blue (1:1 dilution) to determine viability of CTLs; resuspend CTLs in T-cell medium at the concentration of 1×10^6/ml and aliquot 1 ml/well.

2. Add 1 ml of irradiated autologous LCL (40 Gy) resuspended at 2.5×10^5/well in complete medium with or without

the addition of exogenous rhIL-2 (50 U/ml) or rhIL-15 (5 ng/ml).

3. Incubate at 37°C, 5% CO_2.

4. On day 4, remove 1 ml of medium and replace with fresh medium, with or without the addition of exogenous rhIL-2 (50 U/ml) or rhIL-15 (5 ng/ml).

5. Incubate at 37°C, 5% CO_2.

6. On day 7, collect and count CTLs using Trypan blue to determine viability of CTLs.

7. Repeat weekly stimulation, from steps 1 to 6.

3.2.2. Cytokine Production

1. Collect and count CTLs and resuspend them at 10^6/well in complete medium.

2. Add 1 ml of CTL/well in tissue-culture-treated 24-well plate.

3. Add 1 ml of irradiated (40 cGy) autologous LCL resuspend at 10^6/well in complete medium.

4. Incubate at 37°C, 5% CO_2.

5. Collect 0.5 ml of supernatant after 24, 48, and 72 h and store at −80°C (*see* **Note 2**).

6. Thaw supernatant and analyze for appropriate cytokines using the specific ELISA, following the manufacturer's instruction (*see* **Note 3**).

3.2.3. Functionality of the Suicide Gene

1. Collect and count CTLs. Resuspend them at 1×10^6/ml in complete medium and add 1 ml/well.

2. Add 1 ml of complete medium containing CID (final concentration 50 nM).

3. Incubate at 37°C, 5% CO_2.

4. After 24 and 48 h collect cells and wash cells with $1 \times$ Annexin-V Binding Buffer.

5. Aliquot 10^5 cells/tube.

6. Stain with 5 µl of Annexin-V and 5 µl of 7-AAD.

7. Incubate for 15 min in the dark at RT.

8. Add 200 µl of Annexin-V Binding Buffer and proceed with FACS analysis (*see* **Fig. 8.1**).

3.3. Testing Retained Functionality of Gene Modified CTL

3.3.1. Immunophenotype

1. Collect 1×10^6 CTLs and wash with PBS/1% FBS.

2. Aliquot 1×10^5 CTLs/tube.

3. Add 5 µl of appropriate antibody combination to each tube.

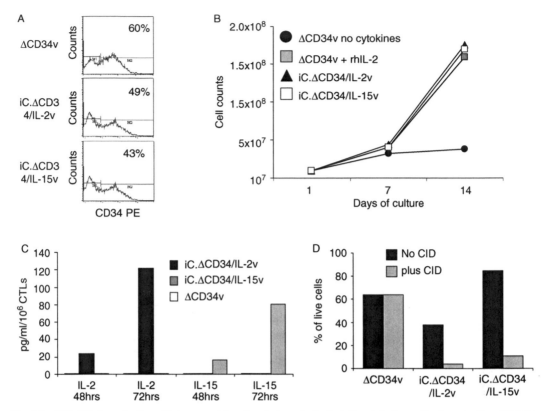

Fig. 8.1. EBV-CTL transduction efficiency and functional characterization. Panel A shows the transduction efficiency of one EBV-specific CTL line. CTLs were transduced with iC.ΔCD34/IL-2v or iC.ΔCD34/IL-15v or ΔCD34v vectors, measured as expression of a truncated form of CD34 (ΔCD34) on the cell surface by FACS analysis. Panel B shows the results of CTLs expanded weekly with autologous LCL in the presence or absence of cytokines. The cell number is illustrated on the x-axes. Both IL-2 and IL-15 transgenic CTLs expanded significantly well as compared to control CTLs (NT or ΔCD34v+ stimulated in the presence of exogenous IL-2) after 35 days of culture. Panel C shows the measurements of cytokines produced by genetically modified CTLs. The specific cytokines were detected after 48 and 72 h post stimulation with autologous LCLs. Panel D shows the evaluation of dead and apoptotic cells after exposure to CID of genetically modified CTL. Significant increase in Annexin-V+ and 7AAD+ cells is observed after addition of increasing concentration of CID for gene-modified CTL but not of control CTLs.

4. Add 5 μl of CD3PerCP, 5 μl of CD8 FITC, 5 μl of CD4APC, and 0.5 μl of the tetramer of interest (**Note 4**).

5. Incubate at 4°C for 20 min.

6. Wash cells.

7. Analyze with FACScan acquiring at least 100,000 events.

3.3.2. Cytotoxic Activity

1. Collect and pellet target cells (at least $2–3 \times 10^6$) (**Note 5**).

2. Resuspend target cells by finger-clicking and perform radio-labeling by adding 100 μCi of ^{51}Chromium in a radioactive safety cabinet. Labeled cells are then incubated for 1 h at 37°C, with a gentle finger flicking every 15 min (*see* **Note 6**).

3. Wash ^{51}Chromium-labeled T lymphocytes by centrifugation at $400 \times g$ for 5 min using 5 ml of complete medium; count cells after the fourth wash, and then resuspend them at the concentration of 5×10^4/ml in complete medium.

4. Collect CTLs, count them, and resuspend at the concentration of 2×10^6/ml in complete medium. Aliquot cells in 96-well plate and perform serial dilutions to obtain triplicate of wells containing cell numbers ranging from 2×10^5/well to 2.5×10^4/well.

5. Add 100 µl of the appropriate target cells to the wells containing 100 µl of the diluted CTLs, 100 µl of medium only (spontaneous release), or 100 µl of Triton-X (maximum release).

6. Incubate the plates for 4–5 h at 37°C, 5% CO_2.

7. Spin plate at $400 \times g$ for 5 min, then collect 100 µl of supernatant, transfer in appropriate tubes, and read using the γ-counter.

8. The percent of killing is calculated as follows: [cpm from experimental wells (target+ CTL) – cpm of target cells in the presence of medium only (spontaneous release)/cpm of target cells in the presence of 1% Triton-X (maximum release) – cpm of target cells in the presence of medium only (spontaneous release)] $\times 100$.

3.3.3. Antigen Specificity

1. Coat plate with 100 µl/well of the filtered primary antibody [Catcher-mAB(1-DIK); working concentration = 10 µg/ml] and incubate overnight at 4°C (**Note 7**).

2. Wash plate with PBS to remove primary antibody and then block plate with medium for 2 h (**Note 8**).

3. Wash plate three times with PBS.

4. Collect CTL, count them, and resuspend them at 1×10^6/ml in Elispot medium.

5. Add 100 µl of CTLs/well.

6. Add appropriate peptides (at concentration of 5 µM in PBS) and incubate for 16–24 h at 37°C, 5% CO_2.

7. Wash plate six times with PBS/0.05% Tween-20.

8. Add 100 µl/well of the secondary antibody [Detector-mAB (7-B6-1-Biotin) working concentration = 1 µg/ml] and incubate for 2 h at 37°C.

9. Wash plate six times with PBS/0.05% Tween-20.

10. Add Avidin-Peroxidase-Complex and incubate for 1 h at room temperature.

11. Wash three times with PBS/0.05% Tween-20 and then three times with PBS.

12. Develop for 4 min using AEC substrate.

13. Stop the reaction by washing with tap water (**Note 9**).

14. Air dry O/N in the dark and then submit for counting.

3.3.4. Polyclonality

1. Collect 1×10^6 CTL and wash with PBS

2. Aliquot 1×10^5 CTLs/tube

3. Add 5 μl of directly conjugated antibody mixes/tube for a total of eight mixes (**Note 10**)

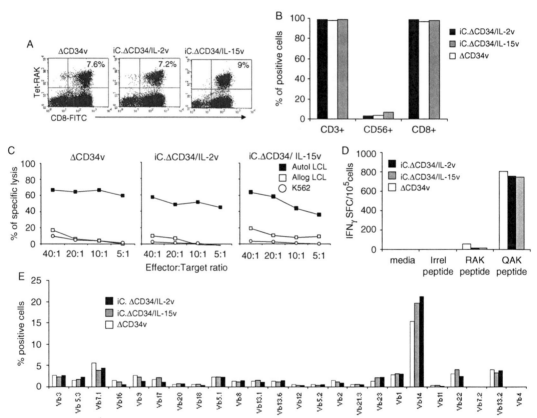

Fig. 8.2. Panel A shows an example of tetramer staining of CTLs: the frequency of EBV-specific tetramer+ CTLs in control and transgenic CTLs was retained and not modified by either IL-2 or IL-15 transgene expression. Panel B shows expression of T-cell markers on EBV-CTLs. The phenotypic profile of CTLs was not altered by cytokine transduction, as most EBV-CTLs remained CD3+/CD8+, while less than 5% were CD3+/CD56+. Panel C shows a typical example of ^{51}Cr cytotoxic assay. The effector: target cell ratio is indicated on the *x*-axis. Figure shows that transgenic and control EBV-CTLs lyse at a significantly higher rate autologous LCLs than allogeneic LCLs, confirming retained MHC restriction. No significant reactivity (< 10%) is observed against the K562 cell lines. Panel D shows an example of IFN-γ Elipost assay. The frequency of EBV-specific T cells in the peripheral blood is measured by the number of IFN-γ secreting PBMCs upon stimulation with EBV peptides. The frequency of EBV-CTLs precursor in control and transgenic CTLs is retained and neither IL-2 nor IL-15 transgenes modified the antigen specificity of the EBV-CTLs. Panel E shows the results of a Vβ repertoire staining in a representative donor. Genetic manipulation of antigen-specific T cells does not generate progressive clonal outgrowth.

4. Incubate at 4°C for 20 min

5. Wash cells

6. Analyze with FACScan

Results of testing the retained functionality of transduced EBV-CTL are shown in **Fig. 8.2**.

4. Notes

1. Keep some Non-Transduced (NT) CTLs as control. These will need to be plated at the same concentration in complete medium containing IL-2 (100 U/ml) in 24-well tissue culture-treated plate.

2. If more cytokines need to be determined, more wells can be prepared to collect more than 0.5 ml at each time point. When collecting supernatant, ensure that cell pellet is not disturbed. It is recommended that supernatants are spin to remove cells before freezing.

3. Avoid multiple thawing and freezing of the supernatants.

4. Tetrameric molecules bind directly to T-cell receptors of a particular specificity, and are generated by combining the Major Histocompatibility Complex (MHC) class I molecules and MHC-class I specific-EBV-peptides. They can be used to detect and separate antigen-specific CD8+ T-cell populations as rare as 0.02% of lymphocytes.

5. To evaluate CTL specificity, autologous LCLs, HLA class I and II mismatched LCLs, and K562 cell lines (that measure natural killer activity) are used as target cells. If CTLs are antigen specific, only autologous LCLs are expected to be significantly lysed.

6. Wear appropriate radio-protection equipments and monitor the work area using a survey meter; label and dispose of radioactive waste according to approved guidelines; personnel monitoring with thermoluminescence dosimeter is recommended.

7. The IFN-γ ELISpot assay exhibits a high level of sensitivity that permits detection of as few as 1 responding cell per 1×10^5 cells. Bound cytokine is visible through color development.

8. Do not touch the bottom of the ELISpot plate to avoid artifacts.

9. Areas of color development form spots that represent single cell that had secreted cytokine in response to the

recognition of the antigen added during the assay. The spot number per well denotes an estimate of the frequency of antigen-specific T cells among the plated cells.

10. Vβ regions can be grouped into 24 mutually exclusive families (covering about 70% of normal human TCR Vβ repertoire). The detection of three Vβ expressions in the same tube is possible by combining three monoclonal antibodies (mAb) with only two fluorophores.

References

1. Waldmann, T. A., Dubois, S., and Tagaya, Y. (2001) Contrasting roles of IL-2 and IL-15 in the life and death of lymphocytes: implications for immunotherapy. *Immunity. 14,* 105–110.

2. Nakamura, Y., Russell, S. M., Mess, S. A., Friedmann, M., Erdos, M., Francois, C., Jacques, Y., Adelstein, S., and Leonard, W. J. (1994) Heterodimerization of the IL-2 receptor beta- and gamma-chain cytoplasmic domains is required for signalling. *Nature 369,* 330–333.

3. Fehniger, T. A., Suzuki, K., VanDeusen, J. B., Cooper, M. A., Freud, A. G., and Caligiuri, M. A. (2001) Fatal leukemia in interleukin-15 transgenic mice. *Blood Cells Mol Dis 27,* 223–230.

4. Lin, J. X., Migone, T. S., Tsang, M., Friedmann, M., Weatherbee, J. A., Zhou, L., Yamauchi, A., Bloom, E. T., Mietz, J., John, S., and Leonard W J. (1995) The role of shared receptor motifs and common Stat proteins in the generation of cytokine pleiotropy and redundancy by IL-2, IL-4, IL-7, IL-13, and IL-15. *Immunity 2,* 331–339.

5. Lotze, M. T., Matory, Y. L., Ettinghausen, S. E., Rayner, A. A., Sharrow, S. O., Seipp, C. A., Custer, M. C., and Rosenberg, S. A. (1985) In vivo administration of purified human interleukin 2. II. Half life, immunologic effects, and expansion of peripheral lymphoid cells in vivo with recombinant IL 2. *J Immunol 135,* 2865–2875.

6. Whitehead, R. P., Friedman, K. D., Clark, D. A., Pagani, K., and Rapp, L. (1995) Phase I trial of simultaneous administration of interleukin 2 and interleukin 4 subcutaneously. *Clin Cancer Res 1,* 1145–1152.

7. Rosenberg, S. A., Lotze, M. T., Yang, J. C., Aebersold, P. M., Linehan, W. M., Seipp, C. A., and White, D. E. (1989) Experience with the use of high-dose interleukin-2 in the treatment of 652 cancer patients. *Ann Surg 210,* 474–484.

8. Finnegan, N. M., Redmond, H. P., and Bouchier-Hayes, D. J. (1998) Taurine attenuates recombinant interleukin-2-activated, lymphocyte-mediated endothelial cell injury. *Cancer 82,* 186–199.

9. Ahmadzadeh, M., and Rosenberg, S. A. (2006) IL-2 administration increases CD4+ CD25(hi) Foxp3+ regulatory T cells in cancer patients. *Blood 107,* 2409–2414.

10. Quintarelli, C., Vera, J. F., Savoldo, B., Giordano Attianese, G. M., Pule, M., Foster, A. E., Heslop, H. E., Rooney, C. M., Brenner, M. K., and Dotti, G. (2007) Co-expression of cytokine and suicide genes to enhance the activity and safety of tumor-specific cytotoxic T lymphocytes. *Blood 110,* 2793–2802.

11. Blau, C. A., Peterson, K. R., Drachman, J. G., and Spencer, D. M. (1997) A proliferation switch for genetically modified cells. *Proc Natl Acad Sci USA 94,* 3076–3081.

Chapter 9

Cytokine-FC Fusion Genes as Molecular Adjuvants for DNA Vaccines

Daniel Hirschhorn-Cymerman and Miguel-Angel Perales

Abstract

The use of gene constructs for DNA immunization offers several potential advantages over other commonly used vaccine approaches: (1) full-length cDNA provides multiple potential class I and class II epitopes, thus bypassing limitations of MHC restriction; (2) bacterial plasmid DNA contains immunogenic unmethylated CpG motifs (immunostimulatory sequences) that may act as a potent immunological adjuvant; and (3) DNA is relatively simple to purify in large quantities. The cDNA encoding the antigen of interest is cloned into a bacterial expression plasmid with a constitutively active promoter and this plasmid is injected into the skin or muscle where it is taken up by professional antigen-presenting cells, particularly dendritic cells, either through direct transfection or cross-priming. One can further enhance or modulate the immune response through co-delivery of DNA encoding cytokines or chemokines, including cytokine-Fc fusion molecules. The latter use molecular techniques to fuse a cytokine to the Fc portion of IgG1, creating a chimeric molecule with functional activity. In the present chapter, we will outline the approach to develop cytokine-Fc fusion genes as molecular adjuvants and will use GM-CSF as an example.

Key words: DNA vaccine, GM-CSF, molecular adjuvant, Fc-fusion.

1. Introduction

The use of gene constructs for DNA immunization offers several potential advantages over other commonly used vaccine approaches: (1) full-length cDNA provides multiple potential class I and class II epitopes, thus bypassing limitations of MHC restriction; (2) bacterial plasmid DNA contains immunogenic unmethylated CpG motifs (immunostimulatory sequences) that may act as a potent immunological adjuvant (1, 2);

P. Yotnda (ed.), *Immunotherapy of Cancer*, Methods in Molecular Biology 651,
DOI 10.1007/978-1-60761-786-0_9, © Springer Science+Business Media, LLC 2010

(3) DNA is relatively simple to purify in large quantities; and (4) one can further enhance or modulate the immune response through co-delivery of DNA encoding cytokines or chemokines (3).

The cDNA encoding the antigen of interest is cloned into a bacterial expression plasmid with a constitutively active promoter and this plasmid is injected into the skin or muscle where it is taken up by professional antigen-presenting cells (APCs), particularly dendritic cells (DCs). One proposed mechanism for the activity of DNA vaccines is direct transfection of DCs by the plasmid DNA (4). An alternative mechanism, termed cross-priming, involves transcription and translation of the antigen by non-APCs, such as keratinocytes or myocytes, and release of mature protein antigen through either secretion or cell death (5, 6). The pre-formed antigen is then captured by APCs and presented to naïve T cells in regional draining lymph nodes. Most likely, both mechanisms (direct transfection of APCs and cross-priming) are operative during successful DNA immunization.

In clinical trials for infectious disease, DNA immunization has been shown to be safe and effective in developing immune responses to malaria and human immunodeficiency virus (7–9). Our group has demonstrated significant activity of DNA vaccines in preclinical mouse models of melanoma (10–16), as well as in clinical trials in dogs with melanoma (17, 18), and patients with melanoma (19, 20).

Furthermore, we have also examined the role of molecular adjuvants, including GM-CSF DNA, and demonstrated their ability to modulate immune responses (3, 11, 21, 22). Administration of the murine GM-CSF gene results in recruitment of epidermal dendritic cells and acts as a potent adjuvant for both peptide and DNA vaccines (11, 21, 22). Based on our pre-clinical work, we conducted a phase I/II trial of human GM-CSF DNA in conjunction with a multipeptide vaccine (gp100 and tyrosinase) in stage III/IV melanoma patients (20). Forty-two percent of the 19 patients treated developed $CD8^+$ T-cell responses to tyrosinase or gp100. Human GM-CSF DNA was found to be a safe and effective adjuvant.

We have studied additional molecular adjuvants and tested a series of molecules that will were used either individually or in combination (3). The cytokines and chemokines were tested as DNA and as Fc fusion molecules. The latter use molecular techniques to fuse a cytokine to the Fc portion of IgG1, creating a chimeric molecule with functional activity (23). They were used as adjuvants for hgp100 DNA, which was shown to induce tumor immunity primarily mediated by $CD8^+$ T cells (12, 13). We observed an increased frequency of $CD8^+$ T cells and increased anti-tumor immunity with the addition of most cytokine and cytokine-Fc constructs. Furthermore, for IL-2, IL-12, and IL-15, administration of the cytokine-Fc fusion gene was more potent than the cytokine gene alone.

In the present chapter, we will outline the approach to develop cytokine-Fc fusion genes as molecular adjuvants and will use GM-CSF as an example (24). Readers are referred to our published work for details and applications regarding additional cytokines (3).

2. Materials

2.1. Cloning of GM-CSF and GM-CSF-Fc

1. Cell strainer 40 μm Nylon.
2. Tissue culture sterile polystyrene 6-well plate.
3. cRPMI medium: RPMI 1640 medium supplemented with 10% fetal bovine serum (FBS), penicillin-streptomycin (100 U of penicillin, 50–100 μg of streptomycin), non-essential amino acids (100 μM), glutamine (2 mM), and β-mercaptoethanol (1×, 55 μM).
4. 15-ml polypropylene sterile centrifuge tubes.
5. Red blood cell (RBC) lysis buffer (ACK Lysing Buffer, Lonza BioWhittaker).
6. Tissue culture sterile polystyrene 96-well plate.
7. Functional grade Armenian hamster anti-mouse CD3ε chain (clone 145-2C11).
8. Functional grade Syrian hamster anti-mouse CD28 (Clone 37.51).
9. Phosphate buffered saline (PBS): 137 mM NaCl, 2.7 mM KCl, 4.3 mM Na_2HPO_4, 1.47 mM KH_2PO_4.
10. Trizol reagent (Invitrogen).
11. Chloroform.
12. Molecular biology grade 99% isopropyl alcohol.
13. Nuclease free-water. It is important to keep water as sterile as possible. It is suggested that small aliquots are kept and be discarded after use. For most applications double distilled autoclaved water can be used. However, it is recommended that, for applications where RNA is being handled, nuclease free or diethyl pyrocarbonate (DEPC)-treated water should be used.
14. 75% Ethanol: 3 part of 100% ethanol is diluted in 1 part of nuclease-free water.
15. Spectrophotometer.

16. 0.2 ml Thin-Walled polymerase chain reaction (PCR) Tubes. Unless the tubes are sterile and nuclease-free, the tubes should be autoclaved prior to use.

17. M-MLV recombinant Reverse Transcriptase (RT) with 5× reaction buffer (Invitrogen).

18. 10 mM deoxynucleotides triphosphate (dNTP) Mix, PCR Grade.

19. Oligo(dT)$_{20}$ Primer.

20. Recombinant RNAse Inhibitor 40 units/μl.

21. Platinum® Pfx DNA polymerase with 10× buffer and 50 mM MgSO$_4$ (Invitrogen) (*see* **Note 1**).

22. Agarose HS molecular biology grade high melt.

23. Ethidium bromide molecular biology grade 10 mg/ml used at final concentration of 0.5 μm/ml.

24. Agarose gel apparatus with power supply.

25. Razor blades.

26. PCR purification kit.

27. Restriction endonuclease: EcoRI, BamHI, KpnI, and XbaI 20,000 U/ml (*see* **Note 2**).

28. DNA loading buffer, 10×.

29. T4 DNA Ligase with 10× reaction buffer (Invitrogen).

30. One Shot® TOP10 chemically competent *Escherichia coli* (Invitrogen).

31. SOC medium: 2% bacto tryptone, 0.5% bacto yeast extract, 10 mM NaCl, 2.5 mM KCl, 10 mM MgCl$_2$, 10 mM MgSO$_4$, and 20 mM glucose in double distilled water. Autoclave all components in 950 ml of water except for glucose. Sterilize a 20× glucose solution by filtration through a 0.2-μm filter and add 50 ml to the final solution. Adjust to pH 7 dropwise with 1 M NaOH.

32. Luria-Bertani (LB) medium: 1% bacto tryptone, 0.5% bacto yeast extract. 1% NaCl. Autoclave components in 1 L of double distilled water and adjust the pH to 7 with 1 M NaOH. For DNA plasmid propagation 50 μg/ml of ampicillin should be added.

33. LB agar plates: Add 15 g/L of agar powder with LB components described in #32 in 1 L of double distilled water to a 2 L Flask. Include an autoclave-resistant magnetic stirrer. Autoclave and let the flask cool down to 40–50°C while stirring. Add 50 μg/ml of ampicillin (prepared as 1000× concentration in water). Aseptically pour LB-agar in 100 × 15 mm polystyrene plates and leave to solidify at room temperature. Store the plates at 4°C until use.

34. Sterilized solid glass beads, 3 mm diameter.

35. QIAprep Spin Miniprep Kit for plasmid purification (Qiagen).

2.2. Testing Constructs In Vitro

2.2.1. Transfection of GM-CSF Constructs to Check Expression of Constructs

1. Human embryonic kidney 293 cells.

2. Tissue culture sterile polystyrene 6-well plate.

3. cDMEM medium. DMEM medium supplemented with 7.5% FBS, penicillin-streptomycin (100 U of penicillin, 50–100 μg of streptomycin), non-essential amino acids (100 μM), glutamine (2 mM).

4. FuGENE 6® Transfection Reagent (Roche Biochemicals).

2.2.2. FACS Staining of Transfected Cells

1. PBS

2. BD Cytofix/Cytoperm™ Plus with Perm/Wash buffer (BD Bioscience)

3. Rat anti-mouse GM-CSF PE (clone MP1-22E9)

4. Flow cytometer

2.2.3. Testing Expression of GM-CSF Constructs by Western Blot

1. NuPAGE® SDS Sample Buffer 4× without reducing agent (Invitrogen).

2. NuPAGE® 4–12% Bis-Tris Gel 1.5 mm × 15 well (Invitrogen).

3. XcCell SureLock™ Mini cell apparatus (Invitrogen).

4. NuPAGE® MOPS [3-(N-morpholino) propanesulfonic acid] SDS (Sodium dodecyl sulfate) running buffer pre-prepared to 1× (Invitrogen).

5. Transfer buffer: a 25× solution is 12 mM of Tris Base [tris(hydroxymethyl)aminomethane] and 96 mM g glycine in deionized water. Dilute the buffer to 1× with 20% methanol.

6. XCell II™ Blot Module CE Mark (Invitrogen).

7. Polyvinylidene fluoride (PDVF) Membrane. The membrane should match the size of the gel.

8. 3 MM Chr filter paper.

9. PBST is PBS with 0.1% Tween-20.

10. Bovine serum albumin (BSA) 99% for electrophoresis.

11. Rocking platform.

12. Goat anti-Mouse IgG (Fc) Horseradish peroxidase (HRP) conjugate.

13. Enhanced luminol-based chemiluminescent (ECL) Western blotting substrate.

14. Plastic Saran™ wrap.

15. Radiography film for detection of chemiluminescence 5 × 7 in (Pierce).

16. Tabletop X-ray film processor.

2.3. Testing Constructs In Vivo

2.3.1. Delivery of GM-CSF-Fc Fusion Constructs via Particle Bombardment

2.3.1.1. Preparation of Gene Gun Bullets

1. 1.8-ml microcentrifuge tubes.

2. Spherical gold powder APS 0.8–1.5 μM, 99.96+% (Alfa Aesar).

3. Spermidine ≥98% for molecular biology.

4. Calcium chloride ≥93.0%, anhydrous, granular.

5. Sonicator.

6. 15-ml polypropylene sterile centrifuge tubes.

7. Ethanol 200 Proof. A fresh unopened bottle of ethanol should be used every time a new set of bullets is made.

8. Tubing prep station (Bio-Rad Laboratories).

9. Vortexer.

10. N_2 tank (grade 4.8) with regulator.

11. DNA bullet tubing: Ethylene tetrafluoroethylene (ETFE) Tube, 0.125″ outer diameter X 0.93″ inner diameter (Saint-Gobain Performance Plastics).

12. Adaptor tubing: Tygon tubing 1/8″ inner diameter × 1/4 outer diameter, Wall 1/16″.

13. 5 ml disposable syringes.

14. 18 G 1 1/2″ hypodermic needle.

15. Tube cutter (Bio-Rad).

16. 50 ml polypropylene sterile centrifuge tube.

17. Desiccator.

2.3.1.2. Delivery of GM-CSF Constructs via Gene Gun

1. Mice (C57B/6).

2. Isoflourane, USP.

3. Gene gun with cartridge.

4. Anesthetizing chamber.

5. Nair® depilatory cream.

6. Surgical Gauze 10 × 10 cm.

7. Helium tank with regulator, high purity.

2.3.2. Preparation of Skin Supernatants for Biochemical Analyses

1. Surgical scissors.

2. 2 ml cryovial.

3. Liquid N_2.

4. 5-ml round-bottom polycarbonate tube 12 × 75 mm.

5. Homogenization buffer: PBS + 0.1% Tween-20 supplemented with dissolved Complete Protease Inhibitor Cocktail Tablets (Roche).

6. Tissue homogenizer.

7. Beaker with ice.

2.3.3. Sandwich Enzyme-Linked Immunoabsorbent Assay (ELISA) for Quantification of In Vivo Expression of Cytokines

1. High protein-binding capacity ELISA plates, flat-bottom 96-well plate.

2. 0.1 M Bicarbonate buffer, pH 9.2: Na_2CO_3 4.5 g, sodium bicarbonate $NaHCO_3$ 0.630 g dissolved in 1 L of deionized water. Adjust the pH to 9.2.

3. Parafilm®.

4. Anti-mouse GM-CSF ELISA antibody pair: Purified capture antibody clone MP1-22E9 and biotin detection antibody Clone MP1-31G6.

5. Blocking buffer: 100 mM phosphate buffer, pH 7.2, 1% BSA, 0.5% Tween-20, and 1 mM ethylenediaminetetraacetic acid (EDTA).

6. Wash buffer: 100 mM phosphate buffer, 150 mM NaCl, 0.2% BSA, and 0.05% Tween-20.

7. HRP-Streptavidin: Vectastain® Elite® ABC Kit diluted in wash buffer according to the manufacturer's instructions (Vector Laboratories).

8. 2,2'-azino-bis(3-ethylbenzthiazoline-6-sulphonic   acid (ABTS) Substrate.

9. Microplate ELISA Reader.

2.3.4. Measuring the Levels of DC Recruitment

1. Cell strainer 40 μm Nylon.

2. Tissue culture sterile polystyrene 6-well plate.

3. Dissociation buffer: PBS supplemented with 1 mg/ml collagenase D, and 50 μg/ml DNAase I, grade II.

4. 500 mM EDTA, pH 8.0.

5. 1 ml disposable syringe tuberculin slip tip.

6. 50-ml polypropylene disposable centrifuge tube.

7. FACS buffer: PBS, 0.5% BSA, 1 mM EDTA.

8. Tissue culture sterile polystyrene U-bottom 96-well plate.

9. Purified anti-mouse CD16/32, Clone 2.4 G2.

10. 4′,6-diamidino-2-phenylindole, dihydrochloride (DAPI). A 1000× stock solution is 0.2 mg/ml in PBS and kept frozen at –20°C.

11. Cocktail of diluted fluorescently labeled antibodies: CD11c Fluorescein isothiocyanate FITC (clone HLA3), I-A^b (MHC Class II of C57BL/6) phycoerythrin PE (Clone AF6-120.1), and CD86 Allophycocyanin APC (Clone GL1).

12. Flow cytometer.

3. Methods

In this section we will describe the following steps: (1) cloning of murine GM-CSF-Fc; (2) testing the constructs in vitro by performing FACS analysis of transfected cells or western blot analysis of the supernatants; and (3) testing the constructs in vivo, by measuring protein levels of GM-CSF and secondary cytokines or chemokines after administration of GM-CSF-Fc DNA (22), and by measuring the recruitment of dendritic cells (21, 22). The final in vivo test of potency, which is not described in this chapter, is the demonstration of GM-CSF-Fc DNA's efficacy as a vaccine adjuvant. For these efficacy studies, the reader is referred to our published work of GM-CSF DNA in mouse models (11, 21), and canine (18) and human clinical trials (20).

3.1. Cloning of Murine GM-CSF and GM-CSF-Fc

In vitro activation of naïve splenocytes can be used to clone the cDNA of numerous cytokines and chemokines. Alternative activation of splenocytes can be achieved with LPS (lipopolysaccharide) PMA (phorbol myristate acetate)/Ionomycin (25 ng/ml and 1 μg/ml) stimulation. Under steady-state, there are sufficient B cells in the spleen expressing IgG to enable cloning of the Fc. In addition, splenocytes can be treated with LPS (10 ng/ml) to stimulate B cells and increase the IgG expression. Alternatively, the Fc gene can be cloned from an IgG-secreting hybridoma.

1. Prepare a single-cell suspension of spleens from a naïve mouse by mechanical disruption with the plunge of a

syringe into a cell strainer placed in a 6-well plate containing 5 ml of cRPMI medium.

2. Transfer the cell suspension to a 15 ml tube and centrifuge at 1500 rpm (500 × g) for 5 min at 4°C.

3. Discard the supernatant and resuspend the pellet in 1 ml of RBC lysis buffer. After 5 min incubation at room temperature, add ice-cold cRPMI medium to fill the tube.

4. Centrifuge the sample as described above.

5. Resuspend the pellet in cRPMI medium such that the final cell concentration is 1×10^7 cells/ml. A spleen from a naïve female mouse typically contains 1×10^8 cells. Therefore, adding 10 ml of cRPMI medium will be sufficient to obtain the desired cell concentration.

6. Plate 100 μl of cells into a 96-well U-shaped plate pre-coated with 2 μg/ml anti-mouse CD3 and 2 μg/ml of soluble anti-mouse CD28 (see **Note 3**). Incubate for 24–48 h in a 37°C incubator with 5% CO_2.

7. Centrifuge the plate at 800 × g in a tabletop centrifuge for 1 min at 4°C and remove the supernatant by decantation. Wash with 200 ml ice-cold PBS and transfer the cells to a 1.5-ml tube. Centrifuge at 2000 rpm 800 × g and completely remove the supernatant by aspiration.

8. Resuspend the pellet in 1 ml of Trizol reagent and pipette up and down several times until all the cells are lysed. After a 5-min incubation, add 200 μl chloroform. Shake the suspension vigorously and incubate the sample for 3 min at room temperature. Centrifuge the sample for 15 min at 12,000 × g at 4°C.

9. Transfer the upper clear phase containing the RNA to a fresh tube without disturbing the interface. Add 0.5 ml of isopropyl alcohol and incubate for 30 min at room temperature.

10. Centrifuge the sample for 15 min at 12,000 × g at 4°C. Decant the supernatant and wash with 1 ml of 75% ethanol. Centrifuge at no more than 7500 × g for 5 min at 4°C. Decant the supernatant and dry the RNA pellet for 10–30 min. Resuspend the pellet in 100 μl of nuclease-free water. Measure the concentration and determine the purity using a spectrophotometer. At this point, the RNA solution can be stored at −80°C or one can proceed to the preparation of complementary DNA (cDNA).

11. To prepare a cDNA, set up the following reaction in a nucleotide-free PCR tube on ice:

5× RT buffer	10 μl
10 mM dNTP mix	5 μl
Oligo(dT)	5 μl
RNAse Inhibitor	1 μl
RNA	5 μg or less
RNAase free water	up to 49 μl

Place the tube in a thermocycler and incubate at 65°C for 5 min to denature RNA. Remove the tubes from the thermocycler and allow the tubes to cool down to room temperature for 10 min. Add 1 μl of reverse transcriptase to each tube and incubate in the thermocycler at 37°C for 1 h. Deactivate the reverse transcriptase by heating the reaction to 70°C for 15 min.

12. Obtain cDNA of the cytokines by PCR. Set up the following PCR reaction in a nucleotide-free PCR tube on ice adding the components in the following order:

Autoclaved distilled water	38 μl
10× Pfx amplification buffer	5 μl
10 mM dNTP mix	1.5 μl
50 mM MgSO$_4$	1 μl
cDNA	2 μl of the reaction
10 μM of primer mix	1.5 μl
Platinum Pfx DNA polymerase	1 μl

Place the tube in a thermocycler and set up the following program:

94°C for 30 s

55°C for 30 s

68°C for 90 s

68°C for 10 min

The first three steps should be repeated 35 times.

Keep the tubes at 4°C after the PCR cycles are completed (*see* **Note 4**).

13. Confirm that the cDNA sequence of the GM-CSF or Fc is present by agarose gel electrophoresis.

14. Purify the PCR product using a PCR purification kit according to the manufacturer's instructions and elute the DNA from the column with 50 μl deionized water. Determine the DNA concentration using a spectrophotometer.

Note: if the concentration of the PCR product is high, this step can be avoided; simply add 1–3 µl of the PCR reaction to the digestion reaction.

15. Place in separate tubes up to 1 µg of the PCR product or plasmid and set up the following digestion reaction:

Restriction enzyme 1	1 µl
Restriction enzyme 2	1 µl
10× Digestion buffer	5 µl
Digested DNA	43 µl

Incubate in a 37°C water bath for 2–4 h.
Note: to prevent self-ligation of plasmid DNA in subsequent steps and increase cloning efficiency, 1 µl of shrimp alkaline phosphatase can be added to the digestion reaction 20 min prior to gel purification.

16. Add 5.5 µl of 10× agarose loading gel and load the entire reaction into a 1% agarose gel with 0.5 µg/ml ethidium bromide. Once separation is completed (marker dye is at the bottom of the gel), expose the gel to a UV translumi-nator and cut the band corresponding to either the plasmid or the cDNA with a razor blade. Cut the gel in small pieces and transfer to a 1.8-ml tube.

17. Extract DNA using a Gel Purification Kit. Elute DNA from the column with 50 µl nuclease-free water and quantify the amount of DNA recovered using a spectrophotometer (*see* **Note 5**).

18. Set up the ligation reaction in an PCR tube as follows:

Plasmid DNA	50 ng
PCR product	15–20 ng[a]
10× T4 ligation reaction	2 µl
T4 ligase	1 µl
Water	up to 20 µl

[a]The molar ratio of PCR product to plasmid is typically 3:1.

Incubate overnight in a 17°C water bath or 2 h at room temperature.

19. In a fresh tube, mix 2, 4, and 10 µl of the ligation reaction with 50 µl chemically-competent DH5α *E. coli* cells on ice and incubate for 30 min.

20. "Heat shock" the cells by submerging the tubes for 45 s in a 42°C water bath. Rapidly transfer the tubes to ice and incubate for 2 min.

21. Recover the cells by adding 450 μl SOC medium prewarmed to 37°C. Place the tubes in a 37°C incubator rotating at 250 rpm/min for 1 h.

22. Aseptically transfer 20 and 200 μl of cells to LB agar plates and 50 μg/ml of ampicillin. Distribute the cells throughout the length of the plate using the tip of a sterile glass pipette or sterile glass beads with a "back and forth" motion until the plate is uniformly covered with the cell solution.

23. Incubate the plates in a 37°C incubator for 18–24 h.

24. Pick isolated colonies with a sterile pipette from the plates and transfer to tubes containing 2 ml of LB medium with 50 μg/ml ampicillin. Incubate overnight in a 37°C incubator rotating at 250 rpm/min. We recommend picking at least ten colonies.

25. Extract plasmid DNA using a mini prep kit. Perform digestion described in step 16 but use only 5 μl plasmid and bring the rest of the volume up to 50 μl with water.

26. Verify that the plasmid contains the cDNA of the cloned gene by agarose gel electrophoresis.

27. It is also important to verify the integrity of the sequence cloned by DNA sequencing.

3.1.1. Discussion of Primers and Cloning Strategy

The complete cDNA of GM-CSF is cloned first into pcDNA3.1 using the primers depicted in **Table 9.1**. The upstream 5′ primer contains the Kozak sequence, which ensures adequate ribosome binding to the translation start site and consequently high levels of protein expression. A typical Kozak sequence consists of the following sequence **GCC(G/A)CC**ATG**G**(25). We have successfully engineered several genes with the consensus sequence GCCACCATGG. If the sequence of the coding gene is not a G after start codon ATG, we do not recommend changing this sequence. The primer also contains an EcoRI restriction site used for cloning into pcDNA3.1⁺. Adjacent to the EcoRI site we include a series of up to six random nucleotides that ensures that the restriction enzyme will adequately cleave the PCR product. All the primers where the PCR product will be digested and subsequently cloned will include at least six random nucleotides (or more depending on the enzyme used). The downstream 3′ end primer contains two consecutive stop codon sequences TGATGG and BamHI for cloning into the pcDNA3.1⁺ vector. This construct will express the coding sequence of GM-CSF.

Table 9.1 Primer for cloning GM-CSF and GM-CSF-Fc constructs

GM-CSF pcDNA3.1	
Upstream	5′ NNNNNN<u>GAATTC</u>**GCCACC**ATGGCCCACGAGAGAAAGGC *Restriction site – Kozak sequence*
Downstream	5′ NNNNNN<u>GGATCC</u>**CCATCA**TTTTTGGACTGGTTTTTTGC *BamHI restriction site – 2 consecutive stop codons*
Fc pcDNA3.1	
Upstream	5′ NNNNNN<u>GGTACC</u>CGAGCCCAGAGGGCCCACATTC *KpnI restriction site*
Downstream	5′ NNNNNN<u>TCTAGA</u>**TTATCA**TTTACCAGGAGTCCGGGAGAAG *KpnI restriction site – 2 consecutive stop codons*
GM-CSF-Fc pcDNA3.1	
Downstream	5′ NNNNNN<u>GGTACC</u>**CC**TTTTTGGACTGGTTTTTTGC *KpnI restriction site – 2 additional nucleotides to ensure that GM-CSF will be in frame with the Fc sequence*

The Fc is cloned from mouse IgG1. We cloned the sequence of CH3 and CH2 including the hinge region, which provides flexibility to cytokine-Fc fusion protein. The 5′ upstream primer contains a KpnI restriction site adjacent to the hinge region. Since the Fc plasmid gene is not designed to be expressed, we included no additional sequences.

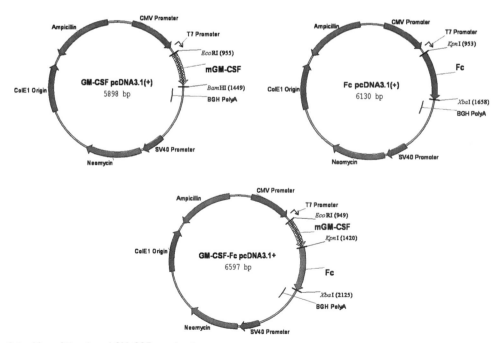

Fig. 9.1. Map of the cloned GM-CSF constructs.

Both genes are cloned into pcDNA3.1$^+$ first as shown in **Fig. 9.1**. To construct GM-CSF-Fc pcDNA3.1$^+$, a PCR is performed on the GM-CSF pcDNA3.1 to amplify the GM-CSF sequence where the stop codons at the 3′ end are substituted with a KpnI restriction site, such that the GM-CSF sequence is in frame with Fc sequence as shown in **Fig. 9.1**.

3.2. Testing Constructs In Vitro

3.2.1. Transfection of Constructs to Test Expression of GM-CSF Constructs

1. The day before transfection, plate 1 X 10^5 and 2 X 10^5 HEK 293 cells per well in a 6-well plate in 2 ml cDMEM. Incubate at 37°C and 5% CO_2 overnight.

2. Remove reagents and allow them to warm to room temperature.

3. Pick a cell dilution where cells are 50–80% confluent.

4. Aliquot DMEM medium (without serum) into sterile 1.8-ml tube.

   Tube 1 = 100 μl (medium only)

   Tube 2 = 97 μl (FuGENE, no DNA)

   Sample 1 = 97 μl

   Sample 2 = 97 μl

5. Mix FuGENE 6 reagent by briefly vortexing (1–2 s).

6. Add to each tube the corresponding volume of FuGENE 6 reagent. It is crucial to add the Fugene 6 reagent directly into the medium being careful not to touch the side of the tube with the tip.

   C1 = 0

   C2 = 3 μl

   Sample 1 = 3 μl

   Sample 2 = 3 μl

7. Incubate at room temperature for 5 min.

8. Add 2 μg of plasmid DNA to each tube. Plasmid concentration should be 0.5–2 μg/μl. If the plasmid concentration is less diluted, the final volume of the DNA/Fugene 6 mix should be adjusted to 100 μl.

9. Mix by vortexing 1 s.

10. Incubate at room temperature for 45 min.

11. Add 100 μl of complex to each corresponding well. Gently tap the plate so the DNA/Fugene 6 mix is distributed throughout the plate.

12. Incubate at 37°C with 5% CO_2 for 48 h.

3.2.2. FACS Staining
of Transfected Cells

1. Harvest cells 48 h (2 days) after transfection. HEK 293 cells are loosely adherent and can be dissociated from the plate by lightly tapping the plate (*see* **Note 6**).

2. Transfer the cells to a 15-ml falcon tube and place it on ice. Count cells and adjust the concentration at 10^6 cells/ml with ice-cold medium.

3. Plate 1×10^5 cells (100 µl) in 96-well plate.

4. Quick-spin the plate down (800 × g for few seconds).

5. Wash cells with 200 µl of PBS and repeat quick spin.

6. Resuspend cells in 100 µl BD Cytofix/Cytoperm™ solution and incubate for 20 min on ice.

7. Wash cells twice with 1× Perm/Wash buffer. Resuspend cells in 50 µl Perm/Wash add 0.5 µl of anti-GM-CSF PE antibody and incubate on ice for 45 min. Keep the plate in the dark by covering with aluminum foil.

8. Wash twice with 1× Perm/Wash solution and resuspend in 120 µl of PBS.

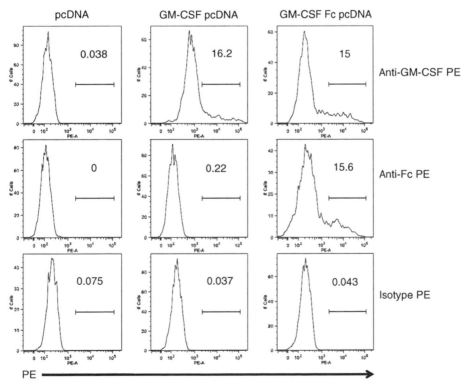

Fig. 9.2. Flow cytometry analysis of HEK 293 cells transfected with GM-CSF constructs. The cells were transfected with the GM-CSF constructs described for 48 h, fixed, permeabilized, and stained with either anti-Fc-PE, anti-GM-CSF-PE or isotype control.

9. Analyze samples by flow cytometry (**Fig. 9.2**). The samples can be analyzed up to 5 days after staining.

3.2.3. Testing Expression of GM-CSF-Fc Constructs by Western Blot

1. Harvest supernatants (about 1 ml) and store at −80°C until ready to use.

2. Thaw samples on ice, transfer to a 1.8-ml tube. Clear supernatants by spinning at 20,800 × *g* for 10 min at 4°C.

3. Transfer 15 μl of supernatants to a fresh tube, add 5 μl of 4× loading buffer without a reducing agent. Boil tubes for 5 min (*see* **Note 7**).

4. While samples are boiling, wash the SDS-polyacrylamide gel electrophoresis (PAGE) gel with deionized water, and place the gel in the running apparatus, fill the apparatus with running buffer without reducing agent and remove the comb from the plate. Wash each well by forcibly pipetting several times with running buffer.

5. Spin quickly and carefully load 20 μl on a SDS-PAGE gel.

6. Close the apparatus, plug into a power supply and run at 200 volts for 60 min or until the tracker dye is at the bottom of the gel.

7. Remove the gel from the container and soak it in transfer buffer.

8. Immerse a PDVF membrane (the membrane must be the exactly the same size as the gel) in 100% methanol for a few seconds. Transfer the membrane to a container with transfer buffer. In the same container, soak six pieces of filter paper the size of the gel.

9. Set up the transfer apparatus by placing 3 filter papers, the gel, the membrane, and an additional three filter papers from bottom to top. Remove any foaming by pressing and rolling the "sandwich" with a Pasteur pipette.

10. Transfer to a blotting apparatus, fill with transfer buffer, and apply 10 volts (100 m Amps) for 1 h.

11. Discard the gel and filter papers and briefly wash the membrane with 5–10 ml of PBST.

12. Place the membrane in a container with 2–3 ml of PBST + 1% BSA over a rocking platform (volume will depend on the size of the container) incubate overnight at 4°C or 1 h at room temperature.

13. Wash the membrane with 5–10 ml of PBST once and add 2–3 ml of anti-mouse Fc-HRP at 1:10,000 dilution in PBST + 1% BSA. Incubate for 1 h at room temperature or 4 h at 4°C on a rocking platform. The antibody dilution

should be carefully titrated if high background or no signal is evident after development.

14. Wash 4× with PBST for 5 min each wash.

15. Develop membrane by incubating with a small amount (enough to completely cover the membrane) of ECL reagent for 5–10 min. Place the membrane in plastic wrap removing extra liquid. Do not let the membrane dry at any time.

16. Expose the membrane to film for 1–2 min. Exposure time will vary depending on the strength of the signal. It is recommended that the membrane is exposed several times varying the exposure time to optimize signal and minimize background.

17. Develop film (**Fig. 9.3**).

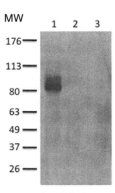

Fig. 9.3. Supernatants of transfected HEK 293 cells analyzed by unreduced 7% polyacrylamide gel electrophoresis. The membrane was probed with an anti-mouse Fc-HRP antibody. Lanes are from cells transfected with: (1) GM-CSF-Fc pcDNA3.1; (2) GM-CSF pcDNA3.1; (3) pcDNA3.1

3.3. Testing Constructs In Vivo

3.3.1. Delivery of GM-CSF-Fc Fusion Constructs via Particle Bombardment

3.3.1.1. Preparation of Gene Gun Bullets

1. Place 75 mg of gold into 1.8-ml tubes.

2. Make a fresh 50 mM spermidine solution (8 µl of pure frozen stock in 1 ml of nuclease free water).

3. Add 200 µl of freshly diluted 50 mM spermidine. Vortex vigorously to resususpend gold particles. Sonicate gold for 30 s to disrupt clumps.

4. Add 100 μg (100 μl) of plasmid DNA. The plasmid DNA solution should be at 1 mg/ml in nuclease-free water. Tap the tube several times to dissolve the plasmid DNA.

5. While slowly vortexing, add 200 μl of 1 M calcium chloride solution dropwise. It is important to deliver the calcium chloride solution very slowly in order to maximize DNA precipitation directly into the gold particles. Close tube and vortex a few seconds.

6. Allow gold to settle for 10 min.

7. While gold settles, label one 15-ml tube for each sample using ethanol resistant pen and add to each 12 ml of ethanol (*see* **Note 8**).

8. Centrifuge 2 min at 2000 × g in a bench top centrifuge. Aspirate off supernatant. Add 1 ml of ethanol and resuspend the gold pellet by vigorously vortexing the tube. Transfer the suspension to corresponding labeled 15-ml tube.

9. Centrifuge for 1 min at 2000 × g. Completely aspirate off the supernatant. Do not decant the supernatant as the pellet might easily detach itself from the tube.

10. Add 10 ml of ethanol and thoroughly resuspend the gold pellet by vortexing. Repeat ethanol wash three more times.

11. After last wash, resuspend the gold pellet in 7 ml of ethanol.

12. Set up the tubing prep station:
    (a) Insert the bullet tubing into the apparatus, cut to 3 inches extra length. Attach short rubber tubing adapter to tube.

    (b) Open the nitrogen tank valves such that a continuous stream of N_2 is flowing. Care should be exercised not to allow the N_2 stream to remove the gold from the tubing.

    (c) Detach the tubing from the N_2 stream. Load ethanol inside the tube and aspirate the ethanol. Dry the tube for at least 2 min before the next step. Pre-washing the tubing with ethanol before introducing the gold removes impurities and improves the quality of bullets.

13. Vortex the 15-ml tube containing the gold/DNA mix and briefly sonicate for 10 s to dissociate clumps of gold. Sonication should be brief as it can fragment plasmid DNA. With a 5-ml syringe and 18″ gauge needle aspirate 3.5 ml of sample. Discard the needle and place the syringe at the end of the adapter tube, slowly push the solution inside

the tube ensuring that the gold is distributed uniformly throughout the tube.

14. Leaving the syringe attached to the tube; allow the gold to settle for 2.5 min.

15. Slowly aspirate the ethanol and remove the syringe.

16. Connect the tube to the N_2 stream and allow the gold to dry.

17. Remove the tube from the apparatus and cut bullets into a 50-ml Falcon tube with a bullet cutter. Store the DNA bullets under vacuum with a desiccant. Atmospheric humidity deteriorates the quality of the bullets.

3.3.1.2. Delivery of GM-CSF Constructs via Gene Gun

1. Anesthetize the mice in a chamber containing isoflourane vaporized at 4% under a biohazard hood. Once the mice are anesthetized the isoflourane level should be reduced to 1–2%.

2. Rub a small amount of nair depilatory cream on the abdomen of the mouse for about 10 s. Place the mouse back in the chamber for 30 s.

3. Remove the abdominal hair with a gauze and clean the area with a second gauze.

4. Load a cartridge with bullets. Plug the gene gun to a high-grade helium gas tank and set up the pressure to 400 psi.

5. Hold the mouse tightly and aim the gun to one corner of depilated abdomen. Trigger the gun discharging the contents of the bullets.

6. Move the cartridge to a new position and aim the gun to the opposite corner. Trigger the gun discharging the contents of the second bullet.

7. Shoot a total of four bullets (1 μg of plasmid/bullet) into each corner of the abdomen.

8. Place the mice back in the cage.

3.3.2. Preparation of Skin Supernatants for Biochemical Analyses

1. Euthanize the mice at different time-points after biobalistic delivery.

2. Carefully remove the skin of the abdomen previously exposed to gold particles with surgical scissors. Certain gene guns or gold particles will leave a mark or "tattoo" at the delivery site.

3. Transfer the skin samples to a 2-ml cryovial and flash-freeze by dropping the vial into liquid N_2. The samples should be stored at −80°C until further use.

4. Weigh the frozen tissue and rapidly transfer to a 5 ml round bottom polycarbonate tube on ice.

5. Add X μl of homogenization buffer (where X= mg of tissue × 8 μl/mg).

6. Mince the tissue with surgical scissors and move the tube into a tissue homogenizer in a beaker containing ice. Homogenize the tissue on an ice bath for short periods (10–15 s) at time. Longer homogenizing periods will increase the sample temperature which can damage the sample. Avoid foaming.

7. Once the sample is completely homogenized, centrifuge the sample in a table top centrifuge at $20{,}800 \times g$ at 4°C for 15 min.

8. Carefully remove the supernatant with a pipette and transfer to a fresh 1.8-ml tube. At this point, the supernatants can be flash-frozen and stored at –80°C or liquid N_2 until further use.

3.3.3. Sandwich ELISA for Quantification of In Vivo expression of cytokines

This approach can be used for the quantification of both primary (cytokine DNA injected) and secondary cytokine or chemokines (proteins produced as a result of cytokine DNA injection) (22) (*see* **Note 9**).

1. Dilute the capture antibody at 10 μg/ml in 0.1 M Bicarbonate buffer, pH 9.2, and add 50 μl to each well of a 96-well microtiter plate.

2. Cover with Parafilm® and incubate at 4°C overnight in a moist box containing a wet paper towel or at room temperature and humidity for 2 h.

3. Aspirate the antibody solution and wash the plate twice with 200 μl of PBS.

4. Block the plate with 100 μl of blocking buffer for 30 min at room temperature.

5. Empty the plate and wash three times with 200 μl of wash buffer.

6. Prepare a standard that consists of recombinant GM-CSF at a range of 10 pg/ml to 5000 ng/ml in serial dilutions. Add the standards and supernatants either undiluted or serially diluted in wash buffer to a total volume of 50 μl per well. Incubate the plate at room temperature for 2 h.

7. Empty the plate and wash with 200 μl of wash buffer at least three times.

8. Add 50 μl of the biotin detection antibody diluted in wash buffer. The appropriate dilution of the detection

antibody should be empirically determined for each antibody in order to maximize detection sensitivity and minimize background. We recommend a starting dilution of 1:1000 or 1:10,000. Incubate at room temperature for 1 h.

9. Empty the plate and wash three times with 200 μl of wash buffer.

10. Add 50 μl of streptavidin-HRP solution. Incubate at room temperature for 20 min.

11. Empty the plate and wash with 200 μl of wash buffer three times.

12. Add 100 μl of ABTS Substrate Incubate at room temperature for color development. Monitor color development with an ELISA plate reader at 405 nm.

3.3.4. Measuring DC Recruitment in Draining Lymph Nodes

1. Deliver GM-CSF constructs via gene gun as described previously (**Section 3.3.1**).

2. Euthanize mice and remove the draining inguinal lymph nodes with surgical scissors and tweezers.

3. Place the lymph node in a 6-well plate with 5 ml of dissociation buffer and incubate for 30 min at 37°C. Gently mix the plate every 5–10 min.

4. Add 100 μl of 500 mM EDTA to deactivate the enzymes.

5. Gently dissociate the lymph node using the plunger of a 1-ml syringe. Transfer the cell suspension to a 50-ml tube containing a cell strainer. Wash plate with 5 ml of iced-cold PBS and transfer to the same tube.

6. Centrifuge tube at $500 \times g$ for 5 min at 4°C.

7. Wash cells twice with 5 ml of FACS buffer centrifuging at $500 \times g$ for 5 min at 4°C between washes.

8. Resuspend cells in 250 μl of FACS buffer and transfer to a U-bottom 96-well plate. Keep plate on ice.

9. Centrifuge at $400 \times g$ for 2 min at 4°C and carefully decant supernatant.

10. Resuspend cell in 50 μl FACS buffer and add 1 μl of anti-mouse CD16/32 to each well and incubate on ice for 15 min.

11. Without washing the plate add 50 μl cocktail of diluted fluorescently labeled antibodies to each well and incubate 40 min. Typically, the markers used for distinguishing DCs are CD11c, MHC class II, and CD86 (*see* **Note 10**).

12. Wash 2× with FACS buffer as described in step 9.

13. Resuspend cells in 100 μl of FACS buffer containing 1× DAPI in order to electronically exclude that dead cells

from subsequent analysis. Other cell-death markers such as 7-ADD or propidium iodide can be used as long as the emission spectrum does not interfere with the spectrum of the markers analyzed.

14. Analyze the samples by flow cytometry (**Fig. 9.4**).

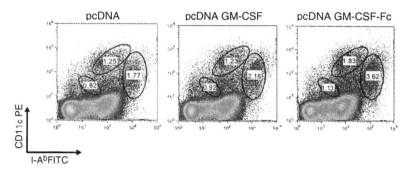

Fig. 9.4. Flow cytometry analysis of dendritic cells' infiltration into draining inguinal lymph node 5 days after gene gunning of GM-CSF constructs.

4. Notes

1. We selected Pfx DNA polymerase over other polymerase because it provides high fidelity and high processivity. Other polymerases provide higher fidelity but lower processivity or alternatively higher processivity but lower fidelity.

2. Enzymes may require different digestion buffers for optimal activity. When double digestions are necessary, it is important to check the compatibility of each enzyme in a specific buffer such that the activity of both enzymes is optimal.

3. To coat a plate with anti-mouse CD3, the antibody is diluted (2 μg/ml) in PBS and 100 μl is added to each well. The plates are incubated at 4°C overnight and washed twice with cRPMI medium before use.

4. It is possible to couple the RT and PCR reactions in one step. For this, set up a PCR reaction as shown in step 12 omitting the cDNA and adding 5 μg of RNA. Incubate the reaction at 65°C for 15 min in the thermocyler. Remove the tubes and add 1 μl of reverse transcriptase to each tube. Place the tubes back in the thermocycler and incubate for 45 min at 42°C, then continue the PCR program. Note that a RT-PCR kit is available to perform this type of one-step reaction (SuperScript® III One-Step RT-PCR System with Platinum® Taq High Fidelity, Invitrogen).

5. Since the DNA concentration may be lower than the detection limits of the spectrophotometer, DNA can also be quantified by agarose gel electrophoresis using a mass ladder to estimate DNA concentration.

6. If adherent cell lines other than HEK 293 are used, the cells can be dissociated with a variety of cell dissociated solutions. We do not recommend the use of a trypsin solution as it can damage the integrity of the recombinant protein.

7. When cytokines-Fc are to be analyzed, we recommend avoiding reducing agents such as β-Mercaptoethanol in order to preserve the integrity of disulfide bonds.

8. Use a new bottle of ethanol for every set of bullets as ethanol needs to be 100% pure. Opened bottles of ethanol absorb moisture from the environment, which compromises the quality of the DNA bullets.

9. Commercial ELISA kits are available for a number of murine cytokines and chemokines including GM-CSF. In addition, this approach can also be used to test the potency of human cytokine DNA constructs. For example, we demonstrated that the human GM-CSF DNA used in our clinical trial lead to detectable human GM-CSF protein levels in the skin of mice injected with the construct (20).

10. The concentration of each antibody needs to be titrated prior to the experiment to obtain optimal results. We recommend a starting titration of 1:50 and serial dilution should be made.

References

1. Klinman, D. M., Yi, A. K., Beaucage, S. L., Conover, J., and Krieg, A. M. (1996) CpG motifs present in bacteria DNA rapidly induce lymphocytes to secrete interleukin 6, interleukin 12, and interferon gamma. *Proc Natl Acad Sci USA* 93, 2879–2883.

2. Sato, Y., Roman, M., Tighe, H., Lee, D., Corr, M., Nguyen, M. D., Silverman, G. J., Lotz, M., Carson, D. A., and Raz, E. (1996) Immunostimulatory DNA sequences necessary for effective intradermal gene immunization. *Science* 273, 352–354.

3. Ferrone, C. R., Perales, M. A., Goldberg, S. M., Somberg, C. J., Hirschhorn-Cymerman, D., Gregor, P. D., Turk, M. J., Ramirez-Montagut, T., Gold, J. S., Houghton, A. N., and Wolchok, J. D. (2006) Adjuvanticity of plasmid DNA encoding cytokines fused to immunoglobulin Fc domains. *Clin Cancer Res* 12, 5511–5519.

4. Porgador, A., Irvine, K. R., Iwasaki, A., Barber, B. H., Restifo, N. P., and Germain, R. N. (1998) Predominant role for directly transfected dendritic cells in antigen presentation to CD8+ T cells after gene gun immunization. *J Exp Med* 188, 1075–1082.

5. Casares, S., Inaba, K., Brumeanu, T. D., Steinman, R. M., and Bona, C. A. (1997) Antigen presentation by dendritic cells after immunization with DNA encoding a major histocompatibility complex class II-restricted viral epitope. *J Exp Med* 186, 1481–1486.

6. Akbari, O., Panjwani, N., Garcia, S., Tascon, R., Lowrie, D., and Stockinger, B. (1999) DNA vaccination: transfection and activation of dendritic cells as key events for immunity. *J Exp Med* 189, 169–178.

7. Wang, R., Doolan, D. L., Le, T. P., Hedstrom, R. C., Coonan, K. M., Charoenvit, Y., Jones, T. R., Hobart, P., Margalith, M., Ng, J., Weiss, W. R., Sedegah, M., de

Taisne, C., Norman, J. A., and Hoffman, S. L. (1998) Induction of antigen-specific cytotoxic T lymphocytes in humans by a malaria DNA vaccine. *Science 282*, 476–480.

8. Boyer, J. D., Cohen, A. D., Vogt, S., Schumann, K., Nath, B., Ahn, L., Lacy, K., Bagarazzi, M. L., Higgins, T. J., Baine, Y., Ciccarelli, R. B., Ginsberg, R. S., MacGregor, R. R., and Weiner, D. B. (2000) Vaccination of seronegative volunteers with a human immunodeficiency virus type 1 env/rev DNA vaccine induces antigen-specific proliferation and lymphocyte production of beta-chemokines. *J Infect Dis 181*, 476–483.

9. Ugen, K. E., Nyland, S. B., Boyer, J. D., Vidal, C., Lera, L., Rasheid, S., Chattergoon, M., Bagarazzi, M. L., Ciccarelli, R., Higgins, T., Baine, Y., Ginsberg, R., Macgregor, R. R., and Weiner, D. B. (1998) DNA vaccination with HIV-1 expressing constructs elicits immune responses in humans. *Vaccine 16*, 1818–1821.

10. Weber, L. W., Bowne, W. B., Wolchok, J. D., Srinivasan, R., Qin, J., Moroi, Y., Clynes, R., Song, P., Lewis, J. J., and Houghton, A. N. (1998) Tumor immunity and autoimmunity induced by immunization with homologous DNA. *J Clin Invest 102*, 1258–1264.

11. Bowne, W. B., Srinivasan, R., Wolchok, J. D., Hawkins, W. G., Blachere, N. E., Dyall, R., Lewis, J. J., and Houghton, A. N. (1999) Coupling and uncoupling of tumor immunity and autoimmunity. *J Exp Med 190*, 1717–1722.

12. Hawkins, W. G., Gold, J. S., Dyall, R., Wolchok, J. D., Hoos, A., Bowne, W. B., Srinivasan, R., Houghton, A. N., and Lewis, J. J. (2000) Immunization with DNA coding for gp100 results in CD4 T-cell independent antitumor immunity. *Surgery 128*, 273–280.

13. Gold, J. S., Ferrone, C. R., Guevara-Patino, J. A., Hawkins, W. G., Dyall, R., Engelhorn, M. E., Wolchok, J. D., Lewis, J. J., and Houghton, A. N. (2003) A single heteroclitic epitope determines cancer immunity after xenogeneic DNA immunization against a tumor differentiation antigen. *J Immunol 170*, 5188–5194.

14. Goldberg, S. M., Bartido, S. M., Gardner, J. P., Guevara-Patino, J. A., Montgomery, S. C., Perales, M. A., Maughan, M. F., Dempsey, J., Donovan, G. P., Olson, W. C., Houghton, A. N., and Wolchok, J. D. (2005) Comparison of two cancer vaccines targeting tyrosinase: plasmid DNA and recombinant alphavirus replicon particles. *Clin Cancer Res 11*, 8114–8121.

15. Engelhorn, M. E., Guevara-Patino, J. A., Merghoub, T., Liu, C., Ferrone, C. R., Rizzuto, G. A., Cymerman, D. H., Posnett, D. N., Houghton, A. N., and Wolchok, J. D. (2008) Mechanisms of immunization against cancer using chimeric antigens. *Mol Ther 16*, 773–781.

16. Engelhorn, M. E., Guevara-Patino, J. A., Noffz, G., Hooper, A. T., Lou, O., Gold, J. S., Kappel, B. J., and Houghton, A. N. (2006) Autoimmunity and tumor immunity induced by immune responses to mutations in self. *Nat Med 12*, 198–206.

17. Bergman, P. J., McKnight, J., Novosad, A., Charney, S., Farrelly, J., Craft, D., Wulderk, M., Jeffers, Y., Sadelain, M., Hohenhaus, A. E., Segal, N., Gregor, P., Engelhorn, M., Riviere, I., Houghton, A. N., and Wolchok, J. D. (2003) Long-term survival of dogs with advanced malignant melanoma after DNA vaccination with xenogeneic human tyrosinase: a phase I trial. *Clin Cancer Res 9*, 1284–1290.

18. Bergman, P. J., Camps-Palau, M. A., McKnight, J. A., Leibman, N. F., Craft, D. M., Leung, C., Liao, J., Riviere, I., Sadelain, M., Hohenhaus, A. E., Gregor, P., Houghton, A. N., Perales, M. A., and Wolchok, J. D. (2006) Development of a xenogeneic DNA vaccine program for canine malignant melanoma at the animal medical center. *Vaccine 24*, 4582–4585.

19. Wolchok, J. D., Yuan, J., Houghton, A. N., Gallardo, H. F., Rasalan, T. S., Wang, J., Zhang, Y., Ranganathan, R., Chapman, P. B., Krown, S. E., Livingston, P. O., Heywood, M., Riviere, I., Panageas, K. S., Terzulli, S. L., and Perales, M. A. (2007) Safety and immunogenicity of tyrosinase DNA vaccines in patients with melanoma. *Mol Ther 15*, 2044–2050.

20. Perales, M. A., Yuan, J., Powel, S., Gallardo, H. F., Rasalan, T. S., Gonzalez, C., Manukian, G., Wang, J., Zhang, Y., Chapman, P. B., Krown, S. E., Livingston, P. O., Ejadi, S., Panageas, K. S., Engelhorn, M. E., Terzulli, S. L., Houghton, A. N., and Wolchok, J. D. (2008) Phase I/II study of GM-CSF DNA as an adjuvant for a multipeptide cancer vaccine in patients with advanced melanoma. *Mol Ther 16*, 2022–2029.

21. Bowne, W. B., Wolchok, J. D., Hawkins, W. G., Srinivasan, R., Gregor, P., Blachere, N. E., Moroi, Y., Engelhorn, M. E., Houghton, A. N., and Lewis, J. J. (1999) Injection of DNA encoding granulocyte-macrophage colony-stimulating factor recruits dendritic cells for immune adjuvant effects. *Cytokines Cell Mol Ther 5*, 217–225.

22. Perales, M. A., Fantuzzi, G., Goldberg, S. M., Turk, M. J., Mortazavi, F., Busam, K., Houghton, A. N., Dinarello, C. A., and Wolchok, J. D. (2002) GM-CSF DNA induces specific patterns of cytokines and chemokines in the skin: implications for DNA vaccines. *Cytokines Cell Mol Ther 7*, 125–133.

23. Barouch, D. H., Santra, S., Schmitz, J. E., Kuroda, M. J., Fu, T. M., Wagner, W., Bilska, M., Craiu, A., Zheng, X. X., Krivulka, G. R., Beaudry, K., Lifton, M. A., Nickerson, C. E., Trigona, W. L., Punt, K., Freed, D. C., Guan, L., Dubey, S., Casimiro, D., Simon, A., Davies, M. E., Chastain, M., Strom, T. B., Gelman, R. S., Montefiori, D. C., Lewis, M. G., Emini, E. A., Shiver, J. W., and Letvin, N. L. (2000) Control of viremia and prevention of clinical AIDS in rhesus monkeys by cytokine-augmented DNA vaccination. *Science 290*, 486–492.

24. Chang, D. Z., Lomazow, W., Joy Somberg, C., Stan, R., and Perales, M. A. (2004) Granulocyte-macrophage colony stimulating factor: an adjuvant for cancer vaccines. *Hematology 9*, 207–215.

25. Kozak, M. (1997) Recognition of AUG and alternative initiator codons is augmented by G in position +4 but is not generally affected by the nucleotides in positions +5 and +6. *EMBO J 16*, 2482–2492.

Chapter 10

Pharmacology of Anti-CD3 Diphtheria Immunotoxin in CD3 Positive T-Cell Lymphoma Trials

Jung Hee Woo, Yu-Jen Lee, David M. Neville, and Arthur E. Frankel

Abstract

Anti-CD3 recombinant diphtheria immunotoxin, A-dmDT$_{390}$-bisFv(UCHT1), consists of the catalytic and translocation domains of diphtheria toxin fused to two single chain Fv fragments of an anti-CD3ε monoclonal antibody (UCHT1). A-dmDT$_{390}$-bisFv(UCHT1) is capable of killing CD3$^+$ T-lymphoma cells and normal T cells specifically in the femtomolar concentration range. To study pharmacology of A-dmDT$_{390}$-bisFv(UCHT1) in patients with CD3$^+$ T-cell lymphoma in a phase I clinical trial, (1) highly sensitive bioassay using Jurkat cells for measuring drug levels, (2) ELISA for measuring anti-DT antibody titer, and (3) 5-color FACS analysis method for measuring changes of subtype T-cell population were developed. In addition to evaluating drug efficacy and pharmacokinetics in patients, it is important to correlate pre-existing anti-DT antibody levels with maximum drug concentration in serum and extent of T-cell depletion because pre-existing anti-DT antibodies due to DPT (Diphtheria, Pertussis, and Tetanus) immunization can neutralize diphtheria immunotoxin. We observed that at the lowest treatment dose (2.5 μg/kg: twice daily for 4 days) A-dmDT$_{390}$-bisFv(UCHT1) depletes greater than 99.0% of normal T cells in all six patients for a short period of time (2–3 days) and that there is no association of C_{max} and extent of T-cell depletion with the pre-existing anti-DT antibody titer.

Key word: UCHT1, immunotoxin, CD3, diphtheria toxin, T-cell depletion, pre-existing anti-DT antibodies.

1. Introduction

T-cell lymphomas are heterogenous and represent 12% of lymphoma cases in the US – a total of 6000 cases/year (1). Conventional therapies (chemotherapies, radiations, monoclonal antibodies, etc.) yield remissions in this diverse set of malignancies,

P. Yotnda (ed.), *Immunotherapy of Cancer*, Methods in Molecular Biology 651,
DOI 10.1007/978-1-60761-786-0_10, © Springer Science+Business Media, LLC 2010

but over half of patients relapse and die with progressive disease (2, 3). Once patients display chemoresistance or relapse, survival is short and treatment options are limited. However, chemoresistant refractory T-lymphoma cells remain sensitive to novel mechanisma of apoptosis including protein synthesis inhibition. Therefore our laboratory has focused on the treatment of such patients with immunotoxins composed of tumor cell-directed ligands covalently linked to protein synthesis inactivating peptide toxin such as diphtheria toxin (DT) and ricin toxin (RT).

Recently we had synthesized clinical grade anti-CD3 recombinant diphtheria immunotoxin, A-dmDT$_{390}$-bisFv(UCHT1) (4), and achieved FDA approval for testing in patients (IND # 100712). A-dmDT$_{390}$-bisFv(UCHT1) consisting of the catalytic and translocation domains of diphtheria toxin fused to two single chain Fv fragments of an anti-CD3ε monoclonal antibody (UCHT1) is capable of killing CD3$^+$ T-lymphoma cells and normal T cells specifically in the femtomolar concentration range.

To study pharmacology of A-dmDT$_{390}$-bisFv(UCHT1) in patients with CD3$^+$ T-cell lymphoma in a phase I clinical trial, (1) highly sensitive bioassay using Jurkat cells for measuring drug levels in patient sera, (2) ELISA for measuring anti-DT antibody titer, and (3) 5-color FACS analysis method for measuring changes of subtype T-cell population were developed. In addition to evaluating drug efficacy and pharmacokinetics in patients, it is important to correlate pre-existing anti-DT antibody levels with maximum drug concentration in serum and extent of T-cell depletion because pre-existing anti-DT antibodies due to DPT (Diphtheria, Pertussis, and Tetanus) immunization can neutralize diphtheria immunotoxins. We observed that at the lowest treatment dose (2.5 μg/kg: twice daily for 4 days) A-dmDT$_{390}$-bisFv(UCHT1) depletes greater than 99.0% of normal T cells in all six patients for a short period of time (2–3 days) and that there is no association of the peak immunotoxin serum level (C_{max}) and extent of T-cell depletion with the pre-existing anti-DT antibody titer (5).

2. Materials

2.1. Cytotoxicity Assay Measuring Drug Levels in Patient Sera

1. Leucine-free RPMI 1640 (LF-RPMI 1640): Dissolve 5.0 g of leucine-free RPMI 1640 (US Biological), 0.5 g of BSA, 150 mg of L-glutamine, 100 mg of sodium bicarbonate (NaHCO$_3$), and 5 ml of 1 M HEPES in 500 ml of water (*see* **Note 1**). Sterile-filter and aliquot 45 ml each into 50-ml centrifuge tubes. Store at –80°C.

2. RPMI 1640/10% FBS/1% PSN: Mix 450 ml RPMI 1640 (ATCC), 50 ml of fetal bovine serum, and 5 ml of penicillin–streptomycin–neomycin antibiotic mixture (GIBCO). Sterile-filter and store it at 4°C.

3. DMSO (dimethylsulfoxide, Hybri-Max, Sigma).

4. Freezing medium: 10% DMSO and 90% of RPMI 1640/10% FBS/1% PSN medium.

5. Jurkat cells (ATCC #TIB-152).

6. A-dmDT$_{390}$-bisFv(UCHT1) (0.8 mg/ml): This recombinant protein was extracellularly expressed in diphtheria toxin-resistant *Pichia patoris* (6–8) and purified by three-step purification procedure (4, 9).

7. Cycloheximide.

8. 96-well cell culture-treated round-bottom plate for drug dilution.

9. 96-well tissue culture-treated flat bottom plate for assay.

10. ^{3}H-leucine (PerkinElmer).

11. Filter mat (Wallac).

12. Sample plastic bag (Wallac).

13. Betaplate Scint (PerkinElmer).

14. Micro96 Harvestor (Molecular Device #0200-3923).

15. Bag heat sealer (PerkinElmer).

16. MicroBeta Trilux detector (PerkinElmer #1450).

2.2. Anti-DT Antibody Titer Assay

2.2.1. Purification of Human Anti-Diphtheria Toxin (DT) Antibodies

1. Coupling buffer: Dissolve 8.6 g sodium bicarbonate (NaHCO$_3$), 20 ml 5 M NaCl into 950 ml of water in a 1.0-L beaker. Adjust the pH with 1 M NaOH to 8.3 and a final volume to 1 L with water. Sterile filter through 0.2-μm filter and store at 4°C.

2. 100 mM Glycine buffer (pH 2.7): Dissolve 1.5 g of glycine into 150 ml of water in a beaker. Adjust the pH with to 2.7 using 1 M HCl and final volume to 200 ml with water. Sterile filter through 0.2 μm filter and store at 4°C.

3. 1× phosphate buffered saline (PBS).

4. 400 mM Tris–HCl, pH 8.0: Mix 20 ml of 1 M Tris–HCl, pH 8.0, and 30 ml water.

5. CNBr-activated Sepharose beads (GE Healthcare).

6. Human normal serum (Valley Biomedical)

7. 30 mg of A-dmDT$_{390}$-bisFv(UCHT1) (0.8 mg/ml).

8. Slide-A-Lyzer dialysis cassette (Pierce).

9. HiTrap Protein G HP 1 ml (GE Healthcare); protein G column.

10. Syringe and needle.

2.2.2.
SDS-Polyacryamide Gel
Electropheresis
(SDS-PAGE)

1. 1× Tris/glycine/SDS running buffer: Dilute 100 ml of 10× Tris/glycine/SDS buffer into 900 ml of water.

2. 6× sample buffer: 35% (v/v) glycerol, 10% (w/v) SDS, 0.012% bromophenol blue, and 350 mM Tris, pH 6.8. Aliquot 0.5 ml each into 1.5 ml microcentrifuge tubes and store them at −80°C.

3. 4–20% Tris–glycine gel, 1.0 mm × 15 well (Invitrogen).

4. Unstained standard Mark12 (Invitrogen).

5. GelCode Blue Stain Reagent (Thermo).

6. XCell SureLock Mini Cell module (Invitrogen).

7. Power supply.

2.2.3. Enzyme-Linked
ImmunoSorbent Assay
(ELISA) for Quantitative
Determination of IgG in
Purified Anti-DT
Antibody

1. ELISA kit (Alpha Diagnostic).

2. Nunc-Immuno wash 8 (Nunc).

3. Microplate reader (Molecular Device, VERSAMAX).

2.2.4. Enzyme-Linked
ImmunoSorbent Assay
(ELISA) for Measuring
Anti-DT Antibody

1. 1× phosphate buffered saline (PBS): Mix 100 ml 10× PBS with 900 ml water. Adjust pH to 7.4 using 1 M HCl. Store at room temperature.

2. PBST washing buffer: Mix 10 ml of 10% Tween-20 and 100 ml of 10× PBS with 850 ml of water. Adjust pH to 7.4 with 1 M NaOH. Store at room temperature.

3. Blocking solution: Dissolve 9.0 g of gelatin in 300 ml of 1× PBS (pH 7.4) while heating at 50°C. Aliquot 25 ml each into twelve 50-ml centrifuge tubes. Store at −80°C.

4. Sample dilution buffer: Mix 5 ml of blocking buffer, 1 ml of fetal bovine serum, 0.5 ml of 10% Tween-20, and 43.5 ml of 1× PBS (pH 7.4). This buffer should be prepared immediately prior to use.

5. Stop solution (1 M HCl): Mix 50 ml of HCl and 550 ml of water. Store at room temperature.

6. Human normal serum (Valley Biomedical): Aliquot 1 ml into 1.5 ml screw cap tubes to use as master aliquots of control serum. Thaw one vial of master stock aliquots of control serum in order to prepare working aliquots. Aliquot 20 μL into 0.2-ml PCR tubes and store at −80°C to use as

working aliquots. Use working aliquots of control serum within 48 h after thawing. Anti-DT antibody concentration of control serum should be determined from at least four independent assay results.

7. 500 μl of A-dmDT$_{390}$-bisFv(UCHT1) (0.8 mg/ml).

8. 96-well EIA/RIA, flat-bottom, high binding plate (Costar).

9. Anti-human IgG-HRP (BD).

10. ABTS peroxidase substrate (KPL, Inc.).

11. Plate washer (ELX50, BioTek).

12. Microplate reader (Molecular Device, VERSAMAX).

2.3. Flow Cytometry for T-Cell Subtyping

1. Sample buffer: Dissolve 0.5 g of BSA in 500 ml of Hanks' balanced salt solution (HBSS). Sterile filter and store at 4°C.

2. Lysing buffer: Mix 2 ml of 10× Lysing reagent (BD) and 18 ml of water. Store in room temperature. This buffer should be prepared immediately prior to use.

3. 1.5-ml microcentrifuge tubes.

4. 12 × 75 polystyrene tubes.

5. Sheath Fluid (Beckman Coulter [BC]) and Cleaning Reagent (BC) are instrument support reagents.

6. Cyto-Trol (BC) and QuickCOMP 4 Kit (BC) for adjusting fluorescence compensation.

7. Flow Check 488 (BC), Flow Set 488 (BC), APC 675 Setup Kit (BC), and PC7 770 Setup Kit (BC) for verifying instrument optical alignment and fluidics.

8. Isotype controls: IOtest IgG1-PC7 (BC), IgG1-APC (BC), Mouse IgG1-PC5 (BC), Mouse IgG2a-FITC (BC), Mouse IgG2a-RD1 (BC), Mouse IgG2a-ECD (BC), Rat IgG2a-PE (BC), Mouse IgG2a-APC (BC), Mouse IgG2b-PE (BC), IOtest Neg control-FITC/PE/ECD (BC).

9. CD marker stain: CD3-FITC (BD), CD26-PE (BD), CD56 N-Cam-PE (BD), CD4-PC7 (BD), CD8-PC7 (BD), CD26-FITC (BD), CD69-APC (BD), CD195-APC (BD), CD19-Alexa488 (BD), CD8-APC (BD), CD27-APC (eBioscience), CD294 (CRTH2)-PE (Miltenyi Biotec), CD3-ECD (BC), CD25-ECD (BC), CD45RA-ECD (BC), CD3-PC5 (BC), CD45-PC7 (BC), CD45-APC (BC).

10. IOTest Beta Mark TCR (BC) for T-cell subtype.

11. Dual laser Flow Cytometry (BC Model #175487).

3. Methods

To determine circulating concentrations of biologically active A-dmDT$_{390}$-bisFv(UCHT1) in the blood, bioassay using Jurkat cells with surface CD3 antigen was developed (10, 11). Bioassays using cell lines have inherent assay variability. The main cause of the assay variability is the variation of cell conditions such as CD3 expression levels. This cell variation was minimized by establishment of master cell bank and a working cell bank of Jurkat cells. After thawing the working cell bank, Jurkat cells, subcultured for less than three passages, were used for the drug level assay. Since diphtheria immunotoxins have a relatively short half life (30–60 min) in the blood, patient serum samples were taken at pre, 5, 15, 30, 60, 90, 120, and 240 min post the first infusion.

For the anti-DT antibody titer assay, human anti-DT antibody standards need to be prepared because they are not commercially available. Therefore, we described how to purify human anti-DT antibodies and how to measure their concentration in the anti-DT antibody titer assay section. The purification procedure of human anti-DT antibodies and anti-DT antibody titer assay procedure were modified from the methods previously described (11, 12). Patient serum samples were obtained at pre, days 1, 2, 3, 4, 5, 8, 10, 12, 14, 21, 30, and at each 30-day follow-up after the first drug infusion.

Five-color flow cytometry was developed to monitor T-cell subset and other lymphocytes (B cells and NK cells) before and after immunotoxin therapy in the clinical trial. T-cell subsets includes CD4$^+$ naïve T cells (CD3$^+$/CD4$^+$/CD26$^+$/CD27$^+$/CD45RA$^+$), CD4$^+$ effector memory T cells (CD3$^+$/CD4$^+$/CD26$^+$/CD27$^-$/CD45RA$^-$), CD4$^+$ central memory T cells (CD3$^+$/CD4$^+$/ CD26$^+$/CD27$^+$/CD45RA$^-$), CD8$^+$ naïve T cells (CD3$^+$/CD8$^+$/CD27$^+$/CD45RA$^+$), CD8$^+$ effector memory T cells (CD3$^+$/CD8$^+$/CD27$^-$/CD45RA$^-$), CD8$^+$ central memory T cells (CD3$^+$/CD8$^+$/CD27$^+$/CD45RA$^-$), and NK T cells (CD3$^+$/CD56$^+$) (13–15). Other lymphocytes include B cells (CD3$^-$/CD19$^+$), CD8$^+$ NK cells (CD3$^-$/CD8$^+$/D56$^+$), and CD8$^-$ NK cells (CD3$^-$/CD8$^-$/CD56$^+$). TCR Vβ repertoire of T lymphocytes was also measured using IOTest Beta Mark TCR Vβ repertoire kit from Beckman Coulter. Data acquisition was done using a Cytomics FC500 flow cytometer and Cellquest software (BD Biosciences). Representative flow data using a healthy volunteer's blood were shown in **Fig. 10.1**.

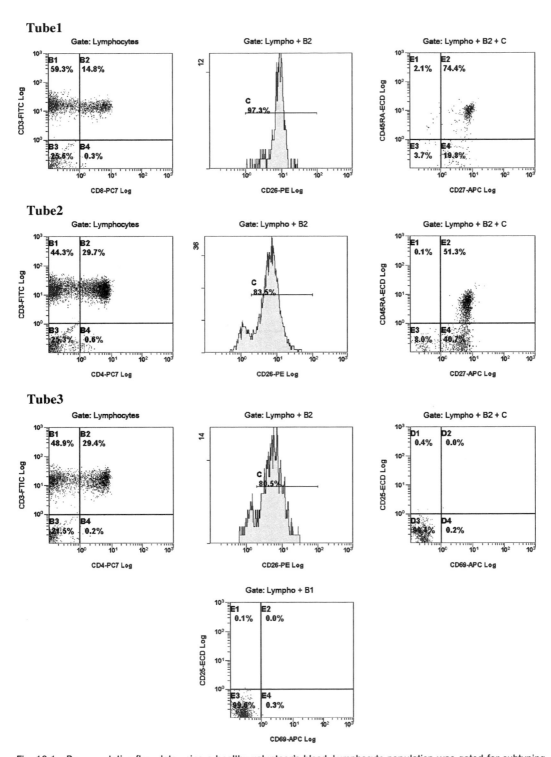

Fig. 10.1. Representative flow data using a healthy volunteer's blood. Lymphocyte population was gated for subtyping analysis. Tube 1: stained lymphocytes with anti-CD3-FITC, anti-CD26-PE, anti-CD45RA-ECD, anti-CD27-APC, and anti-CD8-PC7. Tube 2: stained lymphocytes with anti-CD3-FITC, anti-CD26-PE, anti-CD45RA-ECD, anti-CD27-APC, and anti-CD4-PC7. Tube 3: stained lymphocytes with anti-CD3-FITC, anti-CD26-PE, anti-CD25-ECD, anti-CD69-APC, and anti-CD4-PC7. Tube 4: stained lymphocytes with anti-CD26-FITC, anti-CD2946-PE, anti-CD3-ECD, anti-CD195-APC, and anti-CD4-PC7. Tube 5: stained lymphocytes with anti-CD19-FITC, anti-CD56-PE, anti-CD3-ECD, and anti-CD8-APC.

Tube4

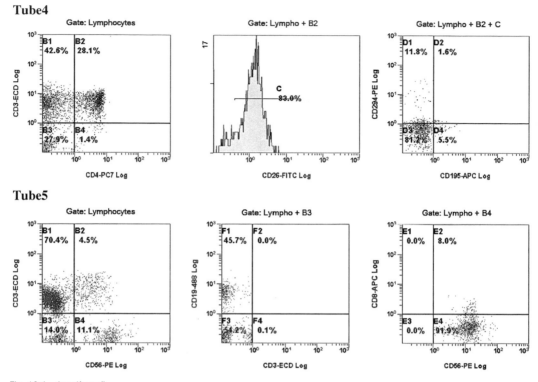

Fig. 10.1. (continued)

3.1. Quantification of A-dmDT₃₉₀-bisFv(UCHT1) Concentration in Patient Serum Post Infusion

3.1.1. Preparation of the Master Cell Bank and the Working Cell Bank

1. Thaw one cryovial of Jurkat cells in order to prepare the master cell bank.

2. Cultivate and expand Jurkat cells using RPMI culture medium at 37°C at 5% CO_2 while maintaining cell density less than 1.5×10^6 cells/ml.

3. Measure cell counts and harvest the expanded cells by centrifuging at $400 \times g$ for 5 min at room temperature.

4. Suspend cells in appropriate volume of freezing medium to make cell density to 2×10^6/ml.

5. Aliquot 1 ml into 81 cryovials and freeze them in Frosty freezing containers at –80°C overnight. The next morning, transfer cryovials to a liquid nitrogen container.

6. Thaw one cryovial of the master cell bank in order to prepare the working cell bank.

7. Cultivate and expand Jurkat cells using RPMI culture medium at 37°C at 5% CO_2 while maintaining cell density less than 1.5×10^6 cells/ml.

8. Measure cell counts and harvest the expanded cells by centrifuging at $400 \times g$ for 5 min at room temperature.

9. Suspend cells in appropriate volume of freezing medium to make the cell density 2×10^6/ml.

10. Aliquot 1 ml into 81 cryovials and freeze them in Frosty freezing containers at −80°C overnight. On next morning transfer cryovials to a liquid nitrogen container.

3.1.2. Quantification of A-dmDT$_{390}$-bisFv(UCHT1) Concentration in Patient Sera

1. Thaw one vial of the working cell bank and cultivate the cells in RPMI culture medium at 37°C at 5% CO_2 for two passages.

2. Harvest cells by spinning down at $400 \times g$ for 5 min at room temperature. Discard supernatant and suspend cells with LF-RPMI 1640. Centrifuge cells at $400 \times g$ for 5 min at room temperature. Discard supernatant and suspend cells in 5 ml of LF-RPMI 1640. Count cell number and then dilute cells with appropriate volume of LF-RPMI 1640 to make cell density to 110,000 cells/ml. Transfer 90 μL of cell suspension to each well of a 96-well flat-bottom plate.

3. Prepare tenfold serial dilutions of A-dmDT$_{390}$-bisFv (UCHT1) drug standard starting from 1.0×10^{-10} M (9610 pg/ml) to 1.0×10^{-16} M (0.0961 pg/ml) using LF-RPMI 1640.

4. Prepare tenfold serial dilutions of serum samples in a 96-well round-bottom plate using LF-RPMI 1640. For 5-, 15-, 30-, and 60-min serum samples; prepare tenfold serial dilutions starting from 1:5 to 1:5000. For 90-, 120-, and 240-min serum samples, start dilution from 1:5 to 1:500 by tenfold serial dilution. Prepare cycloheximide solution (3 mg/ml) by mixing 3 μL of cycloheximide (100 mg/ml) with 97 μL of LF- RPMI 1640.

5. Add 10 μL of the diluted drug standards, serum samples, cycloheximide to designated 90 μl well in the assay plate and incubate for 18 h at 37°C and 5% CO_2. Perform the assay in quadruplicate.

6. Prepare ^{3}H-leucine solution (20 μCi/ml) using LF-RPMI 1640 and dispense 50 μL of ^{3}H-leucine solution into each well. Incubate 2 h at 37°C and 5% CO_2.

7. Harvest cells onto filter mat using a cell harvestor. Allow mat to dry inside the oven. Transfer dry mat into a sample plastic bag and add 6 ml of Betaplate Scint. Remove excess scint solution with a roller and seal the sample plastic bag.

Place bagged filter mat into Betaplate counter cassette and measure leucine incorporation (CPM).

8. Plot the ^{3}H-leucine incorporation vs. the log of the A-dmDT$_{390}$-bisFv(UCHT1) standard concentrations with Sigmoidal dose response nonlinear regression equation of GraphPad Prism V5. Use the CPM readings of patient serum sample dilutions within the standard curve to calculate the A-dmDT$_{390}$-bisFv(UCHT1) levels in sera.

3.2. Measurement of the Anti-DT Antibody Level in Patient Sera

3.2.1. Purification of Human Anti-DT Antibodies by DT-Affinity and Protein G Columns

1. For preparation of DT-affinity resin, immerse two dialysis cassettes (MWCO 10 kDa) into prepared coupling buffer for 30 s.

2. Inject 30 mg of A-dmDT$_{390}$-bisFv(UCHT1) into the cassettes using a syringe attached with an 18-G needle.

3. Dialyze cassettes against coupling buffer pH 8.3 in 4°C for overnight.

4. The next morning, measure 1.0 gram of CNBr-activated Sepharose Beads (swollen volume: 4 ml) and swell the beads in 30 ml of cold water for 2 h at 4°C.

5. Transfer swollen beads into a column or a Buchner funnel to remove water. Suspend beads in 30 ml of 1 mM cold HCl and transfer bead suspension into a conical tube. Rotate the conical tube at 5–10 rpm for 5–10 min at 4°C.

6. Centrifuge the tube at 300× g for 10× min at room temperature. Carefully pour off supernatant without pouring off the beads. Wash the beads with coupling buffer.

7. Add dialyzate to activated beads and allow the conical tube to rotate at 5–10 rpm and 4°C overnight for coupling.

8. Fill the tube with 400 mM Tris–HCl, pH 8.0, and rotate tube at 5–10 rpm and 4°C for 2 h.

9. Pack 4 ml of DT-affinity resin in an Econo-column (1.5 cm × 10 cm).

10. Equilibrate the DT-affinity column with 1× PBS (pH 7.4). Thaw 50 ml of human normal serum and dilute it with four sample volume (200 ml) of 1× PBS (pH 7.4).

11. Load the diluted serum into the DT-affinity column at 3 ml/min and collect sample-flowthrough as 50-ml fractions.

12. Wash the column with 6 column volume of 1× PBS and collect wash-flowthrough.

13. Elute bound anti-DT antibodies with 100 mM glycine buffer (pH 2.7) while collecting 4-ml fractions. Each fraction tube should contain 0.5 ml of 1 M Tris–HCl, pH 9.0, to neutralize pH for prevention from low pH protein degradation/denaturation. Wash column using 50 ml 1× PBS with 0.02% sodium azide for storage. Store column at 4°C.

14. Analyze fractions in the previous step by SDS-polyacrylamide gel electrophoresis (*see* **Section 3.2.2**). Select and pool fractions containing anti-DT antibodies for next Protein G affinity chromatography.

15. For Protein G affinity chromatography, obtain a prepacked HiTrap Protein G HP column (1 ml).

16. Equilibrate the Protein G column with 10 column volume of 1× PBS buffer (pH 7.4) at 1 ml/min.

17. Load the pooled sample in step 14 into the Protein G column at 1 ml/min.

18. Elute bound anti-DT antibodies with 100 mM glycine buffer (pH 2.7) while collecting 1-ml fractions. Each fraction tube should contain 0.1 ml of 1 M Tris–HCl, pH 9.0, to neutralize pH for prevention from low pH protein degradation/denaturation. Wash column using 10 ml 1× PBS with 0.02% sodium azide for storage. Store column at 4°C.

19. Analyze fractions by SDS-polyacrylamide gel electrophoresis (*see* **Section 3.2.2**). Select and pool fractions containing anti-DT antibodies.

20. Quantify antibody concentration of the pooled human anti-DT antibody preparation using human IgG ELISA quantitative kit according to the manufacturer's protocol.

21. Aliquot 0.5 ml of the quantified human anti-DT antibody preparation into 1.5-ml screw cap tubes to use as master aliquots of human anti-DT antibody standard. Store them at –80°C.

22. Thaw one vial of master aliquots in order to prepare working aliquots. Aliquot 50 μL into 0.2-ml PCR tubes and store at –80°C. Use working aliquots of human anti-DT antibodies within 48 h after thawing.

3.2.2. SDS-PAGE Analysis of Purified Human Anti-DT Antibodies

1. Mix 20 μl of each sample with 4 μl of 6× SDS sample buffer. Cook samples at 90°C for 5 min.

2. Load 4–20% Tris–glycine gel into chamber and fill chambers with prepared 1× Tris/Glycine/SDS running buffer.

3. Remove gel teeth carefully and load 12 μl each of the prepared samples.

4. Run gel at 145 V for 100 min.

5. Use a spatula to crack open the cast and cut off the excess of the gel.

6. Wash gel with water for 15 min three times on an orbital shaker at 160 rpm.

7. Stain gel using GelCode Blue Stain Reagent for 1 h in room temperature at 160 rpm.

8. Pour off staining reagent and destain gel with water for 30 min three times.

9. Identify fractions containing human anti-DT immunoglobuins on the Coomassie-stained SDS-polyacrylamide gel.

3.2.3. ELISA for Measuring Anti-DT Antibody Level in Patient Sera

1. Obtain and thaw each working aliquot of A-dmDT$_{390}$-bisFv(UCHT1), anti-DT antibody standard, human control serum, and patient serum samples.

2. Prepare coating protein solution (23 µg/ml) by mixing 431 µL of A-dmDT$_{390}$-bisFv(UCHT1) and 14.569 ml of 1× PBS (pH 7.4).

3. Add 150 µL of coating protein solution to each well of a 96-well microplate and incubate for 2 h at room temperature.

4. While coating the plate, prepare twofold serial dilutions of anti-DT antibody standard starting from 30 ng/ml to 0.94 ng/ml using sample dilution buffer. Prepare twofold serial dilutions (1:50 to 1:400) of patient sera and twofold serial dilutions (1:400–1:1600) of control serum (*see* **Note 3**).

5. Remove liquid by aspiration and wash the plate with 200 µL/well of PBST washing buffer by shaking it for 5 min at 120 rpm at room temperature. Repeat this step two times more.

6. Incubate the plate with 150 µL/well of blocking solution for 1 h at room temperature.

7. Remove liquid by aspiration and wash the plate with 200 µL/well of PBST washing buffer by shaking it for 5 min at 120 rpm at room temperature. Repeat this step two times more.

8. Add 100 µL each of prepared samples, anti-DT antibody standards, and control serum to the designated wells in duplicate. Incubate the plate at 120 rpm at room temperature for 1 h.

9. Remove liquid by aspiration and wash the plate with 200 µL/well of PBST washing buffer by shaking it for 5 min at

120 rpm at room temperature. Repeat this step two times more.

10. Dilute anti-human IgG-HRP 1:1500 in sample dilution buffer. Add 100 μL of the diluted solution to each well. Incubate the plate at room temperature at 120 rpm for 1 h.

11. Remove liquid by aspiration and wash the plate with 200 μL/well of PBST washing buffer by shaking it for 5 min at 120 rpm at room temperature. Repeat this step two times more.

12. Add 100 μL of ABTS peroxidase substrate that has been warmed to room temperature. Incubate at room temperature at 120 rpm for 30 min.

13. Add 100 μL of 1 M HCl and measure absorbance at 405 nm with the microplate reader.

14. Plot absorbance vs. concentration for each standard and obtain a linear regression curve, a regression equation, and a R^2 value using a MS Excel program.

15. Calculate anti-DT antibody levels in samples using the regression equation. To qualify the assay results, (1) absorbance of 30 ng/ml anti-DT antibody standard should be >1.0 $OD_{405\ nm}$ and (2) anti-DT antibody concentration of control serum should be within known value ± 20%.

3.3. Flow Cytometry Analysis for T-Cell Subtypes

3.3.1. Staining Cyto-Trol Cells for Fluorescence Compensation

1. Reconstitute a vial of Cyto-Trol cells with buffer in Cyto-Trol cell kit. Dispense 100 μl each of reconstituted Cyto-Trol cells into 1.5-ml microcentrifuge tubes labeled as #1–#6.

2. Add 10 μL each of anti-CD45-FITC, PE, ECD, APC, PC5, and PC7 to designated tubes #1–#6. Incubate at room temperature in dark for a minimum of 15 min.

3. Add 1 ml cold sample buffer to each tube and mix gently. Centrifuge sample tubes for 5 min at 400×g at 4°C.

4. Carefully aspirate supernatant without disturbing cell pellet. Resuspend cell pellet using 800 μl cold sample buffer and transfer to 5-ml polystyrene tubes. For FITC/PE/ECD/PC5/PC7 compensation, prepare tube 7 by adding 200 μl each of tubes 1, 2, 3, 5, and 6 to tube 7 and mixing gently. For FITC/PE/ECD/APC/PC7 compensation, prepare tube 8 by adding 200 μl each of tube 1, 2, 3, 4, and 6 to tube 8 and mixing gently.

5. Prepare Flow Check mixture by mixing ten drops of Flow Check 488, three drops of Flow Check 675, and three drops

of Flow Check 770 for daily verification of flow cytometer's optical alignment and fluidics system.

6. Prepare Flow Set mixture by mixing ten drops of Flow Set 488, three drops of Flow Set 675, and three drops of Flow Set 770 for standardization of the flow cytometer.

3.3.2. Fluorescence Compensation for FITC/PE/ ECD/PC5/PC7 and FITC/PE /ECD/APC/PC7

1. To perform fluorescence compensation for fluorescence measurement of FITC/PE/ECD/PC5/PC7, run Flow Check mixture. Confirm that the HPCV (half-peak coefficient of variation) of the integral signal intensity values using Flow-Check 448 fluorospheres, Flow-Check 675 fluorospheres, and Flow-Check 770 fluorospheres are <2% for FL1–FL4 from the Argon laser, <2.5% for FL4 from the red laser and, <4% for FL5, respectively. Adjust voltage and gain if necessary.

2. While running Cyto-Trol tube 7 containing anti-CD45-FITC, PE, ECD, PC5, and PC7, set voltage and gain to adjust negative spike under the first decade (10^0) for each fluorescence histogram (FL1–FL5). Record voltage and gain setting for FS, SS, FL1, FL2, FL3, FL4, and FL5.

3. Run Flow Set mixture using the recorded voltage and gain setting in order to obtain acceptable ranges of X-mode of FS, SS, FL1, FL2, FL3, FL4, and FL5.

4. Run automatic procedure using Flow Check mixture, Flow Set mixture, Cyto-Trol tube 1, 2, 3, 5, 6, and 7 in order to obtain optimal compensation for the assay.

5. Record Flow Set setting and Compensation index and use these values for fluorescence measurement of FITC/PE/ECD/PC5/PC7.

6. To perform fluorescence compensation for fluorescence measurement of FITC/PE/ECD/APC/PC7, run Flow Check mixture. Confirm that the HPCV of the integral signal intensity values using Flow-Check 448 fluorospheres, Flow-Check 675 fluorospheres, and Flow-Check 770 fluorospheres are <2% for FL1–FL4 from the Argon laser, <2.5% for FL4 from the red laser, and <4% for FL5, respectively. Adjust voltage and gain if necessary.

7. While running Cyto-Trol tube 8 containing anti-CD45-FITC, PE, ECD, APC, and PC7, set voltage and gain to adjust negative spike under the first decade (10^0) for each fluorescence histogram (FL1–FL5). Record voltage and gain setting for FS, SS, FL1, FL2, FL3, FL4, and FL5.

8. Run Flow Set mixture using the recorded voltage and gain setting in order to obtain acceptable ranges of X-mode of FS, SS, FL1, FL2, FL3, FL4, and FL5.

9. Run automatic procedure using Flow Check mixture, Flow Set mixture, Cyto-Trol tube 1, 2, 3, 4, 6, and 8 in order to obtain optimal compensation for the assay.

10. Record Flow Set setting and Compensation index and use these values for fluorescence measurement of FITC/PE/ECD/APC/PC7.

3.3.3. Staining Patient Samples

1. Obtain whole blood patient samples in K$_2$ EDTA Vacutainers or equivalent (*see* **Note 4**).

2. Add manufacturer's recommended volume of fluorescence-antibody conjugates to designated tubes as follows.

Isotype control 1: IgG1-FITC, IgG1-PE, IgG1-ECD, IgG1-PC5, IgG1-PC7

Isotype control 2: IgG2a-FITC, IgG2b-PE, IgG2a-ECD, IgG2a-APC

Tube 1: anti-CD3-FITC, anti-CD26-PE, anti-CD45RA-ECD, anti-CD27-APC, anti-CD8-PC7

Tube 2: anti-CD3-FITC, anti-CD26-PE, anti-CD45RA-ECD, anti-CD27-APC, anti-CD4-PC7

Tube 3: anti-CD3-FITC, anti-CD26-PE, anti-CD25-ECD, anti-CD69-APC, anti-CD4-PC7

Tube 4: anti-CD26-FITC, anti-CD294-PE, anti-CD3-ECD, anti-CD195-APC, anti-CD4-PC7

Tube 5: anti-CD19-FITC, anti-CD56-PE, anti-CD3-ECD, anti-CD8-APC

Vbeta isotype control: vial A, IgG1-PC5

Vbeta positive control: anti-CD3-PC5

Vbeta tube 1: vial A, anti-CD3-PC5

Vbeta tube 2: vial B, anti-CD3-PC5

Vbeta tube 3: vial C, anti-CD3-PC5

Vbeta tube 4: vial D, anti-CD3-PC5

Vbeta tube 5: vial E, anti-CD3-PC5

Vbeta tube 6: vial F, anti-CD3-PC5

Vbeta tube 7: vial G, anti-CD3-PC5

Vbeta tube 8: vial H, anti-CD3-PC5

---

3. Dispense 100 µl of blood into each 1.5 ml microcentrifuge tube containing antibodies.

4. Incubate microcentrifuge tubes for 30 min in dark at room temperature. Dispense 1 ml of prepared 1× lysing buffer into each sample tubes and vortex. Incubate microcentrifuge tubes in dark for 10 min at room temperature. Vortex again and incubate in dark for another 10 min. Centrifuge sample tubes for 5 min at 400× g at 4°C.

5. Carefully aspirate supernatant without disturbing cell pellet. Resuspend cell pellet using 1.0 ml cold sample buffer. Centrifuge sample tubes for 5 min at $400 \times g$ at 4°C. Resuspend cell pellet using 500 μl cold sample buffer and transfer to designated 5-ml polystyrene tubes for flow analysis.

6. Run stained patient samples.

3.3.4. Analysis of Flow Data (see Note 5)

1. T cells (CD3⁺): Obtain a percentage of CD3 positive population from the lymphocyte population gate in each plot of side scatter vs. forward scatter for tubes 1, 2, 3, 4, and 5. Then calculate mean value of % CD3 positive population.

2. CD4⁺ T cells (CD3⁺/CD4⁺): Set a lymphocyte population gate in each plot of side scatter vs. forward scatter for tubes 2, 3, and 4. Create a histogram with quadstat as CD3 vs. CD4 and then display events from the lymphocyte population gate. Obtain a percentage of CD3⁺/CD4⁺ population. Then calculate mean value of % CD3⁺/CD4⁺ population.

3. CD4⁺ naïve T cells (CD3⁺/CD4⁺/CD26⁺/CD27⁺/CD45RA⁺): Set a lymphocyte population gate in a plot of side scatter vs. forward scatter for tube 2. Create histogram 1 with quadstat as CD3 vs. CD4 and then display events from the lymphocyte population gate. Create CD26 histogram and display events from CD3⁺/CD4⁺ region on histogram 1. Create histogram 2 with quadstat as CD27 vs. CD45RA and then display events from CD26⁺ region on CD26 histogram. Obtain a percentage of CD27⁺/CD45RA⁺ population on histogram 2.

4. CD4⁺ central memory T cells (CD3⁺/CD4⁺/CD26⁺/CD27⁺/CD45RA⁻): Obtain a percentage of CD27⁺/CD45RA⁻ population on histogram 2 in the previous step.

5. CD4⁺ effector memory T cells (CD3⁺/CD4⁺/CD26⁺/CD27⁻/CD45RA⁻): On histogram 2 in the previous step, obtain a percentage of CD27⁻/CD45RA⁻ population.

6. CD4⁺ Th1 effector memory T cells (CD3⁺/CD4⁺/CD26⁺/CD195⁺/CD294⁻): Set a lymphocyte population gate in a plot of side scatter vs. forward scatter for tube 4. Create histogram 1 with quadstat as CD3 vs. CD4 and then display events from the lymphocyte population gate. Create CD26 histogram and display events from CD3⁺/CD4⁺ region on histogram 1. Create histogram 2 with quadstat as CD195 vs. CD294 and then display events from CD26⁺ region on CD26 histogram. Obtain a percentage of CD195⁺/CD294⁻ population on histogram 2.

7. CD4⁺ Th2 effector memory T cells (CD3⁺/CD4⁺/CD26⁺/CD195⁺/CD294⁺): Obtain a percentage of

$CD195^+/CD294^+$ population on histogram 2 in the previous step.

8. $CD4^+$ Tregs cells $(CD3^+/CD4^+/CD25^+/CD26^+/CD69^-)$: Set a lymphocyte population gate in a plot of side scatter vs. forward scatter for tube 3. Create histogram 1 with quadstat as CD3 vs. CD4 and then display events from the lymphocyte population gate. Create CD26 histogram and display events from $CD3^+/CD4^+$ region on histogram 1. Create histogram 2 with quadstat as CD25 vs. CD69 and then display events from $CD26^+$ region on CD26 histogram. Obtain a percentage of $CD25^+/CD69^-$ population on histogram 2.

9. $CD8^+$ T cells $(CD3^+/CD8^+)$: Set a lymphocyte population gate in each plot of side scatter vs. forward scatter for tubes 1 and 5. Create a histogram with quadstat as CD3 vs. CD8 and then display events from the lymphocyte population gate. Obtain a percentage of $CD3^+/CD8^+$ population. Then calculate mean value of % $CD3^+/CD8^+$ population.

10. $CD8^+$ naïve T cells $(CD3^+/CD8^+/CD27^+/CD45RA^+)$: Set a lymphocyte population gate in a plot of side scatter vs. forward scatter for tube 1. Create histogram 1 with quadstat as CD3 vs. CD8 and then display events from the lymphocyte population gate. Create histogram 2 with quadstat as CD27 vs. CD45RA and then display events from $CD3^+/CD4^+$ region on histogram 1. Obtain a percentage of $CD27^+/CD45RA^+$ population on histogram 2.

11. $CD8^+$ central memory T cells $(CD3^+/CD8^+/CD27^+/CD45RA^-)$: Obtain a percentage of $CD27^+/CD45RA^-$ population on histogram 2 in the previous step.

12. $CD8^+$ effector memory T cells $(CD3^+/CD8^+/CD27^-/CD45RA^-)$: On histogram 2 in the previous step, obtain a percentage of $CD27^-/CD45RA^-$ population.

13. $CD8^+$ Tregs cells $(CD3^+/CD4^-/CD25^+/CD69^-)$: Set a lymphocyte population gate in a plot of side scatter vs. forward scatter for tube 3. Create histogram 1 with quadstat as CD3 vs. CD4 and then display events from the lymphocyte population gate. Create histogram 2 with quadstat as CD25 vs. CD69 and then display events from $CD3^+/CD4^-$ region on histogram 1. Obtain a percentage of $CD25^+/CD69^-$ population on histogram 2.

14. NK T cells $(CD3^+/CD56^+)$: Set a lymphocyte population gate in a plot of side scatter vs. forward scatter for tube 5. Create a histogram with quadstat as CD3 vs. CD56 and then display events from the lymphocyte population gate. Obtain a percentage of $CD3^+/CD56^+$ population.

15. B cells (CD3⁻/CD19⁺): Set a lymphocyte population gate in a plot of side scatter vs. forward scatter for tube 5. Create a histogram with quadstat as CD3 vs. CD19 and then display events from the lymphocyte population gate. Obtain a percentage of CD3⁻/CD19⁺ population.

16. NK cells (CD3⁻/CD56⁺): Set a lymphocyte population gate in a plot of side scatter vs. forward scatter for tube 5. Create a histogram with quadstat as CD3 vs. CD56 and then display events from the lymphocyte population gate. Obtain a percentage of CD3⁻/CD56⁺ population.

17. CD8⁺ NK cells (CD3⁻/CD8⁺/CD56⁺): After obtaining NK-cell population in the previous step, create a histogram with quadstat as CD8 vs. CD56 and then display population from the NK-cell region (CD3⁻/CD56⁺). Obtain a percentage of CD8⁺/CD56⁺ population.

18. CD8⁻ NK cells (CD3⁻/CD8⁻/CD56⁺): From the histogram with quadstat as CD8 vs. CD56 in the previous step, obtain a percentage of CD8⁻/CD56⁺ population.

19. CD3⁺ lymphocyte Vβ repertoire: Analyze each Vβ subset according to manufacturer's data analysis procedure.

4. Notes

1. All solutions should be prepared in ultrapure water that has a resistivity of 18.2 MΩ-cm and total organic content of less than 10 ppb (parts per billion).

2. Bioassays using cell lines have inherent assay variability. The main reason for the assay variability is variation of cell culture condition. To minimize the assay variability, master cell bank and working cell bank of Jurkat cells need to be established.

3. Increase dilution ratio (1:800–1:6400) of patient serum samples and repeat the assay, if anti-DT antibody concentration of serial dilutions of patient serum samples is > 30 ng/ml.

4. Whole blood samples in K₂ EDTA Vacutainers should be analyzed within 24 h.

5. To obtain counts/ml of each subset lymphocyte, lymphocyte counts of patient blood are required. The counts can be obtained by multiplying percentage of each subset lymphocyte and lymphocyte counts.

References

1. Rizvi, M. A., Evens, A. M., Tallman, M. S., Nelson, B. P., Rosen, S. T. (2006) T-cell non-Hodgkin lymphoma. *Blood* **107**, 1255–1264.

2. Hymes, K. B. (2007) Choices in the treatment of cutaneous T-cell lymphoma. *Oncology (Williston Park)* **21**, 18–23.

3. Savage, K. J. (2007) Peripheral T-cell lymphomas. *Blood Rev* **21**, 201–216.

4. Woo, J. H., Liu, J. S., Kang, S. H., Singh, R., Park, S. K., Su, Y., Ortiz, J., Neville, D. M., Jr., Willingham, M. C., Frankel, A. E. (2008) GMP production and characterization of the bivalent anti-human T cell immunotoxin, A-dmDT390-bisFv(UCHT1) for phase I/II clinical trials. *Protein Expr Purif* **58**, 1–11.

5. Frankel, A. E., Zuckero, S. L., Mankin, A. A., Grable, M., Mitchell, K., Lee, Y. J., Neville, D. M., Woo, J. H. (2009) Anti-CD3 recombinant diphtheria immunotoxin therapy of cutaneous T cell lymphoma. *Curr Drug Targets* **10**, 104–109.

6. Woo, J. H., Liu, Y. Y., Mathias, A., Stavrou, S., Wang, Z., Thompson, J., Neville, D. M., Jr. (2002) Gene optimization is necessary to express a bivalent anti-human anti-T cell immunotoxin in Pichia pastoris. *Protein Expr Purif* **25**, 270–282.

7. Woo, J. H., Liu, Y. Y., Stavrou, S., Neville, D. M., Jr. (2004) Increasing secretion of a bivalent anti-T-cell immunotoxin by Pichia pastoris. *Appl Environ Microbiol* **70**, 3370–3376.

8. Woo, J. H., Liu, Y. Y., Neville, D. M., Jr. (2006) Minimization of aggregation of secreted bivalent anti-human T cell immunotoxin in Pichia pastoris bioreactor culture by optimizing culture conditions for protein secretion. *J Biotechnol* **121**, 75–85.

9. Woo, J. H., Neville, D. M., Jr. (2003) Separation of bivalent anti-T cell immunotoxin from Pichia pastoris glycoproteins by borate anion exchange. *Biotechniques* **35**, 392–398.

10. Neville, D. M., Jr., Srinivasachar, K., Stone, R., Scharff, J. (1989) Enhancement of immunotoxin efficacy by acid-cleavable cross-linking agents utilizing diphtheria toxin and toxin mutants. *J Biol Chem* **264**, 14653–14661.

11. Thompson, J., Hu, H., Scharff, J., Neville, D. M., Jr. (1995) An anti-CD3 single-chain immunotoxin with a truncated diphtheria toxin avoids inhibition by pre-existing antibodies in human blood. *J Biol Chem* **270**, 28037–28041.

12. Hall, P. D., Virella, G., Willoughby, T., Atchley, D. H., Kreitman, R. J., Frankel, A. E. (2001) Antibody response to DT-GM, a novel fusion toxin consisting of a truncated diphtheria toxin (DT) linked to human granulocyte-macrophage colony stimulating factor (GM), during a phase I trial of patients with relapsed or refractory acute myeloid leukemia. *Clin Immunol* **100**, 191–197.

13. Kivisakk, P., Mahad, D. J., Callahan, M. K., Trebst, C., Tucky, B., Wei, T., Wu, L., Baekkevold, E. S., Lassmann, H., Staugaitis, S. M., Campbell, J. J., Ransohoff, R. M. (2003) Human cerebrospinal fluid central memory CD4+ T cells: evidence for trafficking through choroid plexus and meninges via P-selectin. *Proc Natl Acad Sci U S A* **100**, 8389–8394.

14. Gollob, J. A., Schnipper, C. P., Orsini, E., Murphy, E., Daley, J. F., Lazo, S. B., Frank, D. A., Neuberg, D., Ritz, J. (1998) Characterization of a novel subset of CD8(+) T cells that expands in patients receiving interleukin-12. *J Clin Invest* **102**, 561–575.

15. Soler, D., Chapman, T. R., Poisson, L. R., Wang, L., Cote-Sierra, J., Ryan, M., McDonald, A., Badola, S., Fedyk, E., Coyle, A. J., Hodge, M. R., Kolbeck, R. (2006) CCR8 expression identifies CD4 memory T cells enriched for FOXP3+ regulatory and Th2 effector lymphocytes. *J Immunol* **177**, 6940–6951.

Chapter 11

Construction of Human Antibody Gene Libraries and Selection of Antibodies by Phage Display

Thomas Schirrmann and Michael Hust

Abstract

Recombinant antibodies as therapeutics offer new opportunities for the treatment of many tumor diseases. To date, 18 antibody-based drugs are approved for cancer treatment and hundreds of anti-tumor antibodies are under development. The first clinically approved antibodies were of murine origin or human-mouse chimeric. However, since murine antibody domains are immunogenic in human patients and could result in human anti-mouse antibody (HAMA) responses, currently mainly humanized and fully human antibodies are developed for therapeutic applications.

Here, in vitro antibody selection technologies directly allow the selection of human antibodies and the corresponding genes from human antibody gene libraries. Antibody phage display is the most common way to generate human antibodies and has already yielded thousands of recombinant antibodies for research, diagnostics and therapy. Here, we describe methods for the construction of human scFv gene libraries and the antibody selection.

Key words: scFv, therapeutic antibody, phage display, panning, antibody fragment, antibody gene library.

1. Introduction

In 2006, 18 recombinant antibodies are approved by the FDA (US Food and Drug Administration) for oncology and hematology (1). Rituximab (tradename Rituxan®/MabThera) against non-hodgkin-lymphoma (2) Bevacizumab (tradename Avastin®) primarily against colon cancer (3) and Trastuzumab (tradename Herceptin®) against breast cancer (4) are the top-selling recombinant antibodies in cancer therapy.

P. Yotnda (ed.), *Immunotherapy of Cancer*, Methods in Molecular Biology 651,
DOI 10.1007/978-1-60761-786-0_11, © Springer Science+Business Media, LLC 2010

In 1986, the first antibody muronomab-CD3 (tradename Orthoclone OKT3®) was approved for therapy and was still of murine origin (5). Mouse-derived monoclonal antibodies are problematic as repeated administration of mouse-derived antibodies cause human anti-mouse antibody (HAMA) responses (6). The immunogenicity was step-wise reduced by using chimeric and later humanized antibodies by replacing murine constant and framework regions with the human counterparts, respectively (7). Accordingly, the next therapeutic antibodies were chimeric, e.g. Infliximab (tradename Remicade) (8) or Cetuximab (tradename Erbitux®) (9), and later humanized, e.g. Trastuzumab (4). The use of fully human antibodies is thought to further reduce the immunogenicity. In 2002, the first fully human antibody arrived on the market. Adalimumab (tradename Humira®) was isolated engineered using antibody phage display (10) by guided selection (11).

Currently, two major strategies are used for the generation of human antibodies: transgenic mice and in vitro selection technologies. Transgenic mice contain the human immunoglobulin repertoire instead of the murine, allowing the generation of human antibodies by the hybridoma technology (12–14). An advantage of transgenic mice is the in vivo affinity maturation. Already, transgenic mice yielded a significant number of antibodies that reached clinical studies. The disadvantages are limitations with respect to toxic and conserved antigens (15).

The alternative is the generation of human antibodies by antibody phage display, which is completely independent from any immune system by an in vitro selection process, called "panning." The first antibody gene repertoires in phage were generated and screened by using the lytic phage Lambda (16), however, with limited success. The display method most commonly used today is based on the groundbreaking work of Georg P. Smith (17) on filamentous phage display. Here, the genotype and phenotype of oligopeptides were linked by fusing the corresponding gene fragments to the minor coat protein III gene of the filamentous bacteriophage M13. The resulting peptide::pIII fusion protein is expressed on the surface of phage allowing the affinity purification of the peptide and its corresponding gene. In the same way, antibody fragments fused to pIII can be presented on the surface of M13 phage (18–23). Due to limitations of the *Escherichia coli* folding machinery, complete IgG molecules can only be produced or displayed on the surface of phage in rare cases (24, 25). Mainly, smaller antibody fragments are used for antibody phage display: the Fab fragment or the single chain Fv fragment (scFv). Fab fragments consist of two chains, the variable (V_H) and first constant region of the heavy chain (CH1) and the light chain (LC) of the antibody, both linked by a disulphide bond. In contrast, scFv fragments consist of only one polypeptide chain, composed of the variable region of the heavy chain (VH) and the variable region of the light chain (VL) fused by a short peptide linker. Two different genetic systems have been developed for the expression of the antibody::pIII fusion proteins for phage display. First, the antibody genes can be directly inserted into the phage genome fused to the wildtype pIII gene (18). However, most of the successful systems uncouple antibody expression from phage propagation by providing the genes encoding the antibody::pIII fusion proteins on a separate plasmid (called "phagemid"), containing a phage morphogenetic signal for packaging the vector into the assembled phage particles (19–23). The affinity of antibodies selected by phage display can be increased by additional in vitro affinity maturation steps (26). Despite other in vitro methods like ribosomal display (27, 28), puromycin display (29) or yeast surface display (30), antibody phage display has become the most widely used selection method for human antibodies. An overview about phage display derived human therapeutic antibodies in the clinical development is given by Thie et al. (31).

Depending on the scientific or medical applications, different types of antibody gene libraries can be constructed and used. Immune libraries are constructed from antibody V-genes isolated from IgG secreting plasma cells of immunized donors (20, 32). Immune libraries are typically generated and used in medical research to get an antibody against one particular target antigen, e.g. of an infectious pathogen or an tumor marker. Naive, semi-synthetic and synthetic libraries have been subsumed as "single-pot" libraries, as they are designed to isolate antibody fragments binding to every possible antigen, at least in theory. Naive libraries are constructed from rearranged V genes from B cells (IgM) of non-immunized donors. An example for this library type is the naive human Fab library constructed by de Haard et al. (33). Semi-synthetic libraries are derived from unrearranged V genes from pre B cells (germline cells) or from one antibody framework with genetically randomized complementary determining region (CDR) 3 regions, as described by Pini et al. (34). A combination of naive and synthetic repertoire was used by Hoet et al. (35). They combined light chains from autoimmune patients with a fd fragment containing synthetic CDR1 and CDR2 in the human VH3-23 framework and naive, which originated from autoimmune patients, CDR3 regions. The fully synthetic libraries have a human framework with randomly integrated CDR cassettes (36, 37). All library types – immune, naive, synthetic and their intermediates – are valuable sources for the selection of antibodies for diagnostic and therapeutic purposes. To date, "single-pot" antibody libraries with a theoretical diversity of up to 10^{11} independent clones have been generated (38) to serve as a molecular repertoire for phage display selection procedures. An overview of antibody gene libraries is given by Hust and Dübel (39) and Hust et al. (40).

2. Materials

2.1. Construction of Antibody Gene Libraries

2.1.1. Isolation of Lymphocytes

1. Phosphate buffered saline (PBS), pH 7.4 (8.0 g NaCl, 0.2 g KCl, 1.44 g $Na_2HPO_4 \cdot 2H_2O$, 0.24 g KH_2PO_4 in 1 L)
2. Lymphoprep (Progen, Heidelberg)
3. mRNA isolation Kit (QuickPrep micro mRNA Purification Kit, GE Healthcare, Munich) or Trizol (Invitrogen, Karlsruhe) for total RNA

2.1.2. cDNA Synthesis

1. Superscript II (Invitrogen) + 5 x RT buffer + 0.1 m DTT
2. Random hexamer oligonucleotide primer (dN_6)
3. dNTP mix (2.5 mM each)

2.1.3. /2.1.4 First and Second Antibody Gene PCR

1. Red Taq (Sigma, Hamburg) + 10 x buffer
2. dNTP mix (10 mM each)
3. Oligonucleotide primer (*see* **Table 11.1**)
4. Agarose (Serva, Heidelberg)
5. TAE-buffer 50 x (2 M Tris–HCl, 1 M acetic acid, 0.05 M EDTA, pH 8)
6. Nucleospin Extract 2 Kit (Macherey-Nagel, Düren)

2.1.5. First Cloning Step – VL

1. MluI (NEB, Frankfurt)
2. NotI (NEB)
3. Buffer 3 (NEB)
4. BSA (NEB)
5. Calf intestine phosphatase (CIP) (MBI Fermentas, St. Leon-Rot)
6. T4 ligase (Promegq a, Mannheim)
7. 3 M sodium acetate, pH 5.2
8. *E. coli* XL1-Blue MRF`(Stratagene, Amsterdam), genotype: Δ(*mcrA*)*183* Δ(*mcrCB-hsdSMR-mrr*)*173* *endA1 supE44 thi-1 recA1 gyrA96 relA1 lac* [F´ *proAB lac*I^q ZΔM15 Tn10 (Tet^r)]
9. Electroporator MicroPulser (BIO-RAD, München)

Table 11.1
Primers used for first and second PCR of antibody genes for antibody gene library construction using phagemids like pHAL14. Restriction sites are underlined

Primer	5' to 3' sequence
First antibody gene PCR VH	
MHVH1_f	cag gtb cag ctg gtg cag tct gg
MHVH1/7_f	car rts cag ctg gtr car tct gg
MHVH2_f	cag rtc acc ttg aag gag tct gg
MHVH3_f1	sar gtg cag ctg gtg gag tct gg
MHVH3_f2	gag gtg cag ctg ktg gag wcy sg
MHVH4_f1	cag gtg car ctg cag gag tcg gg
MHVH4_f2	cag stg cag ctr cag sag tss gg
MHVH5_f	gar gtg cag ctg gtg cag tct gg
MHVH6_f	cag gta cag ctg cag cag tca gg
MHIgMCH1_r	aag ggt tgg ggc gga tgc act
MHIgGCH1_r	gac cga tgg gcc ctt ggt gga
First antibody gene PCR kappa	
MHVK1_f1	gac atc cag atg acc cag tct cc
MHVK1_f2	gmc atc crg wtg acc cag tct cc
MHVK2_f	gat rtt gtg atg acy cag wct cc
MHVK3_f	gaa atw gtg wtg acr cag tct cc
MHVK4_f	gac atc gtg atg acc cag tct cc
MHVK5_f	gaa acg aca ctc acg cag tct cc
MHVK6_f	gaw rtt gtg mtg acw cag tct cc
MHkappaCL_r	aca ctc tcc cct gtt gaa gct ctt
First antibody gene PCR lambda	
MHVL1_f1	cag tct gtg ctg act cag cca cc
MHVL1_f2	cag tct gtg ytg acg cag ccg cc
MHVL2_f	cag tct gcc ctg act cag cct
MHVL3_f1	tcc tat gwg ctg acw cag cca cc
MHVL3_f2	tct tct gag ctg act cag gac cc
MHVL4_f1	ctg cct gtg ctg act cag ccc
MHVL4_f2	cag cyt gtg ctg act caa tcr yc
MHVL5_f	cag sct gtg ctg act cag cc
MHVL6_f	aat ttt atg ctg act cag ccc ca
MHVL7/8_f	cag rct gtg gtg acy cag gag cc
MHVL9/10_f	cag scw gkg ctg act cag cca cc
MHlambdaCL_r	tga aca ttc tgt agg ggc cac tg
MHlambdaCL_r2	tga aca ttc cgt agg ggc aac tg

(continued)

Table 11.1 (continued)

Primer	5′ to 3′ sequence
Second antibody gene PCR VH	
MHVH1-NcoI_f	gtcctcgca cc atg gcc cag gtb cag ctg gtg cag tct gg
MHVH1/7-NcoI_f	gtcctcgca cc atg gcc car rts cag ctg gtr car tct gg
MHVH2-NcoI_f	gtcctcgca cc atg gcc cag rtc acc ttg aag gag tct gg
MHVH3-NcoI_f1	gtcctcgca cc atg gcc sar gtg cag ctg gtg gag tct gg
MHVH3-NcoI_f2	gtcctcgca cc atg gcc gag gtg cag ctg ktg gag wcy sg
MHVH4-NcoI_f1	gtcctcgca cc atg gcc cag gtg car ctg cag gag tcg gg
MHVH4-NcoI_f2	gtcctcgca cc atg gcc cag stg cag ctr cag sag tss gg
MHVH5-NcoI_f	gtcctcgca cc atg gcc gar gtg cag ctg gtg cag tct gg
MHVH6-NcoI_f	gtcctcgca cc atg gcc cag gta cag ctg cag cag tca gg
MHIgMCH1scFv-HindIII_r	gtcctcgca aag ctt tgg ggc gga tgc act
MHIgGCH1scFv-HindIII_r	gtcctcgca aag ctt gac cga tgg gcc ctt ggt gga
Second antibody gene PCR kappa	
MHVK1-MluI_f1	accgcctcc a cgc gta gac atc cag atg acc cag tct cc
MHVK1-MluI_f2	accgcctcc a cgc gta gmc atc crg wtg acc cag tct cc
MHVK2-MluI_f	accgcctcc a cgc gta gat rtt gtg atg acy cag wct cc
MHVK3-MluI_f	accgcctcc a cgc gta gaa atw gtg wtg acr cag tct cc
MHVK4-MluI_f	accgcctcc a cgc gta gac atc gtg atg acc cag tct cc
MHVK5-MluI_f	accgcctcc a cgc gta gaa acg aca ctc acg cag tct cc
MHVK6-MluI_f	accgcctcc a cgc gta gaw rtt gtg mtg acw cag tct cc
MHkappaCLscFv-NotI_r	accgcctcc gc ggc cgc gaa gac aga tgg tgc agc cac agt
Second antibody gene PCR lambda	
MHVL1-MluI_f1	accgcctcc a cgc gta cag tct gtg ctg act cag cca cc
MHVL1-MluI_f2	accgcctcc a cgc gta cag tct gtg ytg acg cag ccg cc
MHVL2-MluI_f	accgcctcc a cgc gta cag tct gcc ctg act cag cct
MHVL3-MluI_f1	accgcctcc a cgc gta tcc tat gwg ctg acw cag cca cc
MHVL3-MluI_f2	accgcctcc a cgc gta tct tct gag ctg act cag gac cc
MHVL4-MluI_f1	accgcctcc a cgc gta ctg cct gtg ctg act cag ccc
MHVL4-MluI_f2	accgcctcc a cgc gta cag cyt gtg ctg act caa tcr yc
MHVL5-MluI_f	accgcctcc a cgc gta cag sct gtg ctg act cag cc
MHVL6-MluI_f	accgcctcc a cgc gta aat ttt atg ctg act cag ccc ca
MHVL7/8-MluI_f	accgcctcc a cgc gta cag rct gtg gtg acy cag gag cc
MHVL9/10-MluI_f	accgcctcc a cgc gta cag scw gkg ctg act cag cca cc
MHLambdaCLscFv-NotI_r	accgcctcc gc ggc cgc aga gga sgg ygg gaa cag agt gac
Primer for colony PCR and sequencing	
MHLacZ-Pro_f	ggctcgtatgttgtgtgg
MHgIII_r	c taa agt ttt gtc gtc ttt cc
MKpelB_f	g cct acg gca gcc gct gg
MKmyc_r	g atc ctc ttc tga gat gag

10. 2 M Glucose (sterile filtered)

11. 2 M Magnesium solution (1 M MgCl, 1 M MgSO$_4$) (autoclaved)

12. SOC medium, pH 7.0 (2% (w/v) tryptone, 0.5% (w/v) yeast extract, 0.05% (w/v) NaCl, 20 mM Mg solution, 20 mM glucose) (sterilize magnesium and glucose separatetely; add solutions after autoclavation)

13. 2xYT-medium, pH 7.0 (1.6% (w/v) Tryptone, 1% (w/v) Hefe Extrakt, 0.5% (w/v) NaCl)

14. 2xYT-GAT (2xYT + 100 mM Glucose + 100 µg/ml ampicillin + 20 µg/ml tetracycline)

15. Ampicillin (100 mg/ml stock)

16. Tetracycline (10 mg/ml stock)

17. 9-cm petri dishes

18. 25-cm square petri dishes ("pizza plates")

19. 2xYT-GAT agar plates (2xYT-GAT, 1.5% (w/v) agar-agar)

20. Nucleobond Plasmid Midi Kit (Macherey-Nagel)

2.1.6. Second Cloning Step – VH

1. NcoI (NEB)

2. HindIII (NEB)

3. Buffer 2 (NEB)

4. Glycerol of 99.5% (Roth, Karlsruhe)

2.1.7. Colony PCR

1. Oligonucleotide primer (*see* **Table 11.1**)

2.1.8. Library Packaging and scFv Phage Production

1. 2xTY media, pH 7.0 (1.6% (w/v) tryptone, 1% (w/v) yeast extract, 0.5% (w/v) NaCl)

2. 2xTY-GA (2xTY, 100 mM glucose, 100 µg/ml ampicillin)

3. M13K07 Helperphage for monovalent display (Stratagene)

4. Hyperphage for oligovalent display (Progen, Heidelberg)

5. 2xTY-AK (2xTY, containing 100 µg/ml ampicillin, 50 µg/ml kanamycin)

6. Sorval Centrifuge RC5B Plus, rotor GS3 and SS34 (Thermo Scientific, Waltham)

7. Polyethylene glycol (PEG) solution (20% (w/v) PEG 6000, 2.5 M NaCl)

8. Phage dilution buffer (10 mM Tris–HCl, pH 7.5, 20 mM NaCl, 2 mM EDTA)

9. Mouse α-pIII monoclonal antibody PSKAN3 (Mobitec, Göttingen)

10. Goat α-mouse IgG alkaline phosphatase (AP) conjugate (Sigma, Hamburg)

2.2. Antibody Selection (Panning)

2.2.1. Coating of Microtitre Wells

1. Maxisorb microtitre plates oder stripes (Nunc, Langenselbold)
2. PBS (pH 7.4) (8.0 g NaCl, 0.2 g KCl, 1.44 g $Na_2HPO_4 \cdot 2H_2O$, 0.24 g KH_2PO_4 in 1 L)
3. Dimethyl sulfoxide (DMSO)
4. PBST (PBS + 0.1% (v/v) Tween-20)

2.2.2. Panning

1. MPBST (2% skim milk in PBST, prepare fresh)
2. Panning block solution (1% (w/v) skim milk + 1% (w/v) BSA in PBST, prepare freshly)
3. 10 μg/ml Trypsin in PBS
4. *E. coli* XL1-Blue MRF`(Stratagene)
5. M13K07 Helperphage (Stratagene)
6. 2xTY media, pH 7.0 (1.6% (w/v) tryptone, 1% (w/v) yeast extract, 0.5% (w/v) NaCl)
7. 2xTY-T (2xTY, containing 50 μg/ml tetracycline)
8. SOB media, pH 7.0 (2% (w/v) tryptone, 0.5% (w/v) yeast extract, 0.05% (w/v) NaCl, after autoclavation add sterile 1% (v/v) of the 2 M Mg solution)
9. 2 M Mg solution (1 M MgCl + 1 M $MgSO_4$)
10. SOB-GA (SOB, 100 μg/ml ampicilin, 100 mM glucose)
11. SOB-GA agar plates (SOB-GA + 1,5% (w/v) agar-agar)
12. 15-cm petri dishes
13. 2xTY-GA (2xTY, 100 mM glucose, 100 μg/ml ampicillin)
14. Glycerol (99.5%)

2.2.3. Packaging of Phagemids (scFv Phage Production)

1. 2xTY-AK (2xTY, containing 100 μg/ml ampicillin, 50 μg/ml kanamycin)
2. Polyethylene glycol (PEG) solution (20% (w/v) PEG 6000, 2,5 M NaCl)
3. Phage dilution buffer (10 mM Tris–HCl, pH 7.5, 20 mM NaCl, 2 mM EDTA)

2.2.4. Phage Titration

1. 2xTY-GA agar plates (2xTY-GA + 1.5% (w/v) agar-agar)

2.2.5. ELISA of a Polyclonal Antibody Phage Suspension

1. Bovine serum albumin (BSA) (prepare a 10 mg/ml stock solution in PBS)
2. Anti-M13, horse radish peroxidase (HRP) conjugated monoclonal antibody (GE Healthcare)

3. TMB substrate solution A, pH 4.1 (10 g citric acid solved in 100 ml water, add 9.73 g potassium citrate add to 1 L water)

4. TMB substrate solution B (240 mg tetramethylbenzidine, 10 ml acetone, 90 ml ethanol, 907 µl 30% H_2O_2)

5. 1 N H_2SO_4

2.2.6. Production of Soluble Monoclonal Antibody Fragments in Microtitre Plates

1. 96-well U-bottom polypropylene (PP) microtitre plates (Greiner Bio-One, Frickenhausen)

2. AeraSeal breathable sealing film (Excel Scientific, Victorville)

3. Thermoshaker PST60-HL4 (Lab4You, Berlin)

4. Potassium phosphate buffer (2.31% (w/v) (0,17 M) KH_2PO_4 + 12.54% (w/v) (0,72 M) K_2HPO_4)

5. Buffered 2xTY, pH 7.0 (1.6% (w/v) tryptone, 1% (w/v) yeast extract, 0.5% (w/v) NaCl, 10% (v/v) potassium phosphate buffer)

6. Buffered 2xTY-SAI (buffered 2xTY containing 50 mM saccharose + 100 µg/ml ampicillin + 50 µM isopropyl-beta-D-thiogalactopyranoside (IPTG))

2.2.7. ELISA of Soluble Monoclonal Antibody Fragments

1. Mouse α-His-tag monoclonal antibody (α-Penta His, Qiagen, Hilden)

2. Mouse α-myc-tag monoclonal antibody (9E10, Sigma)

3. Mouse α-pIII monoclonal antibody PSKAN3 (Mobitec)

4. Goat α-Mouse IgG serum, (Fab specific) HRP conjugated (Sigma)

5. Oligonucleotide primers (*see* **Table 11.1**)

3. Methods

3.1. Construction of Single-Chain Antibody Gene Libraries

Various methods have been employed to clone the genetic diversity of antibody repertoires. After isolation of mRNA from B lymphocytes and preparation of cDNA, the construction of immune libraries is usually done by a two-step cloning or assembly PCR (*see* below). Very large "single pot" naive antibody gene libraries are generally constructed by two or three separate cloning steps. In the two-step cloning strategy, the amplified repertoire of light chain genes is cloned into the phage display vector first. In the second step the heavy chain gene repertoire – as the heavy chain contributes more to diversity, due to its highly variable CDRH3 – is cloned into the phagemids containing the light chain gene repertoire (32, 41–44). In the three-step cloning strategy, separate heavy and light chain libraries are engineered. The V_H gene repertoire has then to be excised and cloned into the phage display vector containing the repertoire of VL genes (33). Another common method used for the cloning of naive (45, 46), immune (20) or hybridoma (47) scFv phage display libraries is the assembly PCR. The VH and VL genes including the additional linker sequence are amplified separately and fused by assembly PCR, before the scFv encoding gene fragments are cloned into the vector. Since the CDRH3 is a major source of sequence variety in antibodies (48), the assembly PCR can be combined with a randomization of the CDR3 regions, leading to semi-synthetic libraries. Here, oligonucleotide primers encoding various CDR3 and J gene segments were used for the amplication of the V gene segments of human germlines (49). Hoogenboom and Winter (50) as well as Nissim et al. (51) used degenerated CDRH3 oligonucleotide primers to generate a semi-synthetic heavy chain repertoire derived from human V gene germline segments. Afterwards, this VH repertoire was combined with an anti-BSA light chain. In some cases a framework of a well known/robust antibody was used as scaffold for the integration of randomly created CDRH3 and CDRL3 (52, 53). Jirholt et al. (54) and Söderlind et al. (55) amplified all CDR regions derived from B cells before shuffling them into this antibody framework by assembly PCR. An entirely synthetic library was described by Knappik et al. (37) who utilized seven different VH and VL germline master frameworks combined with six synthetically created CDR cassettes. The construction of large naive and semi-synthetic libraries (35, 43, 46, 56–58) requires significant effort to tunnel the genetic diversity through the bottleneck of *E. coli* transformation, e.g. 600 transformations were necessary for the generation of a 3.5×10^{10} phage library (35).

To overcome the bottleneck of *E. coli* transformation, the Cre-lox or lambda phage recombination system has also been employed for library generation (38, 59–61). However, since libraries with more than 10^{10} independent clones have also been accomplished by conventional transformation, most of these complicated methods are rendered unnecessary in particular as they may result in decreased genetic stability.

In summary, antibodies can be selected from either type of library, naive or synthetic (33, 35, 37). If the assembly by cloning or PCR and preservation of molecular complexity is carefully controlled at every step of its construction, libraries of more than 10^{10} independent clones can be generated (35).

The following protocols describe the generation of human naive or immune scFv antibody gene libraries by a two-step cloning strategy already approved for naive (56) and immune libraries (32, 44).

3.1.1. Isolation of Lymphocytes (Peripheral Blood Mononuclear Cells (PBMC))

1. Mix 20 ml fresh blood or EDTA/citric acid-treated blood ($\sim$2 × 10^7 cells) of each donor with 20 ml PBS (*see* **Note 1**).

2. Fill 10 ml Lymphoprep in a 50-ml polypropylen tube. Carefully cover Lymphoprep with 40 ml of the diluted blood using a plastic pipette.

3. Centrifuge the blood with 800×*g* for 20 min at RT (without brake!).

4. The lymphocytes form a distinct layer between the Lymphoprep and the medium, whereas the erythrocytes and granulocytes will be pelleted. Carefully aspirate the lymphocytes using a plastic pipette and transfer to a new 50-ml polypropylen tube.

5. Fill up with 50 ml PBS and pellet the lymphocytes with 250×*g* for 10 min at RT. Discard the supernatant (be careful, the lymphocyte pellet is not solid).

6. Repeat this washing step to remove most of the thrombocytes.

7. Resuspend the lymphocytes pellet in the supplied extraction buffer of the mRNA isolation kit according to the manufacturers instructions or use 0.5 ml Trizol for total RNA isolation (*see* **Note 2**). After resuspension using the mRNA extraction buffer or Trizol, the RNA pellet can be stored at −80°C.

3.1.2. cDNA Synthesis

1. Set up mixture for the first strand cDNA synthesis:

Solution or component	volume	Final concentration
mRNA or total RNA	9 µl	50–250 ng (mRNA) or 2–20 µg (total RNA)
Random hexamer oligonucleotide primer (dN$_6$) (10 µM)	2.5 µl	1.5 µM
dNTP-Mix (2.5 mM each)	5 µl	500 µM

2. Denature the RNA for 5 min at 70°C. Afterwards directly chill down on ice for 5 min.

3. Add following components:

Solution or component	Volume	Final concentration
RT buffer (5×)	5 µl	1×
0.1 M DTT	2,5 µl	10 mM
Superscript II reverse transcriptase (200 U/µl)	1 µl	200 U

4. Incubate the 25 μl mixture for 10 min at 25°C for primer annealing. Afterwards incubate 50 min at 42°C for first strand synthesis.

5. Denature the RNA/DNA hybrids and the enzyme for 15 min at 70°C. Store at −20°C (*see* **Note 3**).

3.1.3. First Antibody Gene PCR

1. The cDNA derived from 50–250 ng mRNA or 2–20 μg total RNA will be used as template to amplify VH and the light chain. Set up the PCR reactions as follows (30× mastermix for 27 PCR reactions):

Solution or component	Volume	Final concentration
dH$_2$O	1230 μl	–
Buffer (10×)	150 μl	1×
dNTPs (10 mM each)	30 μl	200 μM each
cDNA	25 μl	Complete first strand synthesis reaction
RedTaq 1 U/μl	60 μl	2 U

3. Divide the master mix in 450 μl for VH, 350 μl for kappa and 550 μl for lambda.

4. Add to each of the three reactions the corresponding reverse primers (*see* also **Table 11.1**) as follows (use the IgM primer for naive antibody gene libraries or the IgG primer for a immune antibody gene libraries):

Antibody gene	Primer	Volume	Final concentration
VH	MHIgMCH1_r or MHIgGCH1_r (10 μM)	18 μl	0.4 μM
kappa	MHkappaCL_r (10 μM)	14 μl	0.4 μM
lambda	MHlambdaCL_r1/_r2 mix (9:1) (10 μM)	22 μl	0.4 μM

5. Divide the mixture to 9 (VH), 7 (Kappa) and 11 (Lambda) PCR reactions each with 48 μl and add 2 μl (10 μM, 0.4 μM final concentration) of the subfamily-specific forward primer (*see* also **Table 11.1**):

VH:	(1) MHVH1_f, (2) MHVH1/7_f, (3) MHVH2_f, (4) MHVH3_fl, (5) MHVH3_f2, (6) MHVH4_fl, (7) MHVH4_f2, (8) MHVH5_f, (9) MHVH6_f
Vkappa:	(10) MHVK1_fl, (11) MHVK1_f2, (12) MHVK2_f, (13) MHVK3_f, (14) MHVK4_f, (15) MHVK5_f, (16) MHVK6_f
Vlambda:	(17) MHVL1_fl, (18) MHVL1_f2, (19) MHVL2_f, (20) MHVL3_fl, (21) MHVL3_f2, (22) MHVL4_fl, (23) MHVL4_f2, (24) MHVL5_f, (25) MHVL6_f, (26) MHVL7/8_f, (27) MHVL9/10_f

6. Carry out the PCR using the following program:

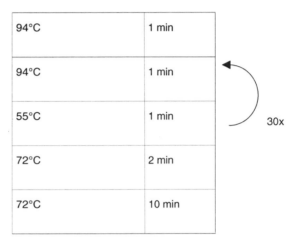

94°C	1 min
94°C	1 min
55°C	1 min
72°C	2 min
72°C	10 min

30x

7. Separate PCR products by 1.5% TAE agarose gel electrophoresis, cut out the amplified antibody genes (VH: ~380 bp, kappa/lambda: ~650 bp) (*see* **Note 4**) and purify the PCR products using a gel extraction kit according to the manufacturers instructions. Pool all VH, kappa and lambda subfamilies separately. Determine the DNA concentration. Store the three purified first PCR pools at −20°C.

3.1.4. Second Antibody Gene PCR

1. In the second PCR the restriction sites for library cloning will be added. Set up the PCR reactions as follows (30× mastermix for 27 PCR reactions) (*see* **Note 5**):

Solution or component	Volume	Final concentration
dH$_2$O	2500 µl	–
RedTaq buffer (10×)	300 µl	1×
dNTPs (10 mM each)	60 µl	200 µM each
RedTaq 1 U/µl	120 µl	2 U

2. Divide the master mix in 900 µl for VH, 700 µl for kappa and 1100 µl for lambda.

3. Add to each of the three reactions the corresponding reverse primers (*see* also **Table 11.1**) as follows:

Antibody gene	Primer	Volume	Final concentration
VH	MHIgMCH1scFv-HindIII_r or MHIgGCH1scFv-HindIII_r (10 µM)	18 µl	0.2 µM
kappa	MHKappaCLscFv-NotI_r (10 µM)	14 µl	0.2 µM
lambda	MHLambdaCLscFv-NotI_r (10 µM)	22 µl	0.2 µM

4. Add the corresponding PCR products of the first PCR as follows:

VH	900 ng
Kappa	700 ng
Lambda	1100 ng

5. Divide the solutions to 9 (VH), 7 (Kappa) and 11 (Lambda) PCR reactions, each with 98 µl and add 2 µl (10 µM, 0.2 µM final concentration) of the subfamily-specific forward primer (*see* also **Table 11.1**):

VH:	(1) MHVH1-NcoI_f, (2) MHVH2-NcoI_f, (3) MHVH1/7-NcoI_f, (4) MHVH3-NcoI_f1, (5) MHVH3-NcoI_f2, (6) MHVH4-NcoI_f1, (7) MHVH4-NcoI_f2, (8) MHVH5-NcoI_f, (9) MHVH6-NcoI_f
Vkappa:	(10) MHVK1-MluI_f1, (11) MHVK1-MluI_f2, (12) MHVK2-MluI_f, (13) MHVK3-MluI_f, (14) MHVK4-MluI_f, (15) MHVK5-MluI_f, (16) MHVK6-MluI_f
Vlambda:	(17) MHVL1-MluI_f1, (18) MHVL1-MluI_f2, (19) MHVL2-MluI_f, (20) MHVL3-MluI_f1, (21) MHVL3-MluI_f2, (22) MHVL4-MluI_f1, (23) MHVL4-MluI_f2, (24) MHVL5-MluI_f, (25) MHVL6-MluI_f, (26) MHVL7/8-MluI_f, (27) MHVL9/10-MluI_f

6. Carry out the PCR using the following program:

94°C	1 min
94°C	1 min
57°C	1 min
72°C	2 min
72°C	10 min

(loop) 20x

7. Separate the PCR products by 1.5% TAE agarose gel electrophoresis, cut out the amplified antibody genes (VH: ~400 bp, kappa/lambda: ~400 bp) and purify the PCR products using a gel extraction kit according to the manufacturers instructions. Pool all VH, kappa and lambda subfamilies separately. Determine the DNA concentration. Store the three purified second PCR pools at −20°C.

3.1.5. First Cloning Step – VL

1. Prepare a plasmid preparation of pHAL14 vector for library cloning.

2. Digest the vector and the VL PCR products (always perform single enzyme digest of the vector in parallel to check whether the digestion is complete, *see* **Notes 5** and **6**):

Solution or component	Volume	Final concentration
dH$_2$O	83-x μl	–
pHAL14 or VL	x μl	5 or 2 μg
NEB buffer 3 (10×)	10 μl	1×
BSA (100×)	1 μl	1×
NEB MluI (10 U/μl)	3 μl	30 U
NEB NotI (10 U/μl)	3 μl	30 U

3. Incubate at 37°C for 2 h. Control the digest of the vector by using a 5 μl aliquot on 1% TAE agarose gel electrophoresis. If the vector is not fully digested, extend the incubation time.

4. Inactivate the enzymes at 65°C for 10 min.

5. Add 0.5 μl CIP (1 U/μl) and incubate at 37°C for 30 min. Repeat this step once.

6. Purify the vector and the PCR product using a PCR purification Kit according the manufacturers instructions and elute with 50 μl elution buffer or water. The short stuffer fragment containing multiple stop codons between MluI and NotI in pHAL14 will be removed. Determine the DNA concentration.

7. Ligate the vector pHAL14 (4255 bp) and VL (~380 bp) as follows (*see* **Note 5**):

Solution or component	Volume	Final concentration
dH$_2$O	89-x-y μl	–
pHAL14	x μl	1000 ng
VL (kappa or lambda)	y μl	270 ng
T4 ligase buffer (10×)	10 μl	1×
T4 ligase (3 U/μl)	1 μl	3 U

8. Incubate at 16°C overnight.

9. Inactivate the ligation at 65°C for 10 min.

10. Precipitate the ligation with 10 μl 3 M sodium acetate, pH 5.2, and 250 μl ethanol, incubate for 2 min at RT and centrifuge for 5 min at 16,000×g and 4°C.

11. Wash the pellet with 500 μl 70% (v/v) ethanol and pellet the DNA for 2 min at 16,000×g and 4°C. Repeat this step once and resolve the DNA pellet in 35 μl dH$_2$O.

12. Thaw 25 μl electrocompetent XL1-Blue MRF' on ice and mix with the ligation reaction.

13. Transfer the 60 μl mix to a prechilled 0.1 cm cuvette. Dry the electrode of the cuvette with a tissue paper.

14. Perform a 1.7 kV pulse using an electroporator (*see* **Note 7**). Immediately, add 1 ml 37°C prewarmed SOC medium, transfer the suspension to a 2 ml cap and shake for 1 h at 600 rpm and 37°C.

15. To determine the amount of transformants, use 10 μl (=10^{-2} dilution) of the transformation and perform a dilution series down to 10^{-6} dilution. Plate out a 10^{-6} dilution on 2xYT-GAT agar plates and incubate overnight at 37°C.

16. Plate out the remaining 990 μl on 2xYT-GAT agar "pizza plate" and incubate overnight at 37°C.

17. Calculate the amount of transformants, which should be $1 \times 10^6 - 5 \times 10^8$ cfu. Control colonies for full-size insert by colony PCR (*see* **Section 3.1.7**).

18. Float off the colonies on the "pizza plate" with 40 ml 2xYT medium using a drigalsky spatula. Use 5 ml bacteria solution for midi plasmid preparation according to the manufacturer's instructions. Determine the DNA concentration.

3.1.6. Second Cloning Step – VH

1. Digest the pHAL14-VL repertoire and the VH PCR products (always perform single enzyme digest of the vector in parallel, *see* **Notes 5** and **6**):

Solution or component	Volume	Final concentration
dH$_2$O	81-x µl	–
pHAL14-VL or VH	x µl	5 or 2 µg
NEB buffer 2 (10×)	10 µl	1×
BSA (100×)	1 µl	1×
NEB NcoI (10 U/µl)	3 µl	30 U
NEB HindIII (20 U/µl)	5 µl	100 U

2. Incubate at 37°C for 2 h (*see* **Note 8**). Control the digest of the vector by using a 5 µl aliquot on 1% agarose gel electrophoresis.

3. Inactivate the digestion at 65°C for 10 min.

4. Add 0.5 µl CIP (1 U/µl) and incubate at 37°C for 30 min. Repeat this step once.

5. Purify the vector and the PCR product using a PCR purification Kit according the manufacturers instructions and elute with 50 µl elution buffer or water. The short stuffer fragment between NcoI and HindII in pHAL14 will be removed. Determine the DNA concentration.

6. Ligate the vector pHAL14-VL (~4610 bp) and VH (~380 bp) as follows (*see* **Note 5**):

Solution or component	Volume	Final concentration
dH$_2$O	89-x-y µl	–
pHAL14	x µl	1000 ng
VH	y µl	250 ng
T4 ligase buffer (10×)	10 µl	1×
T4 ligase (3 U/µl)	1 µl	3 U

7. Incubate at 16°C overnight.

8. Inactivate the ligation at 65°C for 10 min.

9. Precipitate the ligation with 10 µl 3 M, pH 5.2, sodium acetate and 250 µl ethanol, incubate for 2 min at RT and centrifuge for 5 min at 16,000×*g* and 4°C.

10. Wash the pellet with 500 µl 70% (v/v) ethanol and pellet the DNA for 2 min at $16,000 \times g$ and 4°C. Repeat this step once and resolve the pellet in 35 µl dH_2O.

11. Thaw 25 µl electrocompetent XL1-Blue MRF′ on ice and mix with the ligation reaction.

12. Transfer the 60 µl mix to a prechilled 0.1 cm cuvette. Dry the electrode of the cuvette with a tissue paper.

13. Perform a 1.7 kV pulse using a electroporator (*see* **Note 7**). Immediately, add 1 ml 37°C prewarmed SOC medium, transfer to a 2-ml cap and incubate for 1 h at 600 rpm.

14. To determine the amount of transformants, use 10 µl ($=10^{-2}$ dilution) of the transformation and perform a dilution series down to 10^{-6} dilution. Plate out a 10^{-6} dilution on 2xYT-GAT agar plates and incubate overnight at 37°C.

15. Plate out the remaining 990 µl on 2xYT-GAT agar "pizza plate" and incubate overnight at 37°C.

16. Calculate the amount of transformants (1×10^6–5×10^8 should be reached to be included into the final library). Control colonies for full size insert by colony PCR (*see* **Section 3.1.7**).

17. Float off the colonies on the "pizza plate" with 40 ml 2xYT medium using a drigalsky spatula. Use 800 µl bacteria solution ($\sim 1 \times 10^{11}$ bacteria) and 200 µl glycerol for glycerol stocks. Make 5–25 glycerol stocks per sublibrary and store at −80°C.

18. When all transformations are done, thaw one aliquot of each sublibrary on ice, mix all sublibraries (*see* also **Note 5**) and make new aliquots for storage at –80°C (*see* also **Note 9**).

3.1.7. Colony PCR

1. Choose 10–20 single colonies per transformation. Set up the PCR reaction per colonies as follows (*see* **Table 11.1** for primer sequences):

Solution or component	Volume	Final concentration
dH_2O	16,7 µl-x µl	
RedTaq buffer (10×)	2 µl	1×
dNTPs (10 mM each)	0,4 µl	je 200 µM
MHLacZPro_f 10 µM	0,2 µl	0,1 µM
MHgIII_r10 µM	0,2 µl	0,1 µM
RedTag (1 U/µl)	0,5 µl	1 U
template	picked colonie from dilution plate	

2. Control the PCR by 1.5% TAE agarose gel electrophoresis.

3. The PCR products should be ~ 1100 bp when including VH and VL, ~750 bp when including only VL or VH and 375 bp if the vector contains no insert. Each used sublibrary should have more than 80% full-size inserts to be included into the final library.

3.1.8. Library Packaging and scFv Phage Production

1. To package the library, inoculate 400 ml 2xTY-GA in a 1 L Erlenmeyer flask with 1 ml antibody gene library stock. Grow at 250 rpm at 37°C up to an O.D.$_{600\ nm} \sim 0.5$.

2. Infect 25 ml bacteria culture ($\sim1.25 \times 10^{10}$ cells) with 2.5×10^{11} colony forming units (cfu) of the helper phage M13K07 or Hyperphage according to a multiplicity of infection (moi) = 1:20 (*see* **Note 10**). Incubate 30 min without shaking and the following 30 min with 250 rpm at 37°C.

3. To remove the glucose which represses the lac promoter of pHAL14 and therefore the scFv::pIII fusion protein expression, harvest the cells by centrifugation for 10 min at $3200 \times g$ in 50-ml polypropylene tubes.

4. Resuspend the pellet in 400 ml 2xTY-AK in a 1 L Erlenmeyer flask. Produce scFv-phage overnight at 250 rpm and 30°C.

5. Pellet the bacteria by centrifugation for 10 min at $10,000 \times g$ in two GS3 centrifuge tubes. If the supernatant is not clear, centrifuge again to remove remaining bacteria.

6. Precipate the phage from the supernatant by adding 1/5 volume PEG solution in two GS3 tubes. Incubate for 1 h at 4°C with gentle shaking, followed by centrifugation for 1 h at $10,000 \times g$.

7. Discard the supernatant, resolve each pellet in 10 ml phage dilution buffer in SS34 centrifuge tubes and add 1/5 volume PEG solution.

8. Incubate on ice for 20 min and pellet the phage by centrifugation for 30 min at $10,000 \times g$.

9. Discard the supernatant and put the open tubes upside down on tissue paper. Let the viscous PEG solution move out completely. Resuspend the phage pellet in 1 ml phage dilution buffer. Titre the phage preparation (*see* **Section 3.2.4**). Store the packaged antibody phage library at 4°C.

10. The library packaging should be controlled by 10% SDS-PAGE, Western-Blot and anti-pIII immunostain (mouse anti-pIII 1:2000, goat anti-mouse IgG AP conjugate 1:10,000). Wildtype pIII has a calculated molecular mass

of 42.5 kDa, but it runs at an apparent molecular mass of 65 kDa in SDS-PAGE. Accordingly, the scFv::pIII fusion protein runs at about 95 kDa.

3.2. Antibody Selection (Panning)

The in vitro procedure for isolating antibody fragments by their binding activity was called "panning," referring to the gold washers tool (62). The antigen is immobilized to a solid surface, such as nitrocellulose, e.g. (63), magnetic beads, e.g. (64), column matrixes, e.g. (19) or most widely used or plastic surfaces with high protein binding capacity as polystyrole tubes, respectively, microtitre wells, e.g. (65). The antibody phage are incubated with the surface-bound antigen, followed by stringent washing to remove the vast excess of non-binding antibody phage. Subsequently, the bound antibody phage will be eluted and reamplified by infection of *E. coli*. The selection cycle will be repeated by infection of the phagemid bearing *E. coli* colonies from the former panning round with a helperphage to produce new antibody phage, which can be used for further panning rounds until a significant enrichment of antigen specific phage is achieved. The number of antigen-specific antibody phage clones should increase with every panning round. Usually 2–3 panning rounds, sometimes up to 6, are necessary to select specifically binding antibody fragments.

The first step in the evaluation process of potential binders is often done – but not a requisite – by an ELISA of the polyclonal phage preparations from each panning round against the target antigen and control proteins, e.g. BSA. In the next step, antibody clones are isolated from panning rounds showing a significant enrichment of specific antigen binding in the polyclonal phage ELISA. These antibodies clones are produced as soluble monoclonal antibody fragments in microtitre plates followed by an antigen ELISA. An ELISA with monoclonal phage preparations should be omitted because often antibody clones that bind only as scFv-phage or scFv-pIII fusion but not as soluble scFv fragment are identified. The complete panning and screening procedure is given in **Fig. 11.1**.

The following protocols describe the selection of recombinant antibody fragments from antibody gene libraries by phage display and the screening of the selected antibody fragments.

3.2.1. Coating of Microtitre Plate Wells

1. (A) Protein antigen: For the first panning round, use 2–10 μg protein/well per panning; for the following rounds use 0.1–1 μg protein/well for more stringent conditions. Dissolve the antigen in 150 μl PBS and incubate it into a microtitre plate well overnight at 4°C (*see* **Note 11**).
   (B) Oligopeptide antigen: Use 100–500 ng oligopeptide for each panning round. Dissolve the oligopeptide in 150 μl

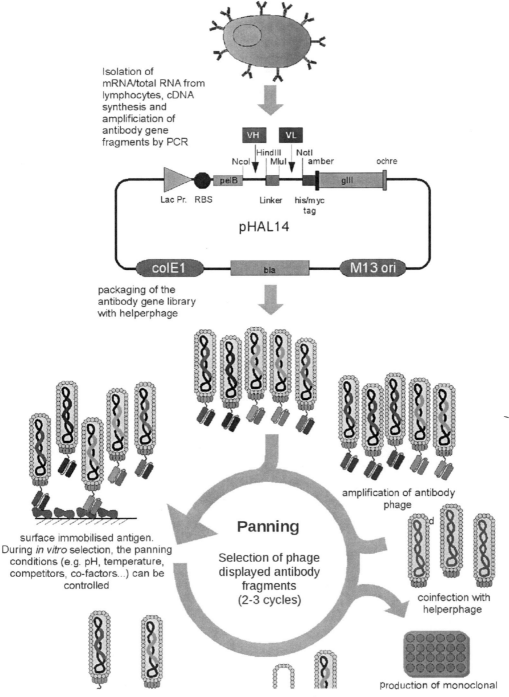

Fig. 11.1. Schematic overview about of the construction of antibody gene libraries and selection of antibodies ("panning") by phage display.

PBS, transfer into the microtitre plate well and incubate overnight at 4°C (*see* **Note 12**).

2. Wash the coated microtitre plate wells 3× with PBST using an ELISA washer (*see* **Note 13**).

3.2.2. Panning

1. (A) Block the antigen coated wells with MPBST for 2 h at RT. The wells must be completely filled. Afterwards, wash the blocked antigen coated wells 3× with PBST (*see* **Note 13**).

   (B) *You need to perform this step only in the first panning round but it also can be done in the following rounds!* In parallel, block an additional well (without antigen!) per panning with MPBST for 1 h at RT for preincubation of the antibody gene library. The wells must be completely filled. Wash 3× times with PBST (*see* **Note 13**). Incubate $10^{11}-10^{12}$ antibody phage from the library in 150 µl panning block for 1 h at RT. This step removes unspecific binders, which often occur from the antibody gene libraries due to incorrect folding of individual antibodies.

2. Carry over the preincubated antibody phage library to the blocked wells or fill $10^{11}-10^{12}$ amplified phage solved in 150 µl panning block from the former panning round in the blocked wells. Incubate at RT for 2 h for binding of the antibody phage.

3. Remove the unspecifically bound antibody phage by stringent washing. Therefore, wash the wells 10× with an ELISA washer in the first panning round. In the following panning rounds increase the number of washing steps (20× in the second panning round, 30× in the third panning round...) (*see* **Note 13**).

4. Elute bound antibody phage with 200 µl Trypsin solution for 30 min at 37°C (*see* **Note 14**).

5. Use 10 µl of the eluted phage for titration (*see* **Section 3.2.4**).

6. Inoculate 50 ml 2xTY-T with an overnight culture of *E. coli* XL1-Blue MRF′ in 100-ml Erlenmeyer flasks and grow at 250 rpm and 37°C.

7. Infect exponential (O.D.$_{600\,nm}$ ∼ 0.5, after 2–3 h) growing 20 ml XL1-Blue MRF′ culture with the remaining 190 µl of the eluted phage. Incubate 30 min at 37°C without shaking and the following 30 min with 250 rpm at 37°C.

8. Harvest the infected bacteria by centrifugation for 10 min at 3200×*g* in 50 ml polypropylene tubes. Resolve the pellet in 250 µl SOB-GA and plate the bacteria suspension on SOB-GA agar plates (15-cm petri dish). Grow overnight at 37°C (*see* **Note 15**).

9. Harvest the grown colonies by suspending in 2.5 ml 2xTY-GA with a Drigalsky spatula.

10. Use 100 µl of the harvested bacteria for the amplification of the eluted phage (*see* **Section 3.2.3**).

11. Make a glycerol stock of the panning round by adding 250 µl glycerol to 750 ml of the harvested bacteria. Mix and store at −80°C.

3.2.3. Packaging of Phagemids (scFv Phage Production)

1. For the next panning round the eluted phage must be packaged and reamplified. Inoculate 30 ml 2xTY-GA in a 100 ml Erlenmeyer flask with 100 µl harvested bacteria (O.D.$_{600}$ < 0.1). Grow at 250 rpm at 37°C up to an O.D.$_{600\ nm}$ ∼ 0.5.

2. Infect 5 ml bacteria culture (∼2.5×10^9 cells) with 5×10^{10} cfu of the helper phage M13K07 (moi = 1:20). Incubate for 30 min without shaking at 37°C and for the following 30 min at 250 rpm at 37°C.

3. To remove the glucose, harvest the cells by centrifugation for 10 min at 3200×g in 50-ml polypropylene tubes.

4. Resuspend the pellet in 30 ml 2xTY-AK and transfer into a 100-ml Erlenmeyer flask. Produce the phage for 16 h at 250 rpm and 30°C.

5. Pellet the bacteria by centrifugation for 10 min at 3200×g in 50-ml polypropylene tubes. If the supernatant is not clear, centrifuge again to remove remaining bacteria.

6. Precipate the phage in the supernatant by adding 1/5 volume PEG solution in 50-ml polypropylene tubes. Incubate for 1 h at 4°C with gentle shaking.

7. Pellet the phage by centrifugation for 1 h at 3200×g and 4°C. Discard the supernatant and put the open tubes upside down on tissue paper. Let the viscous PEG solution move out completely. Resuspend the phage pellet in 500 µl phage dilution buffer. Titre the phage preparation and use it for the next panning round. Store the remaining phage at 4°C.

3.2.4. Phage Titration

1. Inoculate 5 ml 2xTY-T in a 100 ml Erlenmeyer flask with XL1-Blue MRF' and grow overnight at 37°C and 250 rpm.

2. Inoculate 50 ml 2xTY-T with 500 µl overnight culture and grow at 250 rpm at 37°C up to O.D.$_{600}$ ∼ 0.5 (*see* **Note 16**).

3. Make serial dilutions of the phage suspension in PBS. The number of eluted phages depends on several parameters (e.g. antigen, library, panning round and washing stringency). In case of a successful enrichment, the titre of eluted phage usually is 10^3–10^5 phage per well after the first panning round

and increases two to three orders in magnitude per additional panning round (*see* **Note 17**). The phage preparation after reamplification of the eluted phage have a titre of about $10^{12}-10^{14}$ phage/ml.

4. Infect 50 μl bacteria with 10 μl phage dilution and incubate 30 min at 37°C (*see* **Note 18**).

5. You can perform titrations in two different ways:
   (A) plate the 60 μl infected bacteria on 2xTY-GA agar plates (9 cm petri dishes).
   (B) pipette 10 μl (in triplicate) on 2xTY-GA agar plates. Here, about 20 titering spots can be placed on one 9-cm petri dish. Dry drops under workbench.

6. Incubate the plates overnight at 37°C.

7. Count the colonies and calculate the cfu or cfu/ml titre according to the dilution.

3.2.5. ELISA of a Polyclonal Antibody Phage Suspension

1. To investigate the enrichment of antigen specific antibody phage after a panning round, coat microtitre plate wells with 100–1000 ng antigen per well for each panning round (for method *see* **Section 3.1**). As a control, coat other wells with 100–1000 ng BSA in 150 μl PBS overnight at 4°C (*see* **Note 19**).

2. Wash the coated microtitre plate wells 3× with PBST using an ELISA washer (for washing procedure *see* **Section 3.2** and **Note 13**).

3. Block the antigen-coated wells with MPBST for 2 h at RT. The wells must be completely filled.

4. Wash the coated microtitre plate wells 3× with PBST (for washing procedure *see* **Section 3.2** and **Note 13**).

5. Resuspend 10^9 and 10^{10} cfu/well antibody phage from each panning round in 150 μl 2%MPST and incubate them for 1.5 h on the antigen and the BSA control, respectively.

6. Wash the microtitre plate wells 3× with PBST (for washing procedure *see* **Section 3.2** and **Note 13**).

7. Incubate each well with 100 μl HRP-conjugated anti-M13 antibody 1:5000 diluted in 2% MPBST for 1.5 h.

8. Wash the microtitre plate wells 3× with PBST (for washing procedure *see* **Section 3.2** and **Note 13**).

9. Shortly before use, mix 19 parts TMB substrate solution A and 1 part TMB substrate solution B. Add 100 μl of this TMB solution to each well and incubate for 1–15 min.

10. Stop the substrate reaction by adding 100 μl 1 N sulphuric acid. The colour turns from blue to yellow.

11. Measure the extinction at 450 nm using an ELISA reader.

*3.2.6. Production
of Soluble Monoclonal
Antibody Fragments in
Microtitre Plates*

1. Fill each well of a 96-well U-bottom polypropylene microtitre plate with 150 μl 2xTY-GA.

2. Pick 92 clones with sterile tips from the desired panning round (*see* **Note 20**) and inoculate each well (*see* **Note 21**). Seal the plate with a breathable sealing film.

3. Incubate overnight in a microtitre plate shaker at 37°C and 1000 rpm.

4. (A) Fill a new 96-well polypropylene microtitre plate with 150 μl 2xTY-GA and add 10 μl of the overnight cultures. Incubate for 2 h at 37°C and 1000 rpm.
(B) Add 30 μl glycerol solution to the remaining 140 μl overnight cultures. Mix by pipetting and store this master-plate at −80°C.

5. Pellet the bacteria in the microtitre plates by centrifugation for 10 min at 3200×*g* and 4°C. Remove 180 μl glucose containing media by carefully pipetting (do not disturb the pellet).

6. Add 180 μl buffered 2xTY-SAI (containing saccharose, ampicillin and 50 μM IPTG) and incubate overnight at 30°C and 1000 rpm (*see* **Note 22**).

7. Pellet the bacteria by centrifugation for 10 min at 3200×*g* in the microtitre plates. Transfer the antibody fragment containing supernatant to a new polypropylene microtitre plate and store at 4°C.

*3.2.7. ELISA of Soluble
Monoclonal Antibody
Fragments*

1. To analyse the antigen specificity of the monoclonal soluble antibody fragments, coat 100–1000 ng antigen per well overnight at 4°C. As control coat 100–1000 ng BSA per well (*see* **Section 3.1, Note 19**).

2. Wash the coated microtitre plate wells 3× with PBST (for washing procedure *see* **Section 3.2** and **Note 3**).

3. Block the antigen coated wells with MPBST for 2 h at RT. The wells must be completely filled.

4. Fill 50 μl MPBST in each well and add 50 μl of antibody solution (*see* **Section 3.6**). Incubate for 1.5 h at RT (or overnight at 4°C).

5. Wash the microtitre plate wells 3× with PBST (for washing procedure *see* **Section 3.2** and **Note 3**).

6. Incubate 100 μl mouse 9E10 α-myc tag antibody solution for 1.5 h (appropriate dilution in MPBST).

7. Wash the microtitre plate wells 3× with PBST (for washing procedure *see* **Section 3.2** and **Note 13**).

8. Incubate 100 μl goat α-mouse HRP conjugate (1:10,000 in MPBST).

9. Wash the microtitre plate wells 3× with PBST (for washing procedure *see* **Section 3.2** and **Note 3**).

10. Shortly before use, mix 19 parts TMB substrate solution A and 1 part TMB substrate solution B. Add 100 μl of this TMB solution into each well and incubate for 1–15 min.

11. Stop the colour reaction by adding 100 μl 1 N sulphuric acid. The colour turns from blue to yellow.

12. Measure the extinction at 450 nm using an ELISA reader.

13. Identify positive candidates with a signal (on antigen) 10× over noise (on control protein, e.g. BSA) (*see* **Note 23**).

14. DNA sequencing of binders is performed with appropriate oligonucleotide primers (MKpelB_f and MKmyc_r or with MHLacZ-Pro_f). The antibody sequences can be analysed by VBASE2 (www.vbase2.org) (66).

4. Notes

1. Be careful with human blood samples since it is potentially infectious (HIV, hepatitis, etc.)!

2. Both methods, mRNA or total RNA isolation, work well.

3. Check the cDNA quality using standard glyceraldehyde 3-phosphate dehydrogenase (GAPDH) oligonucleotide primers. Do not use cDNA preparations if the GAPDH fragment could not be amplified by PCR.

4. The VH amplifications of VH subfamilies sometimes results also in longer PCR products. Cut out only the ~380 bp fragment. The amplifications of kappa subfamilies should always give a clear ~650 bp fragment. When amplifying lambda subfamilies often other PCR products are generated, especially the amplification of the lambda2 subfamily results often in slushy bands. If some subfamilies are bad amplified and no clear ~650 bp fragment is detectable, use only the ~650 bp fragments from the well amplified subfamilies. Additional comment: since the first PCR amplifies the full LC, it can be used also to construct a Fab or scFab (67) libraries from this material.

5. For a very large naive antibody gene library perform as many PCRs as sufficient to perform 20 light chains ligations/transformations and about 100 VH ligations. For an immune library 4 light chains ligations/transformations and 8 VH ligations are usually sufficient. Prepare and digest

also adequate amounts of pHAL14 and VL for the first cloning step and pHAL14-VL library and VH for the second cloning step. Keep kappa and lambda in all steps (cloning, packaging) separately and mix only after phage production before panning.

6. Always perform single digests using only one enzyme in parallel to control the success of the restriction reaction. Analyse the digestion by TAE agarose gel electrophoresis by comparing with the undigested plasmid. Use only material where both single digests are successful and where no degradation is visible in the double digest.

7. The pulse time should be between 4 and 5 ms for optimal electroporation efficiency.

8. Often the HindIII digestion is incomplete after 2 h. Then, inactivate the enzymes by heating up to 65°C for 10 min, add additional 5 μl of HindIII and incubate overnight. You can use also higher concentrated HindIII. Alternatively, perform the NcoI digest first for 2 h, inactive the digest and afterwards perform the HindIII digest.

9. To minimize loss of diversity, avoid to many freeze and thaw steps, e.g. when constructing an immune library make eight transformations in parallel and directly package the immune library.

10. The use of Hyperphage as helperphage instead of M13K07 offers oligovalent phage display, facilitates the selection of specific binders in the first and most critical panning round by avidity effect (32, 44, 68, 69). The Hyperphage should be only used for library packaging. For the following panning rounds use M13K07 to enhance the stringency of the panning process.

11. If the protein is not binding properly to the microtitre plate surface, try bicarbonat buffer (50 mM NaHCO₃, pH 9.6).

12. More hydrophobic oligopeptides may need to be dissolved in PBS containing 5% DMSO. If biotinylated oligopeptide is used as antigen for panning, dissolve 100 ng Streptavidin in 150 μl PBS and coat overnight at 4°C. Coat two wells for each panning, one well is for the panning, the second one for the preincubation of the library to remove streptavidin binders! Sometimes it is necessary to use free streptavidin during panning for competition to remove streptavidin binders. Pour out the wells and wash 3× with PBST. Dissolve 100–500 ng biotinylated oligopeptide in PBS and incubate for 1 h at RT. Alternatively, oligopeptides with a terminal cysteine residue can be coupled to BSA and coated overnight at 4°C.

13. The washing should be performed with an ELISA washer
(e.g. TECAN Columbus Plus) to increase the stringency
and reproducibility. To remove antigen or blocking solutions wash 3× with PBST ("standard washing protocol"
for TECAN washer). If no ELISA washer is available, wash
manually 3× with PBST.
After binding of antibody phage, wash 10× with PBST
("stringent bottom washing protocol" in case of TECAN
washer). If no ELISA washer is available, wash manually
10× with PBST and 10× with PBS. For stringent off-rate
selection increase the number of washing steps or additionally incubate the microtitre plate in 1 L PBS for several
days.

14. Phagemids like pSEX81 (41) or pHAL14 (32, 44, 56)
have coding sequences for a trypsin specific cleavage
site between the antibody fragment gene and the gIII.
Trypsin also cleaves within antibody fragments but does
not degrade the phage particles including the pIII that
mediates the binding of the phage to the F pili of *E. coli*
required for the infection. We observed that proteolytic
cleavage of the antibody fragments from the antibody::pIII
fusion by trypsin not only increases the elution but also
enhances the infection rate of eluted phage particles, especially when using Hyperphage as helperphage (68–70).

15. The high concentration of glucose is necessary to efficiently
repress the lac promoter controlling the antibody::pIII
fusion gene on the phagemid. Low glucose concentrations
lead to an inefficient repression of the lac promoter and
background expression of the antibody::pIII fusion protein. Background antibody expression is a strong selection pressure frequent causing mutations in the phagemid,
especially in the promoter region and the antibody::pIII
fusion gene. Bacteria with this kind of mutations in
the phagemids proliferate faster than bacteria with non-
mutated phagemids. Therefore, the 100 mM glucose must
be included in every step of *E. coli* cultivation except during
the phage production!

16. If the bacteria have reached O.D.$_{600}$ ∼ 0,5 before they are
needed, store the culture immediately on ice to maintain
the F pili on the *E. coli* cells for several hours. M13K07
helperphage (kan$^+$) or other scFv-phage (amp$^+$) can be
used as positive control to check the infectibility of the *E.
coli* cells.

17. If the antibody gene library is packaged using Hyperphage,
the titre of the eluted phage after the second panning may

not increase as strongly or even decreases slightly due to the change from oligovalent to monovalent display.

18. Check all solutions for phage contamination. To check the PBS or PEG solutions use 10 µl of these solution for *E. coli* "infection." In parallel plate out non-infected XL1-Blue MRF' to check the bacteria. We recommend to clean the working place each time with virus inactivating solutions (e.g. Barrycidal 36, BIO-HIT, Germany) and to use filter tips for pipetting!

19. Antibody phage which bind unspecifically are usually enriched during panning. These unspecific binding often results from misfolded or incomplete antibodies. They often bind to BSA, Streptavidin and plastic surfaces.

20. Use the polyclonal antibody phage ELISA to select the suitable panning round for picking monoclonals.

21. We recommend picking only 92 clones. Use the wells H3, H6, H9 and H12 for controls. H3 and H6 are negative controls – these wells will not be inoculated and not used for the following ELISA with soluble antibodies. We inoculate the wells H9 and H12 with a clone containing a phagemid encoding a known antibody fragment. In ELISA, the wells H9 and H12 are coated with the antigen corresponding to the control antibody fragment in order to check scFv production and ELISA.

22. The appropriate IPTG concentration for induction of antibody or antibody::pIII expression depends on the vector design. A concentration of 50 µM was well suited for vectors with a Lac promoter like pSEX81 (41), pIT2 (71), pHENIX (72) and pHAL14 (32, 44, 56). The method for the production of soluble antibodies works with vectors with (e.g. pHAL14) and without (e.g. pSEX81) an amber stop codon between antibody fragment and gIII. If the vector has no amber stop codon the antibody::pIII fusion protein will be produced (73). Buffered culture media and the addition of saccharose enhances the production of many but not all scFvs. We observed that antibody::pIII fusion proteins and antibody phage sometimes show differences in antigen binding in comparison to soluble antibody fragments because some antibodies can bind the corresponding antigen only as pIII fusion. Therefore, we recommend to perform the screening procedure only by using soluble antibody fragment, to avoid false positive binders.

23. The background (noise) signals should be about $O.D._{450}$ ~ 0.02 after 5–30 min TMB incubation time.

Acknowledgements

We thank Stefan Dübel and Torsten Meyer for discussion and corrections on the manuscript. We gratefully acknowledge the financial support by the German ministry of education and research (BMBF, SMP "Antibody Factory" in the NGFN2 program).

References

1. Dübel, S. (2007) Recombinant therapeutic antibodies. *Appl Microbiol Biotechnol 74*, 723–729.
2. Coiffier, B. (2008) Monoclonal antibodies in the treatment of malignant lymphomas. *Adv Exp Med Biol 610*, 155–176.
3. Cao, Y. (2008) Molecular mechanisms and therapeutic development of angiogenesis inhibitors. *Adv Cancer Res 100*, 113–131.
4. Jones, S. E. (2008) Metastatic breast cancer: the treatment challenge. *Clin Breast Cancer 8*, 224–233.
5. Chatenoud, L., and Bluestone, J. A. (2007) CD3-specific antibodies: a portal to the treatment of autoimmunity. *Nat Rev Immunol 7*, 622–632.
6. Courtenay-Luck, N. S., Epenetos, A. A., Moore, R., Larche, M., Pectasides, D., Dhokia, B., and Ritter, M. A. (1986) Development of primary and secondary immune responses to mouse monoclonal antibodies used in the diagnosis and therapy of malignant neoplasms. *Cancer Res 46*, 6489–6493.
7. Moroney, S., and Plückthun, A. (2005) Modern antibody technology: the impact on drug development. In: Knäblein, J. (ed.) *Modern Biopharmaceuticals*. Wiley-VCH, Weinheim, pp. 1147–1186.
8. Moss, M. L., Sklair-Tavron, L., and Nudelman, R. (2008) Drug insight: tumor necrosis factor-converting enzyme as a pharmaceutical target for rheumatoid arthritis. *Nat Clin Pract Rheumatol 4*, 300–309.
9. Dalle, S., Thieblemont, C., Thomas, L., and Dumontet, C. (2008) Monoclonal antibodies in clinical oncology. *Anti-Can Agents Med Chem 8*, 523–532.
10. Alonso-Ruiz, A., Pijoan, J. I., Ansuategui, E., Urkaregi, A., Calabozo, M., and Quintana, A. (2008) Tumor necrosis factor alpha drugs in rheumatoid arthritis: systematic review and metaanalysis of efficacy and safety. *BMC Musculoskeletal Disord 9*, 52.
11. Osbourn, J., Groves, M., and Vaughan, T. (2005) From rodent reagents to human therapeutics using antibody guided selection. *Methods 36*, 61–68.
12. Fishwild, D. M. et al. (1996) High-avidity human IgG kappa monoclonal antibodies from a novel strain of minilocus transgenic mice. *Nat Biotechnol 14*, 845–851.
13. Lonberg, N., and Huszar, D. (1995) Human antibodies from transgenic mice. *Int Rev Immunol 13*, 65–93.
14. Jakobovits, A. (1995) Production of fully human antibodies by transgenic mice. *Curr Opin Biotechnol 6*, 561–566.
15. Winter, G., and Milstein, C. (1991) Man-made antibodies. *Nature 349*, 293–299.
16. Huse, W. D., Sastry, L., Iverson, S. A., Kang, A. S., Alting-Mees, M., Burton, D. R., Benkovic, S. J., and Lerner, R. A. (1989) Generation of a large combinatorial library of the immunoglobulin repertoire in phage lambda. *Science 246*, 1275–1281.
17. Smith, G. P. (1985) Filamentous fusion phage: novel expression vectors that display cloned antigens on the virion surface. *Science 228*, 1315–1317.
18. McCafferty, J., Griffiths, A. D., Winter, G., and Chiswell, D. J. (1990) Phage antibodies: filamentous phage displaying antibody variable domains. *Nature 348*, 552–554.
19. Breitling, F., Dübel, S., Seehaus, T., Klewinghaus, I., and Little, M. (1991) A surface expression vector for antibody screening. *Gene 104*, 147–153.
20. Clackson, T., Hoogenboom, H. R., Griffiths, A. D., and Winter, G. (1991) Making antibody fragments using phage display libraries. *Nature 352*, 624–628.
21. Hoogenboom, H. R., Griffiths, A. D., Johnson, K. S., Chiswell, D. J., Hudson, P., and Winter, G. (1991) Multi-subunit proteins on the surface of filamentous phage: methodologies for displaying antibody (Fab) heavy and light chains. *Nucleic Acids Res 19*, 4133–4137.
22. Marks, J. D., Hoogenboom, H. R., Bonnert, T. P., McCafferty, J., Griffiths, A. D., and Winter, G. (1991) By-passing immunization.

Human antibodies from V-gene libraries displayed on phage. *J Mol Biol* 222, 581–597.

23. Barbas, C. F., Kang, A. S., Lerner, R. A., and Benkovic, S. J. (1991) Assembly of combinatorial antibody libraries on phage surfaces: the gene III site. *Proc Natl Acad Sci USA* 88, 7978–7982.

24. Mazor, Y., Van Blarcom, T., Mabry, R., Iverson, B. L., and Georgiou, G. (2007) Isolation of engineered, full-length antibodies from libraries expressed in Escherichia coli. *Nat Biotechnol* 25, 563–565.

25. Simmons, L. C. et al. (2002) Expression of full-length immunoglobulins in Escherichia coli: rapid and efficient production of aglycosylated antibodies. *J Immunol Methods* 263, 133–147.

26. Thie, H., Voedisch, B., Dübel, S., Hust, M., and Schirrmann, T. (2009) Affinity maturation by phage display. *Methods Mol Biol* 525, 309–322.

27. Hanes, J., and Plückthun, A. (1997) In vitro selection and evolution of functional proteins by using ribosome display. *Proc Natl Acad Sci USA* 94, 4937–4942.

28. He, M., and Taussig, M. J. (1997) Antibody-ribosome-mRNA (ARM) complexes as efficient selection particles for in vitro display and evolution of antibody combining sites. *Nucleic Acids Res* 25, 5132–5134.

29. Roberts, R. W., and Szostak, J. W. (1997) RNA-peptide fusions for the in vitro selection of peptides and proteins. *Proc Natl Acad Sci USA* 94, 12297–12302.

30. Boder, E. T., and Wittrup, K. D. (1997) Yeast surface display for screening combinatorial polypeptide libraries. *Nat Biotechnol* 15, 553–557.

31. Thie, H., Meyer, T., Schirrmann, T., Hust, M., and Dübel, S. (2008) Phage display derived therapeutic antibodies. *Curr Pharm Biotechnol* 9, 439–446.

32. Pelat, T., Hust, M., Laffly, E., Condemine, F., Bottex, C., Vidal, D., Lefranc, M., Dübel, S., and Thullier, P. (2007) High-affinity, human antibody-like antibody fragment (single-chain variable fragment) neutralizing the lethal factor (LF) of Bacillus anthracis by inhibiting protective antigen-LF complex formation. *Antimicrob Agents Chemother* 51, 2758–2764.

33. de Haard, H. J., van Neer, N., Reurs, A., Hufton, S. E., Roovers, R. C., Henderikx, P., de Bruïne, A. P., Arends, J. W., and Hoogenboom, H. R. (1999) A large non-immunized human Fab fragment phage library that permits rapid isolation and kinetic analysis of high affinity antibodies. *J Biol Chem* 274, 18218–18230.

34. Pini, A., Viti, F., Santucci, A., Carnemolla, B., Zardi, L., Neri, P., and Neri, D. (1998) Design and use of a phage display library. Human antibodies with subnanomolar affinity against a marker of angiogenesis eluted from a two-dimensional gel. *J Biol Chem* 273, 21769–21776.

35. Hoet, R. M. et al. (2005) Generation of high-affinity human antibodies by combining donor-derived and synthetic complementarity-determining-region diversity. *Nat Biotechnol* 23, 344–348.

36. Hayashi, N., Welschof, M., Zewe, M., Braunagel, M., Dübel, S., Breitling, F., and Little, M. (1994) Simultaneous mutagenesis of antibody CDR regions by overlap extension and PCR. *Biotechniques* 17, 310–315.

37. Knappik, A., Ge, L., Honegger, A., Pack, P., Fischer, M., Wellnhofer, G., Hoess, A., Wölle, J., Plückthun, A., and Virnekäs, B. (2000) Fully synthetic human combinatorial antibody libraries (HuCAL) based on modular consensus frameworks and CDRs randomized with trinucleotides. *J Mol Biol* 296, 57–86.

38. Sblattero, D., and Bradbury, A. (2000) Exploiting recombination in single bacteria to make large phage antibody libraries. *Nat Biotechnol* 18, 75–80.

39. Hust, M., and Dübel, S. (2004) Mating antibody phage display with proteomics. *Trends Biotechnol* 22, 8–14.

40. Hust, M., Dübel, S., and Schirrmann, T. (2007) Selection of recombinant antibodies from antibody gene libraries. *Methods Mol Biol* 408, 243–255.

41. Welschof, M., Terness, P., Kipriyanov, S. M., Stanescu, D., Breitling, F., Dörsam, H., Dübel, S., Little, M., and Opelz, G. (1997) The antigen-binding domain of a human IgG-anti-F(ab')2 autoantibody. *Proc Natl Acad Sci USA* 94, 1902–1907.

42. Johansen, L. K., Albrechtsen, B., Andersen, H. W., and Engberg, J. (1995) pFab60: a new, efficient vector for expression of antibody Fab fragments displayed on phage. *Protein Eng* 8, 1063–1067.

43. Little, M. et al. (1999) Generation of a large complex antibody library from multiple donors. *J Immunol Methods* 231, 3–9.

44. Kirsch, M., Hülseweh, B., Nacke, C., Rülker, T., Schirrmann, T., Marschall, H., Hust, M., and Dübel, S. (2008) Development of human antibody fragments using antibody phage display for the detection and diagnosis of Venezuelan equine encephalitis virus (VEEV). *BMC Biotechnol* 8, 66.

45. McCafferty, J., Fitzgerald, K. J., Earnshaw, J., Chiswell, D. J., Link, J., Smith, R., and

Kenten, J. (1994) Selection and rapid purification of murine antibody fragments that bind a transition-state analog by phage display. *Appl Biochem Biotechnol 47*, 157–171.

46. Vaughan, T. J., Williams, A. J., Pritchard, K., Osbourn, J. K., Pope, A. R., Earnshaw, J. C., McCafferty, J., Hodits, R. A., Wilton, J., and Johnson, K. S. (1996) Human antibodies with sub-nanomolar affinities isolated from a large non-immunized phage display library. *Nat Biotechnol 14*, 309–314.

47. Krebber, A., Bornhauser, S., Burmester, J., Honegger, A., Willuda, J., Bosshard, H. R., and Plückthun, A. (1997) Reliable cloning of functional antibody variable domains from hybridomas and spleen cell repertoires employing a reengineered phage display system. *J Immunol Methods 201*, 35–55.

48. Shirai, H., Kidera, A., and Nakamura, H. (1999) H3-rules: identification of CDR-H3 structures in antibodies. *FEBS Lett 455*, 188–197.

49. Akamatsu, Y., Cole, M. S., Tso, J. Y., and Tsurushita, N. (1993) Construction of a human Ig combinatorial library from genomic V segments and synthetic CDR3 fragments. *J Immunol 151*, 4651–4659.

50. Hoogenboom, H. R., and Winter, G. (1992) By-passing immunisation. Human antibodies from synthetic repertoires of germline VH gene segments rearranged in vitro. *J Mol Biol 227*, 381–388.

51. Nissim, A., Hoogenboom, H. R., Tomlinson, I. M., Flynn, G., Midgley, C., Lane, D., and Winter, G. (1994) Antibody fragments from a 'single pot' phage display library as immunochemical reagents. *EMBO J 13*, 692–698.

52. Desiderio, A., Franconi, R., Lopez, M., Villani, M. E., Viti, F., Chiaraluce, R., Consalvi, V., Neri, D., and Benvenuto, E. (2001) A semi-synthetic repertoire of intrinsically stable antibody fragments derived from a single-framework scaffold. *J Mol Biol 310*, 603–615.

53. Barbas, C. F., Bain, J. D., Hoekstra, D. M., and Lerner, R. A. (1992) Semisynthetic combinatorial antibody libraries: a chemical solution to the diversity problem. *Proc Natl Acad Sci USA. 89*, 4457–4461.

54. Jirholt, P., Ohlin, M., Borrebaeck, C. A., and Söderlind, E. (1998) Exploiting sequence space: shuffling in vivo formed complementarity determining regions into a master framework. *Gene 215*, 471–476.

55. Söderlind, E. et al. (2000) Recombining germline-derived CDR sequences for creating diverse single-framework antibody libraries. *Nat Biotechnol 18*, 852–856.

56. Schütte, M., Thullier, P., Pelat, T., Wezler, X., Rosenstock, P., Hinz, D., Kirsch, M.I., Hasenberg, M., Frank, R., Schirrmann, T., Gunzer, M., Hust, M., and Dübel, S. (2009) Identification of a putative Crf splice variant and generation of recombinant antibodies for the specific detection of Aspergillus fumigatus. *PLoS ONE 4*, e6625.

57. Løset, G. A., Løbersli, I., Kavlie, A., Stacy, J. E., Borgen, T., Kausmally, L., Hvattum, E., Simonsen, B., Hovda, M. B., and Brekke, O. H. (2005) Construction, evaluation and refinement of a large human antibody phage library based on the IgD and IgM variable gene repertoire. *J Immunol Methods. 299*, 47–62.

58. Sheets, M. D. et al. (1998) Efficient construction of a large nonimmune phage antibody library: the production of high-affinity human single-chain antibodies to protein antigens. *Proc Natl Acad Sci USA 95*, 6157–6162.

59. Waterhouse, P., Griffiths, A. D., Johnson, K. S., and Winter, G. (1993) Combinatorial infection and in vivo recombination: a strategy for making large phage antibody repertoires. *Nucleic Acids Res 21*, 2265–2266.

60. Griffiths, A. D., Williams, S. C., Hartley, O., Tomlinson, I. M., Waterhouse, P., Crosby, W. L., Kontermann, R. E., Jones, P. T., Low, N. M., and Allison, T. J. (1994) Isolation of high affinity human antibodies directly from large synthetic repertoires. *EMBO J 13*, 3245–3260.

61. Geoffroy, F., Sodoyer, R., and Aujame, L. (1994) A new phage display system to construct multicombinatorial libraries of very large antibody repertoires. *Gene 151*, 109–113.

62. Parmley, S. F., and Smith, G.,P. (1988) Antibody-selectable filamentous fd phage vectors: affinity purification of target genes. *Gene 73*, 305–318.

63. Hawlisch, H., Müller, M., Frank, R., Bautsch, W., Klos, A., and Köhl, J. (2001) Site-specific anti-C3a receptor single-chain antibodies selected by differential panning on cellulose sheets. *Anal Biochem 293*, 142–145.

64. Moghaddam, A., Borgen, T., Stacy, J., Kausmally, L., Simonsen, B., Marvik, O. J., Brekke, O. H., and Braunagel, M. (September 2003) Identification of scFv antibody fragments that specifically recognise the heroin metabolite 6-monoacetylmorphine but not morphine. *J Immunol Methods 280*, 139–155.

65. Hust, M., Maiss, E., Jacobsen, H., and Reinard, T. (2002) The production of a genus-specific recombinant antibody (scFv)

using a recombinant potyvirus protease. *J Virol Methods 106*, 225–233.

66. Retter, I., Althaus, H. H., Münch, R., and Müller, W. (2005) VBASE2, an integrative V gene database. *Nucleic Acids Res 33*, D671-D674.

67. Hust, M., Jostock, T., Menzel, C., Voedisch, B., Mohr, A., Brenneis, M., Kirsch, M. I., Meier, D., and Dübel, S. (2007) Single chain Fab (scFab) fragment. *BMC Biotechnol 7,*14.

68. Rondot, S., Koch, J., Breitling, F., and Dübel, S. (2001) A helper phage to improve single-chain antibody presentation in phage display. *Nat Biotechnol 19*, 75–78.

69. Soltes, G., Hust, M., Ng, K. K. Y., Bansal, A., Field, J., Stewart, D. I. H., Dübel, S., Cha, S., and Wiersma, E. J. (2007) On the influence of vector design on antibody phage display. *J Biotechnol 127*, 626–637.

70. Hust, M., Meysing, M., Schirrmann, T., Selke, M., Meens, J., Gerlach, G., and Dübel, S. (2006) Enrichment of open

reading frames presented on bacteriophage M13 using hyperphage. *Biotechniques 41*, 335–342.

71. Goletz, S., Christensen, P. A., Kristensen, P., Blohm, D., Tomlinson, I., Winter, G., and Karsten, U. (2002) Selection of large diversities of antiidiotypic antibody fragments by phage display. *J Mol Biol 315*, 1087–1097.

72. Finnern, R., Pedrollo, E., Fisch, I., Wieslander, J., Marks, J. D., Lockwood, C. M., and Ouwehand, W. H. (1997) Human autoimmune anti-proteinase 3 scFv from a phage display library. *Clin Exp Immunol 107*, 269–281.

73. Mersmann, M., Schmidt, A., Tesar, M., Schöneberg, A., Welschof, M., Kipriyanov, S., Terness, P., Little, M., Pfizenmaier, K., and Moosmayer, D. (1998) Monitoring of scFv selected by phage display using detection of scFv-pIII fusion proteins in a microtiter scale assay. *J Immunol Methods 220*, 51–58.

Chapter 12

Identification of Immunogenic Peptides of the Self-Tumor Antigen: Our Experience with Telomerase Reverse Transcriptase

Xochitl Cortez-Gonzalez and Maurizio Zanetti

Abstract

The general approach, termed reverse immunology, to predict and identify immunogenic peptides from the sequence of a gene product of interest has been postulated to be a particularly efficient, high-throughput approach to discover tumor antigens. This laboratory has successfully identified immunogenic peptides of the human telomerase reverse transcriptase (hTERT), a self-tumor antigen, by using a multi-step approach. These steps include the following: the use of predictive bioinformatics algorithms, molecular methods to identify tumor-specific transcripts, prediction of proteasomal cleavage sites, peptide-binding prediction to HLA molecules and experimental validation, assessment of the in vitro and in vivo immunogenic potential of selected peptide antigens, isolation of specific cytolytic T lymphocyte clones, and final validation in functional assays of tumor cell recognition. This laboratory, and others have used similar methods to identify immunogenic peptides of self-tumor antigens, and many of those peptides are included in vaccines currently tested in clinical trials.

Key words: Telomerase, MHC I, immunogenicity, affinity, peptides.

1. Introduction

The concept of vaccination against cancer comes from the observation that immune responses, albeit weak, have been detected in cancer patients against overexpressed self-tumor antigens; therefore, these antigens have become ideal targets for active and passive immunotherapy.

P. Yotnda (ed.), *Immunotherapy of Cancer*, Methods in Molecular Biology 651,
DOI 10.1007/978-1-60761-786-0_12, © Springer Science+Business Media, LLC 2010

Adaptive responses are mediated by CD8 and CD4 T cells and are based on the recognition of peptide epitopes derived from tumor antigens expressed in association with major histocompatibility complex (MHC) molecules or human leukocyte antigen (HLA) on the surface of tumor cells. CD8 T cells recognize antigen presented through MHC Class I molecules expressed at the surface of every nucleated cell after antigen peptides have been processed inside the cell and exported to the cell surface through the endogenous pathway. Through this pathway an antigen-presenting cell (APC) or a tumor cell can activate CD8 T cells and induce cytotoxic T lymphocytes (CTL) responses. CTL constitute the main effector arm of the adaptive responses against tumors, while CD4 T cells provide help for the development of efficient CTL responses. In animals, control of tumor growth in vivo through CTL specific for tumor antigens has been documented in many systems.

Vaccines to induce T-cell responses against self-tumor antigens need to overcome a variety of barriers. Among them are two prominent obstacles. One is the ability to identify antigens that could help in the widest variety of tumors. The second is the possibility of selecting antigen peptides that can be used in the widest spectrum of MHC specificities.

The large degree of MHC polymorphism is an important factor to be taken into account in the identification and selection of these antigen peptides for the development of epitope-based vaccines. The HLA polymorphism tends to concentrate in hypervariable regions that correspond to MHC-binding pockets engaging specific "anchor" residues of their peptide ligands. Different HLA molecules are characterized by different ligand specificities, revealing allele-specific motifs. Sette et al. has revealed a way to simplify epitope selection by identifying peptides capable of binding multiple HLA molecules: grouping HLA alleles into large supertype families. A HLA supertype is defined by the ability of a peptide to bind to multiple HLA molecules (supermotif). The HLA allelic variants that bind peptides possessing a particular HLA supermotif are referred to as an HLA supertype (1, 2). For instance, peptides that bind to supertypes A2, A3, and B7 cover 86% of the human population. Thus, utilizing the supertype working model the generation of peptide-based vaccines for the human population becomes a feasible task.

Telomerase is a ribonucleoprotein complex that preserves the end of chromosomes during replication, to ensure genomic integrity during cell division. Its gradual loss is implicated in cell senescence and differentiation. Its maintenance is crucial to cell renewal of stem cells. Telomerase activity is detected in > 80% of all cancers, regardless of origin or type, but not in normal tissue.

For this reason, we and others proposed telomerase reverse transcriptase as the first universal cancer antigen. This laboratory has successfully identified HLA-A2 and HLA-B7 restricted telomerase peptides. Thus, demonstrating that although telomerase is per se a self antigen, the human CD8 T repertoire possesses precursors for it. CTL induced by in vitro immunization using PBMC from cancer patients recognize and kill tumor cells representative of different types of cancers in a MHC-restricted fashion (3). HLA-A2 restricted CTL against the same high-affinity hTRT peptide identified in this laboratory have been confirmed by other groups (4). Finally, this laboratory has used the available tools to generate and identify repertoire selection in vivo (5, 6). Using a similar approach analogous findings have been made by others (7).

These studies have materialized in a selection of candidate peptides for inclusion in the first genetic vaccine against HLA-A2 restricted hTRT peptides in humans in prostate cancer (8). Several other human phase 1 clinical trials have been completed in cancer patients of different types, demonstrating that hTRT-specific immune responses can be safely induced in patients and impact on clinical outcomes (9–11).

This chapter describes the multi-step approach (*see* **Fig. 12.1**) taken by this laboratory in order to identify immunogenic peptides restricted to MHC class I from human telomerase reverse transcriptase (3, 5, 12).

Multi-step approach to select immunogenic peptides of tumor antigens

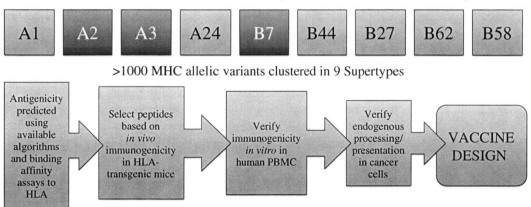

Fig. 12.1. Multi-step approach described herein used to identify immunogenic peptides of tumor antigens for vaccine design. The boxes of supertypes A2, A3, and B7 constitute together 86% of the human population.

2. Materials

2.1. Predictive Algorithms

2.1.1. HLA-Restricted Peptide Predictive Algorithms

1. *BIMAS,* which is based upon on highly favorable and unfavorable dominant anchor residues, as well as auxiliary anchor residues, scores peptides according to a coefficient (13) (access via: www-bimas.cit.nih.gov/molbio/hla_bind/).

2. *SYFPEITHI,* which is based on known T-cell epitopes and MHC ligands (14, 15) (access via: www.syfpeithi.de).

2.1.2. Proteasome Cleavage Predictive Algorithms

PAProC, prediction database for proteasomal cleavages, a computer-based theoretical model for the cleavage of substrate proteins by yeast and human 20S proteasomes (16, 17) (access via: www.paproc.de/).

2.2. Synthetic Peptides

1. Synthetic peptides can be purchased from several companies. This laboratory has purchased peptides from the Peptide Synthesis Core Facility of Ohio State University (Columbus, OH) and Proimmune (Oxford, UK).

2.3. In Vivo Immunization of HLA Transgenic Mice

1. HLA transgenic mice (HLA-A2: Jackson Laboratories, Barharbord, Maine; HLA-B7: Francois Lemmonier, Institut Pasteur, Paris, via Charles River, Lyon, France; and other laboratories for the other HLA transgenic mice).

2. Synthetic peptide diluted in dimethyl sulfoxide (DMSO) or 1× phosphate buffered saline (PBS) (depending on peptide solubility).

3. Incomplete Freund's adjuvant (Sigma, St Louis, MO).

2.4. Generation of Mouse CTL

1. RPMI-1640 medium containing 10% heat inactivated fetal bovine serum, 2 mM glutamine, 5×10^{-5} M 2-mercaptoethanol, 50 µg/ml streptomycin, and 50 µg/ml penicillin (complete medium).

2. Bacterial lipopolysaccharides, cell culture grade (Sigma, St Louis, MO).

3. Dextran, cell culture grade (Sigma, St Louis, MO).

4. hr IL-2.

5. Gamma irradiator.

6. Autologous HLA transgenic mouse splenocytes, for restimulations and CTL maintenance.

2.5. In Vitro Immunization of Human PBMC

1. RPMI 1640 medium containing 10% heat-inactivated human AB$^+$ serum, 2 mM glutamine, 50 μg/ml strepto-mycin, and 50 μg/ml penicillin (complete human media).

2. Ficoll hypaque (Sigma, St Louis, MO).

3. Synthetic peptide (product information found in **Section 2.2**).

4. HLA-matching human PBMC.

5. Gamma Irradiator.

6. hr IL-2.

2.6. CTL Assay

1. Target cells: mouse HLA-matching RMAS or RMA cells; HLA-matching human T2 cells, and HLA-matching human cancer cells (ATCC, Manassas, VA).

2. Synthetic peptide (product information found in **Section 2.2**).

3. ^{51}Cr (Perkin Elmer, Waltham, MA).

4. Scintillation cocktail buffer, OptiPhase "supermix" (Perkin Elmer, Waltham, MA).

5. Tween.

6. LKB Wallac beta plate Counter (Perkin Elmer, Waltham, MA).

2.7. Generation of Human CTL

1. hr IL-2 (use fresh).

2. hr IL-7 (use fresh).

2.8. Tetramer Staining

1. Tetramer (product information found in **Section 3.3.8**).

2. Anti-human CD8a mAb.

3. Hank's balanced saline solution.

4. Bovine serum albumin (BSA).

5. FACS Calibur, Bekton Dickinson (BD Biosciences, San Jose, CA).

3. Methods

3.1. Selection of Peptides with Predictive Algorithms

To limit the number of candidate peptides from the full length of a self-tumor antigen to a manageable panel, it is recommended to select a pool of ten peptides for each HLA molecule based on their binding affinity and proteasome cleavage (*see* **Note 1**).

3.1.1. Select a Pool of ten candidate Peptides by HLA Binding Affinity Algorithms

Our laboratory has used BIMAS and SYFPEITHI.

1. For SYFPEITHI, follow the website's instructions (*see* materials for website):

    1. Select "epitope prediction."

    2. Enter the full protein sequence of the selected tumor antigen, the HLA type, and the preferred peptide size (8-, 9-, and 10-mer) and proceed to run the prediction (*see* **Note 2**).

    3. For a 400 amino acid protein, the best peptides are within the top eight scored peptides (*see* **Note 3**).

2. For BIMAS, follow the website's instructions (*see* materials for website):

    1. Enter the full protein sequence of the selected tumor antigen, the HLA type, peptide size, and proceed to run the prediction.

    2. Compare the top ten predicted peptides with the top eight predicted by SYFPEITHI, and make a list of ten peptides.

3.1.2. For Complete Peptide Selection

For a more complete peptide selection, we also consider the proteasome cleavage of the protein of interest, by predicting if the selected peptides (by binding affinity, *see* **Section 3.1.1.**) would be cleaved at the C-terminus. To date, an updated proteasome algorithm is available as a neural network (access via: www.cbs.dtu.dk/services/NetChop/) (18).

1. Follow PAProC website's instructions (*see* materials for website access).

2. Enter the full protein sequence.

3. Select human proteasome wild type III (*see* website description for each proteasome model type) and run the prediction.

4. Find whether or not the candidate predicted peptides C-terminus are cleaved (*see* **Note 4**).

3.2. MHC Binding Assays

3.2.1. Relative Avidity Measurements

By measuring the avidity of the selected peptides to the HLA type of interest, one can narrow the list to only those that have actual high avidity.

1. Synthesize top 8–10 list of predicted peptides.

2. Measure their relative avidity using a MHC stabilization assay on HLA$^+$ (e.g. T2, T2-B7) cells in comparison with

a reference peptide as described in (19). However, we recommend using the following assay, described by Sidney et al (20, 21).

3. Incubate 1–10 nM of radiolabeled peptide with 1 µM to 1 nM of purified MHC in the presence of 1–3 µM human β2-microglobulin, and a cocktail of protease inhibitors.

4. Incubate for 48 h at room temperature. Binding of the radiolabled peptide to the corresponding MHC class I molecule is determined by capturing MHC/peptide complexes on Greiner Lumitrac 600 microplates coated with the W6/32 antibody, and measuring bound cpm using the TopCount microscintillation counter.

3.2.2. Supertype Binding Analysis

This analysis is recommended to broaden the HLA spectrum to which the select peptides can theoretically bind. This competition assay is described in detail by Sidney et al. (22), in which the concentration of peptide yielding 50% inhibition of the binding (IC_{50}) of the radiolabeled peptide is calculated. In summary:

1. Peptides are tested at different concentrations covering a 100,000-fold dose range, and in three or more independent assays.

2. Measure of the radiolabeled MHC/peptide complex is performed as previously described in **Section 3.2.1**, Step 4.

3. Based on the peptide concentration added to the competition assays, where [label]<[MHC] and IC_{50} U$\geq$ [MHC], the measured IC50 values are reasonable approximations of the true K_d values.

3.3. In Vivo Mouse Immunization Procedures

The first concrete step in assessing the potential immunogenicity of a selected peptide is the choice of the most effective epitopes that may be recognized by T cells to effect a cellular response. This enables one to correlate each peptide's immunogenicity to the binding characteristics and the scores of the predictive algorithms.

3.3.1. Peptide Immunization

1. Prepare an emulsion containing 100 µg of the selected peptides (dissolved in DMSO) along with 120 µg of I-A^b MHC Class II helper peptide 128–140 of the hepatitis B virus core protein in incomplete Freund's adjuvant (oil fraction – comprehending 50% of the total volume), adding 1× PBS to make up to the total volume. For subcutaneous (s.c.) injections, we recommend a total volume of 100 µl per mouse.

2. Inject HLA-transgenic mice s.c. at the base of the tail.

3.3.2. Generation of CTL Lines from Peptide Immunized HLA-Transgenic Mice

To generate a CTL line from peptide-immunized mice, prepare LPS stimulated syngeneic splenocytes (stimulators) as follows:

1. Prepare stimulators: Three days before harvesting peptide immunized mouse spleens, bring autologous HLA-mice splenocytes up to 1×10^6 cells/ml in complete RPMI with 2.5 mg/ml LPS and 0.7 mg/ml dextran sulfate. Incubate these LPS blasts for three days in T75 flasks, adding up to 40 ml in each, keeping them in upright position.

2. Pool cells and wash twice in plain RPMI. Resuspend cells in ~ 10–20×10^6 cells/ml in conical tubes.

3. Irradiate cell suspension at 3000 rads. Wash twice with plain RPMI, and resuspend in 0.8 ml complete RPMI.

4. Add 5 mg of peptide to each tube. Incubate for 1 h, at 37°C. Wash twice and resuspend in complete RPMI. Bring them up to 3×10^6 cells/ml. These cells will be added to the responders at **Section 3.3.2**, Step 7.

5. Prepare responders: After 9–10 days of peptide immunization, sacrifice mice and harvest spleen.

6. Wash single cell suspension twice with complete RPMI, and bring cells up to 7×10^6 cells/ ml in complete RPMI.

7. In a 24-well plate, add 1 ml of responders at 7×10^6 cells/ml (**Section 3.3.2**, Step 6) and 1 ml of stimulators at 3×10^6 cells/ml (**Section 3.3.2**, Step 4).

8. Incubate at 37°C in a 5% CO_2 incubator. Long-term CTL lines are maintained in culture by weekly re-stimulation, *see* **Section 3.3.3**.

3.3.3. Maintenance and/or Re-stimulation of Peptide-Specific Mouse CTL Line

1. Prepare stimulators: 6–7 days after setting up the primary culture (**Section 3.3.2.**), harvest autologous HLA transgenic mouse spleens (1 spleen is enough for 30–40 wells).

2. Bring spleens into a single cell suspension in complete RPMI and wash once. Resuspend each spleen in 10 ml of complete RPMI, irradiate at 3000 rads, wash once, resuspend splenocytes in 0.8 ml of complete RPMI.

3. Add peptide (5 μg), and incubate for 1 h at 37°C in a 5% CO_2 incubator.

4. Wash twice with plain RPMI, resuspend cells at $\sim 3 \times 10^6$ cells/ml in complete RPMI.

5. Dilute freshly thawed hrIL-2 in complete RPMI, final concentration 40 U/ml. Prepare enough to add 1 ml to each well (*see* **Note 5**).

6. Add 1 ml of Stimulators (from **Section 3.3.3**, Step 4.) and 1 ml of the IL-2 supplemented RPMI (from **Section 3.3.3**, Step 5) to each well using a new 24-well plate.

7. Prepare responders: From **Section 3.3.2**, Step 8 set up (peptide specific CTL line), gently remove supernatant (media) ~1.2 ml from each well with a pipette.

8. Using a sterile disposable flexible Pasteur (transfer) pipette, resuspend gently the cells in each well, and transfer CTL to one or two wells of the new 24-well plate (from **Section 3.3.2**, Step 6) (*see* **Note 6**).

3.3.4. CTL Assay

To measure the specificity and lysis capability of the mouse CTL line generated in **Section 3.3.2.**, we suggest a 96-well plate based ^{51}Cr release assay by days 5–6 after weekly restimulation.

1. Prepare target cells: Use HLA transgenic mouse RMA cell line (described in **Section 3**). Start with a number of cells enough to have 5000 cells per well. Wash cells and resuspend them in approximately 100 μl.

2. Add 50 μCi and 2 μg of the peptide to which the CTL line is specific to; prepare another tube with target cells loaded with ^{51}Cr and an unspecific peptide (control).

3. Incubate cells for 1.5 h at 37°C.

4. While target cells are incubating, prepare effectors cells (CTL line); from their original setting (24-well plate), harvest the cells by pipetting up and down gently, and wash once.

5. For a maximum of 100:1 (effector to target) ratio, prepare effectors cells (CTL) at 5×10^6 cells/ml. In a 96-well round-bottom plate, dispense 200 μl of effector cells into the 100:1 ratio dedicated well (triplicate for each condition: specific and unspecific peptide loaded target cells). Dilute CTL 1:1 with complete medium in the 96-well plate, to obtain a serial of lower E:T ratios, i.e., 100 μl of the 100:1 into 1:1 will make a 50:1 E:T ratio (*see* **Note 7**).

6. Wash peptide-loaded/^{51}Cr labeled target cells (from **Section 3.3.4**, Step 3) twice and resuspend at 50,000 cells/ml in complete medium. Add 100 μl (5000 cells) per well on the already plated effector cells (from **Section 3.3.4**, Step 5). In addition, dispense 100 μl of target cells per well (six wells) for maximal cell lysis control (adding 100 μl of 2% triton in plain RPMI), and another six wells for spontaneous release control (adding 100 μl of complete media). Incubate plate for 4 h at 37°C.

7. Centrifuge plates at 500 rpm/5 min. Add 120 μl of scintillation buffer into a flexible 96-well microplate. Transfer 25 μl supernatant into the plate, seal, and vortex. Read plates using a LKB wallac betaplate.

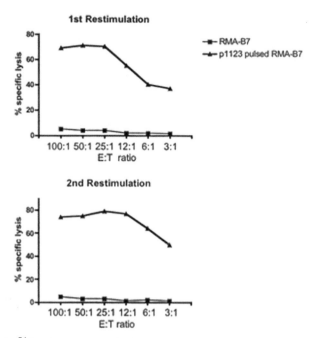

Fig. 12.2. ^{51}Cr release assay using human telomerase peptide p1123 specific mouse CTL line. CTL line was generated from peptide immunized HLA-B7 transgenic mice, as described in **Section 3.3.1**. CTL killing assays were performed 4–5 days as described in **Section 3.3.3**, after the first and second restimulation (described in **Section 3.3.2**).

8. Determine the percentage lysis based on ^{51}Cr-release compared to spontaneous and maximal release using the formula: experiment lysis – spontaneous lysis/maximallysis × 100. An example of CTL activity using telomerase peptide p1123 specific HLA-B7 transgenic mouse CTL line is shown in **Fig. 12.2**.

3.3.5. In Vitro Immunization Procedures

To further assess the immunogenicity of the selected peptide candidates as well as their ability to expand precursor CD8 T cell in HLA matching human PBMC (from normal donors or cancer patients), we suggest a miniature in vitro sensitization assay (MISA).

1. Plate 2×10^5 irradiated (6000 rads) human PBMC in 96 (flat)-well plate in 100 µl of complete human medium with 100 µg/ml of peptide. A total of 12 wells per peptide are recommended per patient/normal donor.

2. Add 2×10^5 PBMC in 100 µl of complete human medium into each well. Four days later, gently (without disturbing the bottom of the wells) replace 100 µl of medium with 100 µl of fresh complete human medium containing 80 U/ml of hrIL-2.

3. On days 6–7, split each well into two, setting up an identical 96-well plate. Add a 100 U/ml of hrIL-2 to each well.

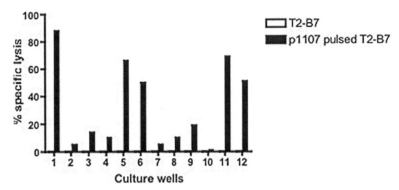

Fig. 12.3. Example of CTL induction in a miniature in vitro sensitization assay using normal donor PBMC. HLA-B7+ human PBMCs were immunized in vitro in a 96-well plate assay, and tested for specific lysis of T2-B7 pulsed with peptide on days 10–11. The micro-CTL assay was performed as described in **Section 3.3.5**.

4. On days 10–11, perform a micro-cytotoxicity assay, where the effector cells are the identical 96-well plate (from **Section 3.3.5**, Step 3), and target cells are HLA-matched peptide-loaded-T2 cells or HLA-matched human tumor cells (with no peptide). Effector cells cannot be counted based on the small number; therefore, it is recommended to split them into two, one for unspecific and specific loaded target cells. Include maximum release and spontaneous release controls, as detailed in **Section 3.3.4**.

5. Determine CTL specific lysis by comparing with spontaneous and maximum release, as well as the negative control (unspecific peptide loaded-target cells) (*see* **Note 8**). For an example of MISA results, *see* **Fig. 12.3**. Testing more than one patient/normal donor through this method helps ranking peptides based on their human immunogenicity and/or CTL repertoire (*see* **Table 12.1**).

3.3.6. Generation of Human CTL by In Vitro Peptide Immunization of Human Peripheral Blood Mononuclear Cells (PBMC)

To further confirm (1) the existence of peptide specific CTL in cancer patients or in normal donors and (2) the endogenous presentation of the peptide by tumor cells, we generate a stable human CTL line. This line is used to analyze their specificity and lysis capability toward HLA-matching-antigen+ tumor human cells.

1. Separate human PBMC by centrifugation using Ficoll-Hypaque gradient (follow manufacturer instructions). Wash twice with complete human media.

2. Plate the responders, by dispensing 5×10^5 cells/ml per well in a 24-well plate. Set apart in the incubator, while preparing stimulators (**Section 3.3.6**, Step 3).

Table 12.1
CTL response in vitro following immunization of normal donors PMBC with HLA-B7-restricted hTRT peptides

hTRT peptide	Donor 1	Donor 2	Donor 3	Donor 4	Donor 5	Donor 6	Donor 7	Donor 8	High responders/ Total	Low responders/ Total
p277	>50%	>50%	>50%	>50%	>50%	<25%	<25%	<25%	5/8	0/8
p342	>25%	>25%	>25%	>50%	0	<25%	>25%	0	1/8	4/8
p444	ND	ND	<25%	>25%	0	0	0	<25%	0/6	1/6
p464	>50%	>50%	0	>25%	<25%	<25%	<25%	0	2/8	1/8
p966	ND	ND	ND	ND	ND	ND	ND	ND	ND	ND
p1107	>50%	>50%	0	>50%	>25%	<25%	>25%	0	3/8	2/8
p1123	>50%	>50%	>50%	<25%	>50%	>50%	>50%	>50%	7/8	0/8

PBMC from HLA-B7$^+$ normal blood donors were pulsed with the candidate peptide in 96-well plate assay, called Miniature in vitro Sensitization Assay (MISA), as described in **Section 3.3.5**. Each well was tested for lysis of T2-B7 pulsed with peptide on days 10–11. A micro ^{51}Cr-release assay was performed as described in **Sections 3.3.5** and **3.3.4**. High and low responders were considered at >50 or >25% specific CTL lysis, respectively. CTL assays were performed at an approximate E:T ratio of 10:1. ND = not done.

3. Prepare stimulators, using autologous PBMC. Pulse them at 10 μg/ml of peptide for 3 h at 37°C. Irradiate at 5000 rads, wash once, and add to responder cells (**Section 3.3.6**, Step 2) at a responder to stimulator ratio ranging between 1:1 and 1:4.

4. The next day, add 12 units/ml of hrIL-2 and 30 units/ml of hrIL-7 to the culture.

5. Days 6–7 after setting the culture, CTL line needs to be re-stimulated as described in **Section 3.3.7**.

3.3.7. Maintenance or Re-stimulation of Human CTL Line

CTL line generated in **Section 3.3.6**. requires weekly restimulations with peptide-pulsed autologous adherent cells as follows:

1. Incubate autologous PBMC with 10 μg/ml of peptide in complete human media for 3 h at 37°C. Remove non-adherent cells by washing gently.

2. Incubate the non-adherent cells obtained above (**Section 3.3.7**, Step 2) with 10 μg/ml of peptide in complete human media for an additional 3 h at 37°C.

3. Harvest responders from original setting or previous stimulation (**Section 3.3.6**), wash once, and add to peptide-pulsed adherent cells at a concentration of 5×10^5 cells/ml (2 ml/well) in complete human media without peptide.

4. Add hrIL-2 and IL7 (12 and 30 U/ml, respectively) the following day. Use freshly thawed cytokines.

5. ^{51}Cr-release assay to test CTL line specificity can be done by day 4 or day 5 after re-stimulation, as described in **Section 3.3.4**; however, this time besides using HLA matching T2 cells or human target cells, use HLA matching-human cancer cells expressing the tumor antigen studied. Use at least two different cancer cell lines to assess the processing and presentation of the peptide by cancer cells.

3.3.8.
Tetramer/Pentamer
Staining of CD8 T Cells

The number and affinity of peptide specific CTL in human PBMCs can be characterized by tetramer staining.

1. HLA-pentamers containing the tumor antigen peptides can be obtained from ProImmune (UK). HLA-tetramers can be purchased from Beckman Coulter Immunomics, the NIH-sponsored Tetramer Core Facility, or other company/Institution.

2. On day 4 or day 5 after stimulation, incubate 0.5×10^6 cells from human CTL line obtained from **Section 3.3.6** with 20 µg/ml of fluorochrome-conjugated-HLA-peptide tetramer and 2 µg/ml fluorochrome-conjugated anti-human CD8a mAb in Hank's balanced saline solution containing 0.1% bovine serum albumin (BSA) and 0.05% sodium azide for 30 min at 4°C.

3. Samples are washed twice.

4. Analyze samples using a FACS Calibur Flow Cytometer, collecting 100,000 events for CD8 positive cells.

5. Report result as tetramer and CD8 double positive cells.

4. Notes

1. To date, there are mathematic models in which algorithms for peptide prediction takes into account MHC binding, proteasome cleavage, and TAP transport simultaneously (23).

2. This laboratory used HLA binding affinity algorithms to predict 9-mers, based on the fact that 9-amino-acid-long peptides are the best fit size for most HLA class I molecules (i.e., HLA-A2 and HLA-B7). Nonetheless, other groups suggest doing 8- or 10-mer peptide predictions for HLA molecules, from which naturally "occurring" 8- or 10-mer peptides have been identified.

3. SYFPEITHI has a greater predictive advantage over BIMAS for HLA-B7 restricted peptides.

4. Proteasome cleavage algorithm is used to have another point of comparison, in order to rank the peptides.

5. We use hrIL-2, since it is biologically active in human and mouse cells. We highly recommend to aliquot IL-2 in single-use vials and store them at −70°C.

6. The ratio at which CTL lines are split during re-stimulations depends on how much they have grown at the time of re-stimulation. If with naked eye cell clusters (in the bottom of the wells) can be seen, and the medium looks acidic, this will be an indication that cells are growing well, and each well needs to be split at least 1:2, in other words, 1 CTL well (responder) into two wells of stimulators. On the other hand, if there are not many cells by microscope inspection, one may want to pool two CTL (responder) wells into one (stimulator) well, or just do 1:1.

7. Decision making regarding the working E:T ratio in a CTL assay depends on the CTL specificity and ability to lyse target cells. For a new experiment we recommend to start at 100:1 and 50:1, 25:1, 12:1, and so on. Nonetheless, one can use other E:T ratios, such as 90:1, 60:1, 30:1, and 10:1. Highly specific CTL lines can kill 100% peptide loaded target cells at a 10:1 E:T ratio, or lower.

8. This assay draws positive or negative results, regarding the human immunogenicity of the investigated peptide. It is not intended as a quantitative method to determine CTL ability to kill target cells. Based on these results, one can speculate how frequent is the peptide-specific CD8 T cell repertoire in one or among all tested donors.

References

1. Sette, A., and Sidney, J. (1999) Nine major HLA class I supertypes account for the vast preponderance of HLA-A and -B polymorphism. *Immunogenetics* 50, 201–212.

2. Sette, A., Keogh, E., Ishioka, G., Sidney, J., Tangri, S., Livingston, B., McKinney, D., Newman, M., Chesnut, R., and Fikes, J. (2002) Epitope identification and vaccine design for cancer immunotherapy. *Curr Opin Investig Drugs* 3, 132–139.

3. Minev, B., Hipp, J., Firat, H., Schmidt, J. D., Langlade-Demoyen, P., and Zanetti, M. (2000) Cytotoxic T cell immunity against telomerase reverse transcriptase in humans. *Proc Natl Acad Sci U S A* 97, 4796–4801.

4. Vonderheide, R. H., Schultze, J. L., Anderson, K. S., Maecker, B., Butler, M. O., Xia, Z., Kuroda, M. J., von Bergwelt-Baildon, M.

S., Bedor, M. M., Hoar, K. M., Schnipper, D. R., Brooks, M. W., Letvin, N. L., Stephans, K. F., Wucherpfennig, K. W., Hahn, W. C., and Nadler, L. M. (2001) Equivalent induction of telomerase-specific cytotoxic T lymphocytes from tumor-bearing patients and healthy individuals. *Cancer Res* 61, 8366–8370.

5. Hernandez, J., Garcia-Pons, F., Lone, L. C., Firat, H., Schmidt, J. D., Langlade-Demoyen, P., and Zanetti, M. (2002) Identification of a human telomerase reverse transcriptase peptide of low affinity for HLA-A2.1 that induces CTL and mediates lysis of tumor cells. *Proc Natl Acad Sci U S A* 99, 12275–12280.

6. Hernandez, J., Schoeder, K., Blondelle, S. E., Pons, F. G., Lone, Y. C., Simora,

A., Langlade-Demoyen, P., Wilson, D. B., and Zanetti, M. (2004) Antigenicity and immunogenicity of peptide analogues of a low affinity peptide of the human telomerase reverse transcriptase tumor antigen. *Eur J Immunol 34*, 2331–2341.

7. Gross, D. A., Graff-Dubois, S., Opolon, P., Cornet, S. S., Alves, P., Bennaceur-Griscelli, A., Faure, O., Guillaume, P., Firat, H. H., Chouaib, S., Lemonnier, F. A., Davoust, J., Miconnet, I., Vonderheide, R. H., and Kosmatopoulos, K. (2004) High vaccination efficiency of low-affinity epitopes in antitumor immunotherapy. *J Clin Invest 113*, 425–433.

8. Zanetti, M. (2003) Protocol #0207-545: a phase I, escalating dose, open-label evaluation of safety, feasibility, and tolerability of transgenic lymphocyte immunization (TLI) vaccine subjects with histologically proven prostate adenocarcinoma. *Hum Gene Ther 14*, 301–302.

9. Cortez-Gonzalez, X., and Zanetti, M. (2007) Telomerase immunity from bench to bedside: round one. *J Transl Med 5*, 12.

10. Zanetti, M., Hernandez, X., and Langlade-Demoyen, P. (2005) Telomerase reverse transcriptase as target for anti-tumor T cell responses in humans. *Springer Semin Immunopathol 27*, 87–104.

11. Vonderheide, R. H., Domchek, S. M., Schultze, J. L., George, D. J., Hoar, K. M., Chen, D. Y., Stephans, K. F., Masutomi, K., Loda, M., Xia, Z., Anderson, K. S., Hahn, W. C., and Nadler, L. M. (2004) Vaccination of cancer patients against telomerase induces functional antitumor CD8+ T lymphocytes. *Clin Cancer Res 10*, 828–839.

12. Cortez-Gonzalez, X., Sidney, J., Adotevi, O., Sette, A., Millard, F., Lemonier, F., Langlade-Demoyen, P., and Zanetti, M. (2006) Immunogenic HLA-B7 restricted peptides of hTRT. *Int Immunol 18*, 1707–1718.

13. Parker, K. C., Bednarek, M. A., and Coligan, J. E. (1994) Scheme for ranking potential HLA-A2 binding peptides based on independent binding of individual peptide side-chains. *Journal of Immunology 152*, 163–175.

14. Rammensee, H. G., Friede, T., and Stevanoviic, S. (1995) MHC ligands and peptide motifs: first listing. *Immunogenetics 41*, 178–228.

15. Rammensee, H., Bachmann, J., Emmerich, N. P., Bachor, O. A., and Stevanovic, S. (1999) SYFPEITHI: database for MHC ligands and peptide motifs. *Immunogenetics 50*, 213–219.

16. Kuttler, C., Nussbaum, A. K., Dick, T. P., Rammensee, H. G., Schild, H., and Hadeler, K. P. (2000) An algorithm for the prediction of proteasomal cleavages. *J Mol Biol 298*, 417–429.

17. Nussbaum, A. K., Kuttler, C., Hadeler, K. P., Rammensee, H. G., and Schild, H. (2001) PAProC: a prediction algorithm for proteasomal cleavages available on the WWW. *Immunogenetics 53*, 87–94.

18. Nielsen, M., Lundegaard, C., Lund, O., and Kesmir, C. (2005) The role of the proteasome in generating cytotoxic T-cell epitopes: insights obtained from improved predictions of proteasomal cleavage. *Immunogenetics 57*, 33–41.

19. Firat, H., Garcia-Pons, F., tourdot, S., Pascolo, S., Scardino, A., Garcia, Z., Michel, M.-L., Jack, R., Jung, G., Kostmatopoulos, K., Mateo, L., Suhrbrier, A., Lemonnier, F., and Langlade-Demoyen, P. (1999) H-2 class I knockout, HLA-A2.1-transgenic mice: a versatile animal model for preclinical evaluation of antitumor immunotherapeutic strategies. *Eur. J. Immunol. 29*, 3112–3121.

20. Sidney, J., del Guercio, M. F., Southwood, S., Engelhard, V. H., Appella, E., Rammensee, H. G., Falk, K., Rotzschke, O., Takiguchi, M., Kubo, R. T., and et al. (1995) Several HLA alleles share overlapping peptide specificities. *J Immunol 154*, 247–259.

21. Sidney, J., Southwood, S., del Guercio, M. F., Grey, H. M., Chesnut, R. W., Kubo, R. T., and Sette, A. (1996) Specificity and degeneracy in peptide binding to HLA-B7-like class I molecules. *J Immunol 157*, 3480–3490.

22. Sidney, J., Southwood, S., Oseroff, C., del Guercio, M. F., Sette, A., and Grey, H. M. (2001) Measurement of MHC/peptide interactions by gel filtration. *Curr Protoc Immunol Chapter 18*, Unit 18 13.

23. Schiewe, A. J., and Haworth, I. S. (2007) Structure-based prediction of MHC-peptide association: algorithm comparison and application to cancer vaccine design. *J Mol Graph Model 26*, 667–675.

Chapter 13

Rescue, Amplification, Purification, and PEGylation of Replication Defective First-Generation Adenoviral Vectors

Michael A. Barry, Eric A. Weaver, and Sean E. Hofherr

Abstract

Adenoviral gene therapy vectors have been widely studied and used. Their extremely high transduction efficiency and gene delivery in vivo make them attractive for cancer gene therapy approaches. While they are robust, they are also very immunogenic. One approach to mitigate the immunogenicity of adenoviruses and to evade neutralizing antibodies is to coat the virus with the hydrophilic polymer polyethylene glycol (PEG) (1). This chapter details the steps involved when going from recombinant adenoviral vector plasmid all the way to validated PEGylated adenovirus product.

Key words: PEG, adenovirus, gene therapy, vector production, Ad5, polyethylene glycol, PEGylation.

1. Introduction

Human adenoviral vectors (Ad5) have been widely studied and utilized for gene therapy. Ad5 vectors when injected systemically transduce the liver at extremely high levels (2–4). The limitations of adenoviral vectors are the high toxicity and immune response of the host. Various methods have been developed to address these shortcomings. One such technique, PEGylation, is described in this chapter.

PEGylation involves the chemical conjugation of reactive polyethylene glycol (1) molecules to the virus capsid (1). The reaction is based on the chemistry of PEG molecules that are activated for covalent modification by addition of an N-hydroxysuccinimide (NHS) group. This NHS group reacts with free

P. Yotnda (ed.), *Immunotherapy of Cancer*, Methods in Molecular Biology 651,
DOI 10.1007/978-1-60761-786-0_13, © Springer Science+Business Media, LLC 2010

amines on the virus capsid proteins, mostly with lysine residues. Recent work in preclinical models has demonstrated that PEGylated vectors have a variety of advantages over the unmodified vector, including evasion of neutralizing antibodies, reduced antibody and T-cell responses against modified cells, reductions in innate immune responses and thrombocytopenia, and reduced cytokine release (5–11).

The studies performed in our lab typically utilize a 5 kDa PEG; however, multiple sizes of PEG molecules are commercially available. For example, we recently demonstrated variations in liver tropism after PEGylation with different-sized PEGs (12) and variations in the ability of Ad to drive vaccine responses (13).

This chapter details the process of PEGylating a replication defective recombinant Ad5 virus, but can be applied to any Ad5 vector. We begin with a recombinant Ad5 vector plasmid, and detail the specific techniques and methodology that our lab uses to rescue the virus from the plasmid. Next, the protocol to generate a large-scale preparation of the vector is described, followed by the purification of the virus from the cell lysate (adapted from (14)). We then discuss the process of PEGylation as well as the determination of the quality of the PEGylated Ad5. These quality control measures: CBQCA assay, particle sizing, loss if in vitro activity, and retention of systemic in vivo activity, all together ensure the virus is PEGylated. Finally, the limitations and problems we experience when PEGylating the virus are specifically mentioned with common solutions.

2. Materials

1. DNase Solution (10 mg/ml): 200 μl 1 M Tris, pH 7.4, 100 μl 5 M NaCl, 10 μl 1 M dithiothreitol (DTT), 100 μl of 10 mg/ml BSA, 4.6 ml DDI H_2O, and 100 mg DNase 1 are combined then filter sterilized. 5 ml of sterile glycerol is added and the solution is aliquoted and stored at −20°C.

2. DOC 5%: To reduce potential toxicity, this must be made in a chemical hood. 5 g of deoxycholic acid are dissolved in 100 ml of DDI H_2O in a 250-ml graduated cylinder, filter sterilized, and stored at room temperature.

3. 10X KPBS: 500 ml DDI H_2O, 80 g NaCl, 2 g KCl, 17.7 g K_2HPO_4, 2.4 g KH_2PO_4 are dissolved in up to 1 L of DDI H_2O, adjusted to a pH of 8.0, filter sterilized, and stored at room temperature.

4. 1X KPBS 0.5 M sucrose: Dissolve 171.5 g of sucrose in 10X KPBS, and up to 1 L DDI H_2O. pH to 8.0, filter sterilize, and store at 4°C.

5. CsCl Heavy: 87 ml of 1X KPBS, 53 g CsCl are combined, filter sterilized, and stored at 4°C.

6. CsCl Light: 92 ml of 1X KPBS and 26.8 g CsCl are combined, filter sterilized, and stored at 4°C.

7. 1X DPBS: 800 ml DDI H_2O, 0.2 g KCl, 0.2 g KH_2PO_4, 8.0 g NaCl, and 1.15 g Na_2HPO_4 are combined, the volume adjusted to 1 L, pH adjusted to 9.3, filter sterilized, and stored at room temperature.

8. KNO_3: 1.01 g KNO_3 in 1 L DDI H_2O is filter sterilized and stored at room temperature.

9. Pac 1: Catalog # R0547 (NEB, Ipswich, MA, USA).

10. QiaexII: 20021 (Qiagen, Valencia, CA, USA).

11. Lipofectamine 2000 (Invitrogen, Carlsbad, CA, USA).

12. DMEM High Glucose (Invitrogen, Carlsbad, CA, USA).

13. Fetal bovine serum (FBS) (Invitrogen, Carlsbad, CA, USA).

14. RNase A (Qiagen, Valencia, CA, USA).

15. 10-DG desalting column (BioRad, Hercules, CA, USA).

16. Sephadex g50 (GE Healthcare, Piscataway, NJ, USA).

17. Dextran Blue 2000 (GE Healthcare, Piscataway, NJ, USA).

18. Proteinase K (Qiagen, Valencia, CA, USA).

19. Quantitech Sybr Green Master Mix (Qiagen, Valencia, CA, USA).

20. CBQCA Protein Quantitation Kit (Invitrogen, Carlsbad, CA, USA).

21. Plate Reader: Beckman Coulter DTX 880 Multimode Detector (Beckman Coulter, Fullerton, CA).

22. 5X Reporter Lysis Buffer (Promega, Madison, WI, USA).

23. Luciferase Assay Reagent (Promega, Madison, WI, USA).

24. Particle Sizer: Brookhaven Instruments 90Plus/BI-MAS Multi Angle Particle Sizer.

3. Methods

3.1. Rescuing Virus and Generating Low Passage Stock

1. Plate 293 cells in a T25 flask for 60–80% confluency the next day (see **Note 1**).

2. Digest recombinant Ad-Easy-based plasmid with Pac1.

3. Purify DNA using QiaexII.

4. Transfect Pac I-linearized Ad genome per Lipofectamine 2000 protocol (steps 5–12) (*see* **Notes 2** and **3**).

5. Replace media in flask with 3 ml of DMEM supplemented only with 5% FBS (no antibiotic or antimycotic).

6. Add 3 μg of DNA to 500 μl of incomplete DMEM in 1.5 ml sterile microfuge tube.

7. In a separate tube, add 9 μl of Lipofectamine 2000 reagent to 500 μl of incomplete DMEM.

8. Incubate for 5 min at room temperature.

9. Combine tubes 1 and 2 together.

10. Incubate for 20 min at room temperature.

11. Add step 10 contents dropwise to flask.

12. Replace media 1 day later with complete DMEM 5% FBS with antibiotics and antimycotics.

13. Observe transfection efficiency of reporter virus; it must be ~50–70% or start over if not (*see* **Note 4**).

14. Maintain cells by removing 2/3 to 3/4 of media and replacing with DMEM with 5% FBS every 3–4 days.

15. Check cells for cytopathic effect (CPE) or virus foci regularly. Passage when significant viral spreading has occurred (*see* **Note 5**).

16. To passage, harvest cells by disrupting the monolayer with a pipette and resuspend pellet in 1 ml of 5% complete media.

17. Distribute this cellular lysate to two 1.5-ml microfuge tubes and freeze each at –80°C. One tube is backup and one tube is used for next passage (*see* **Note 6**).

18. Freeze–thaw prior passage 3X, spin in microfuge for 5 min at 750 rcf, and apply supernatant to one T25 flask with 60–80% confluent 293 cells.

19. Passage (repeat steps 16–18) onto T25 flasks until complete CPE in 2–3 days is observed.

20. When complete CPE in 2–3 days is observed, repeat steps 5.3–5.4. Freeze–thaw 3X, remove debris, and save supernatant as low-passage stock.

3.2. Amplification from Low-Passage Stock

1. Plate T25 flask with 293 or N3S cells (*see* **Note 7**).

2. Infect flask with 100–200 μl of virus stock.

3. Wait for complete cytopathic effect (CPE) (should be 2–3 days, if not repeat).

4. Harvest cells, pellet, and resuspend in 1 ml of with DMEM with 5% FBS.

5. Infect a T75 flask with supernatant; wait for CPE.

6. Harvest cells, pellet, and resuspend in 2 ml of with DMEM with 5% FBS.

7. Infect T225 with supernatant; wait for CPE.

8. Harvest cells, pellet, and resuspend in 5 ml of with DMEM with 5% FBS.

9. Infect five T225 flasks with supernatant, wait for CPE.

10. Harvest cells, pellet, and resuspend in 5 ml of with DMEM with 5% FBS.

11. Seed cell factory or spinner flask with 6–8 T225 flasks (*see* **Note 8**).

12. Infect confluent cell factory or spinner flask with cell free lysate of (5) T225 infected as described above.

13. After 72 h harvest cells and spin down at 500 rcf for 15 min.

14. Remove supernatant and resuspend the cell pellet in with DMEM with 5% FBS totaling a 15-ml volume in a 50-ml conical tube.

15. Freeze this tube or band virus using protocol (*see* **Note 9**).

3.3. CsCl Purification of Large Scale Ad

1. Add 2 ml of 5% deoxycholine (DOC) solution to sample from 2.15, invert 4–6 times to mix completely.

2. Incubate room temperature 30 min inverting every 5 min. Solution should become viscous and snotty.

3. Add 15 μl of 100 mg/ml RNase A, 150 μl of DNase 1 Solution, and 170 μl 2 M $MgCl_2$.

4. Incubate at 37°C for 30 min and invert periodically.

5. Solution should become a smooth milky texture.

6. Spin for 10 min in a 50-ml conical tube at 4500 rcf.

7. Form step gradient by adding 10 ml of light CsCl to a ultracentrifuge tube and then underlaying 10 ml of heavy CsCl.

8. Load supernatant (up to 18 ml) on CsCl step gradient.

9. Spin 2 h at 115,000 rcf.

10. Collect band (up to 4 ml) load on smaller CsCl step gradient 6 ml light, then underlay with 6 ml heavy to bottom.

11. Spin overnight 115,000 rcf (*see* **Note 8**).

3.4. If Not PEGylating: Buffer Exchange to Remove CsCl

1. Use EconoPac 10-DG desalting columns to remove CsCl and Tris (steps 2–6).

2. Remove buffer from column.

3. Run KPBS 0.5 M sucrose through column two times (*see* **Note 10**).

4. Add (X) ml of virus in CsCl to desalting column let drain. (X)= the amount of virus collected from gradient (≈ 1.5 ml).

5. Add 3.3 ml–(X) ml of column buffer to column and let it drain.

6. Elute column with (X) ml of column buffer.

7. Check concentration of virus using spectrophotometer.

8. Using equation ($OD_{260} \times 10^{12} =$ Viral Particles/ml) calculate concentration.

3.5. PEGylation Protocol

1. Starting with virus in CsCl or Tris buffer (start with at least four times the needed particle number). Tris must be removed prior to PEGylation, since it has amines that can react with NHS (*see* **Notes 11, 12,** and **13**).

2. Buffer exchange with 10 DG Econopac columns (steps 3–6).

3. 2 column volumes of KPBS to column. Then add starting virus (X) ml let drip without collection.

4. Add KPBS (3.3 ml–(X) ml) let drip without collection.

5. Add KPBS ((X) ml+0.2 ml), collect this fraction.

6. O.D.260 to determine number of viral particles (v.p.) unless the starting virus is in Tris buffer. If this is the case, repeat step 2 to ensure removal of all Tris.

7. Remove PEG from freezer.

8. Let PEG equilibrate to room temp to avoid condensation of humidity onto powder (*see* **Note 14**).

9. Open PEG and add 10 mg/1 e12 v.p. to 15-ml conical tube ≈ 1.0 ml final volume (V) ml.

10. Store PEG at –20°C (*see* **Note 15).**

11. Incubate virus + PEG by rotation at room temp for 1–2 hrs.

12. Make 2 Sephadex G50 columns (steps 13–24) (*see* **Note 16**).

13. Add 5–10 g of G50 to 300 ml of H_2O.

14. Autoclave on short 10-min cycle to allow beads to swell.

15. Let slurry cool and settle.

16. Remove excess liquid and add 300 ml of fresh H_2O.

17. Allow slurry to settle and pour excess H_2O.

18. Add 300 ml fresh H_2O.

19. Repeat steps 17 and 18.

20. Degas overnight in a vacuum-rated flask or bottle.

21. Next day add slurry to empty columns.

22. Fill so that the packed slurry reaches the 10-ml line (and looks like packed 10DG columns).

23. Add frit to surface of resin carefully without disturbing column.

24. Wash with 2 column volumes of KPBS 0.5 M sucrose without collecting flow through making sure to not let the resin dry out.

25. Calculate void volume for each G50 column using blue dextran 2000 (steps 26–37).

26. Make solution of blue dextran 2000 (2 mg/ml) in KPBS.

27. Take G50 column and tape to 15-ml conical tube.

28. Add volume of blue dextran solution equal to volume you have of PEG + virus (V) ml to column and allow to drip into 15-ml conical tube.

29. Add an excess of KPBS 0.5 M sucrose to column and collect in same 15-ml conical tube.

30. Keep a close eye on the drip and when the color begins to become blue move column to second 15-ml conical tube and collect this fraction.

31. Allow this blue color to drip and collect, but as soon as the color is no longer blue remove the column from the 15-ml conical tube.

32. The first 15-ml tube without the blue color is the void volume of the column (Z) ml.

33. Write void volume on column (so that you do not forget).

34. The second 15-ml tube with the blue color is the elution volume (Y).

35. Write elution volume on column (so that you do not forget).

36. Run 1 column volume of KPBS 0.5 M sucrose through column.

37. Leave some KPBS 0.5 M sucrose in column and put on stopper supplied and cover without pushing in cap until you use the column (use parafilm and store at 4°C if more than a few hours).

38. Use column to remove free PEG (steps 39–41).

39. Apply (V) ml of virus + PEG to column and let drip without collection.

40. Add KPBS 0.5 M sucrose (Z) ml–(V) ml let drip without collection.

41. Add KPBS 0.5 M sucrose (Y) ml. This fraction is your PEGylated virus.

42. Store at PEGylated virus at 4°C for up to 2 weeks (*see* **Note 17**).

43. Perform quantitative PCR to determine viral genome quantitation (*see* **Note 18**).

3.6. Quantitative PCR of Viral Genomes for Titering

1. Release viral DNA from virions (steps 2–5).

2. Add 94 μl of nuclease-free water to 1.5-ml microfuge tube.

3. Add 1 μl Proteinase K.

4. Add 5 μl of purified virus preparation.

5. Incubate 55°C for 1 h.

6. Heat-inactivate the Proteinase K at 95°C for 20 min.

7. Dilute 1/1000 to fall within the standards (300–300,000,000).

8. Set up standard curve with control plasmid (p-cmvi-Hexon).

9. Calculate mass of a single plasmid molecule (m) using the equation $m =(n)(1.096e{-}21$ g/bp). Where $n=$ plasmid size (bp), $m=$ mass, and e-21$= x10^{-21}$.

10. Calculate the mass of plasmid containing copy # of interest (300–300,000,000) using equation (copy # of interest × (m) = mass needed).

11. Calculate final concentration of DNA needed for each standard (300–300,000,000) by dividing values from step 10 by the number of μl of standard that will be applied for each PCR reaction (typically 3—5 μl).

12. Using equation($Ci \times Vi = Cf \times Vf$) prepare serial dilution of plasmid DNA. Where $Ci=$ initial concentration (based on Abs260 of plasmid DNA), $Vi=$ initial volume (unknown), $Cf=$ final concentration (calculated above for each dilution), and $Vf=$ final volume (500 μl).

13. Design primers. For Ad5 hexon use following primers [(forward-GAACAAGCGAGTGGTGGCTC) and (reverse-GCATTGCGGTGGTGGTTAA)].

14. Set up and run Q-PCR reaction (steps 15 and 16).

15. Setup reaction in 384 well plates: 5 μl DNA, (1 μl) 3 μM forward primer, (1 μl) 3 μM 3′ oligo, and 7 μl SYBR Green.

16. Run reaction with the following conditions: step 1 (1 cycle – 95°C 15 min), step 2 (40 cycles – 95°C 15 sec, 55°C 30 sec, 72°C 30 sec), and to check for specificity of reaction add dissociation step.

3.7. Quantitation of Free Amines by CBQCA Assay

1. Ensure all buffers and reagents are free of Tris (*see* **Notes 19** and **20**).

2. Modified viruses are diluted in 135 µl of reaction buffer (Dulbecco's phosphate-buffered saline (DPBS), pH 9.3) to a final concentration of 1×10^{12} v.p./ml in a 96-well black plate.

3. Add 5.0 µl of 20 mmol/L KCN and 10 µl of 5 mmol/L CBQCA.

4. Cover the plate with aluminum foil to protect from light and incubate at RT with shaking for 1 h.

5. Fluorescence emission is then detected at 550 nm with excitation at 465 nm using a plate reader.

6. The percentage of free amines is determined relative to a standard curve of unmodified virus and the inverse is expressed as the percentage of PEG-conjugated free amines. Saturation of amines by PEGs generally occurs near 70% of CBQCA-reactive sites.

3.8. In Vitro Transduction (for Luciferase-Expressing Viruses)

1. Grow 293 and A549 cells in 96-well plate in DMEM 10% FBS to 80% confluency.

2. Add 1×10^4 viral particles to each well of plate.

3. Incubate the plate at 37°C for 20 min.

4. Wash cells to remove excess virus.

5. Incubate 24 h at 37°C.

6. Add 25 µl of 5X Reporter Lysis Buffer to each well.

7. Freeze–thaw plate at −80°C.

8. Add 50 µl of Luciferase Assay Reagent to each well.

9. Detect luminescence using a plate reader.

10. The percent transduction determined by comparison to unmodified virus.

3.9. Particle Sizing (by Dynamic Light Scattering)

1. Dilute viruses in 10 mmol/l KNO3 to a final concentration of 1×10^{11} v.p./ml.

2. Measure on a particle sizer at three 3-min runs.

3. Polydispersity is calculated by the instrument and is proportional to the variance of the intensity weighted diffusion coefficient distribution.

4. Molecular weights are calculated using the Mark–Houwink–Sakadura equation.

4. Notes

1. Adenoviruses are treated as biosafety level 2 (BL2) agents
   in the United States and require biocontainment. If they
   encode dangerous transgene products, they will be given
   an even higher BL level with more stringent containment
   procedures. Work with these viruses cannot be performed
   without prior approval by your institution's biosafety com-
   mittees. This includes work with the viral plasmids and
   with the viruses themselves. All steps must be carried out
   under the biocontainment protocols designated by your
   institutions biosafety committee. Likewise the use of any
   chemicals and instruments described below must be performed as designated by each institution's safety guidelines.
   Note also that production of E1-deleted viruses in 293
   cells will result in the production of replication-competent
   Ad, since there is overlap in the E1 sequences embedded
   in the cells and with the vectors. The use of alternate cell
   lines that avoid this problem is recommended. However,
   most of these are impossible to obtain from the companies that own them. If 293 cells are used, large scale virus
   production should always start from a transfection or an
   early lysate to reduce the fraction of replication-competent
   virus that is in the preparation. If virus is produced serially
   from large scale preparations, the replication-competent
   contaminant will take over the population and increase side
   effects.

2. If the Adenovirus vector in question does not have a
   reporter gene like GFP or dsRed, generate a parallel DNA
   prep of a viral genome with reporter gene as a positive
   control for producing virus. Use of a small reporter gene
   plasmid is misleading as its transfection efficiency will be
   substantially higher than a 36-kbp Ad plasmid.

3. Transfection of the linearized vector plasmid should be performed in T25 flasks to reduce the potential for cross-
   contamination. If a T25 is not an option, a 60-mm dish
   can be substituted; however, there is a higher chance of
   contamination. 6-well plates should be avoided especially if
   different genomes are being transfected on the same dish.
   This will avoid the potential for cross contamination.

4. With a first-generation Ad5 vector, following a successful
   transfection (50–70%), the rescue of the virus typically will
   take 2–3 weeks. The method for rescuing the virus does
   not include the plaque purification method, so the resulting
   virus should be verified by PCR and sequencing. Plaque

purification may be favored and is detailed in alternative protocols.

5. Virus foci are recognized by two methods determined by the presence or absence of a detectable transgene like GFP. If a detectable transgene is in your virus, the foci can be observed as a spreading of transgene expression to neighboring cells. These foci will be hard to focus on and will likely for a comet shape with a focused body and a streaming tail. If there is no detectable transgene available, the foci can be observed by looking at the monolayer of cells with a low power microscope or the naked eye and the cells will begin to die in clusters that also will likely have a comet shape. For highly efficient viruses, foci may not be observed, but rather, in the first 2 weeks the virus will begin to kill the cells. This is known as cytopathic effect (cpe), and if complete cytopathic effect is observed, the cells will all be detached from the flask surface.

6. As passaging the virus continues, it is very important to always save half of the cell lysate at −80°C. This is essential so if contamination occurs you have a backup.

7. Large-scale virus preparations from low passage stocks should be a rapid process that, if planned correctly, can be done in 2–3 weeks. This is dependent on the continuous maintenance, carrying, and expansion of cells to infect.

8. Cell Factories or Spinner flasks are both useful means to grow large scale preparations of Adenovirus. If using a cell factory, adherent cells are required, such as HEK 293 cells. Whereas, if a spinner flask is used a suspension adapted cell line is required, such as N3S cells.

9. Virus in cell lysate can be stored at −80°C for a long duration without losing large degrees of activity.

10. If not PEGylated, the virus can be stored at −80°C in KPBS with 0.5 M sucrose for months without reducing the activity. The virus will retain its activity for longer, but it may be decreased. It should be noted that sucrose is an excellent carbon source for microbes. So, maintaining sterility is critical to avoid contamination.

11. If the virus is to be PEGylated, Tris containing buffers should be avoided since they react with the NHS group of the PEG molecule. If the virus has already been stored in Tris buffer, the Tris should be removed by performing two buffer exchanges. In our experience, dialysis has been problematic; however, if this is used in your lab it should work in theory.

12. It is important to use an unmodified virus that has been "mock PEGylated" as a negative control. This virus is

treated exactly as the PEGylated virus, but without the addition of the PEG.

13. The optimal conditions for PEGylation are for the virus to be a fresh preparation that has not been frozen. In addition, the more starting virus to be PEGylated, the better the yield. This is likely due to the loss of virus and the increase in volume that occur with the size exclusion chromatography column.

14. The NHS group on the PEG molecule loses its activity as it is exposed to air. In addition, the activity is reduced with each freeze thaw. To avoid these problems, the PEG should be purchase in small aliquots if available. If this is not an option the PEG should be stored at −20°C and once opened, overlayed with nitrogen. When the PEG is used, equilibrate the reagent to room temperature before exposing it to air.

15. Prior to freezing, partially close PEG bag and gently overlay with N_2 gas in a chemical hood. Be careful to not blow the powder out of the bag onto yourself or elsewhere with excess gas flow. The goal here is to remove oxygen from the bag to maximize the stability of the water-sensitive NHS reactive group.

16. When making the size exclusion column to remove the excess PEG, the protocol is designed for 5 kDa PEG. This uses a Sephadex g50 column, but if a larger PEG is used, the protocol for PEGylation remains the same except for the use of a Sephadex g100 column instead.

17. Once again it should be noted that sucrose is an excellent carbon source for bacteria and other microbes, so sterility must be maintained.

18. This step is necessary, since PEGylation can perturb the accuracy of OD260 estimates of virus particle concentrations. This is most likely seen with small 5 kDa PEG.

19. The premise of the kit is essentially to detect any remaining reactive amines on the virus with the amine-reactive CBQCA reagents. Since this agent is smaller than PEG, it can react not only with exposed amines, but also with amines that may be unavailable to PEG due to steric hindrance. It is therefore essential that the virus you are testing as well as the "mock" PEGylated control have not been in contact with Tris-containing buffers.

20. The CBQCA assay used to measure percent PEGylation has caused problems in the past perhaps due to aging of the reagent. To ensure the PEGylation has occurred, we

use the loss of in vitro activity as a quality control measure. We also use the particle sizing to show that as the virus is PEGylated the size increases. To ensure the PEGylation did not kill the activity of the virus, we test the in vivo activity following intravenous injection into mice. These four methods compare the PEGylated virus to an unmodified virus. It is important to use an unmodified virus that has been "mock PEGylated." This virus is treated exactly as the PEGylated virus, but without the addition of the PEG.

References

1. Lorimer, I. A., Keppler-Hafkemeyer, A., Beers, R. A., Pegram, C. N., Bigner, D. D., and Pastan, I. (1996) Recombinant immunotoxins specific for a mutant epidermal growth factor receptor: targeting with a single chain antibody variable domain isolated by phage display. *Proc Natl Acad Sci USA* **93**, 14815–14820.

2. Huard, J., Lochmuller, H., Acsadi, G., Jani, A., Massie, B., and Karpati, G. (1995) The route of administration is a major determinant of the transduction efficiency of rat tissues by adenoviral recombinants. *Gene Therapy* **2**, 107–115.

3. Morral, N., Parks, R. J., Zhou, H., Langston, C., Schiedner, G., Quinones, J., Graham, F. L., Kochanek, S., and Beaudet, A. L. (1998) High doses of a helper-dependent adenoviral vector yield supraphysiological levels of a1-antitrypsin with neglible toxicity. *Hum Gene Ther* **9**, 2709–2716.

4. Tang, D., Johnston, S. A., and Carbone, D. P. (1994) Butyrate-inducible and tumor-restricted gene expression by adenovirus vectors. *Cancer Gene Ther* **1**, 15–20.

5. Chillon, M., Lee, J. H., Fasbender, A., and Welsh, M. J. (1998) Adenovirus complexed with polyethylene glycol and cationic lipid is shielded from neutralizing antibodies in vitro. *Gene Ther* **5**, 995–1002.

6. O'Riordan, C. R., Lachapelle, A., Delgado, C., Parkes, V., Wadsworth, S. C., Smith, A. E., and Francis, G. E. (1999) PEGylation of adenovirus with retention of infectivity and protection from neutralizing antibody in vitro and in vivo. *Hum Gene Ther* **10**, 1349–1358.

7. Croyle, M. A., Chirmule, N., Zhang, Y., and Wilson, J. M. (2001) "Stealth" adenoviruses blunt cell-mediated and humoral immune responses against the virus and allow for significant gene expression upon readministration in the lung. *J Virol* **75**, 4792–4801.

8. Zhang, Y., Chirmule, N., Gao, G. P., Qian, R., Croyle, M., Joshi, B., Tazelaar, J., and Wilson, J. M. (2001) Acute cytokine response to systemic adenoviral vectors in mice is mediated by dendritic cells and macrophages. *Mol Ther* **3**, 697–707.

9. Croyle, M. A., Chirmule, N., Zhang, Y., and Wilson, J. M. (2002) PEGylation of E1-deleted adenovirus vectors allows significant gene expression on readministration to liver. *Hum Gene Ther* **13**, 1887–1900.

10. Mok, H., Palmer, D. J., Ng, P., and Barry, M. A. (2005) Evaluation of polyethylene glycol modification of first-generation and helper-dependent adenoviral vectors to reduce innate immune responses. *Mol Ther* **11**, 66–79.

11. Hofherr, S. E., Mok, H., Gushiken, F. C., Lopez, J. A., and Barry, M. A. (2007) Polyethylene glycol modification of adenovirus reduces platelet activation, endothelial cell activation, and thrombocytopenia. *Hum Gene Ther* **18**, 837–848.

12. Hofherr, S. E., Shashkova, E. V., Weaver, E. A., Khare, R., and Barry, M. A. (2008) Modification of Adenoviral Vectors With Polyethylene Glycol Modulates In Vivo Tissue Tropism and Gene Expression. *Mol Ther* **7**, 1276–1282

13. Weaver, E. A., and Barry, M. A. (2008) Effects of Shielding Adenoviral Vectors with Polyethylene Glycol (PEG) on Vector-specific and Vaccine-mediated Immune Responses. *Hum Gene Ther* **433**, 55–78

14. Palmer, D. J., and Ng, P. (2008) Methods for the production of first generation adenoviral vectors. *Methods Mol Biol* **433**, 55–78.

Chapter 14

Adenovirus-Mediated Interleukin (IL)-24 Immunotherapy for Cancer

Rajagopal Ramesh, Constantine G. Ioannides, Jack A. Roth, and Sunil Chada

Abstract

Interleukin-24 (IL-24) is a member of the IL-10 cytokine family. IL-24, also known as melanoma differentiation associated gene 7 (mda-7), is a unique cytokine in that it has cytokine properties and functions as a novel tumor suppressor gene. Studies by us and other investigators using viral and non-viral vectors have demonstrated IL-24 overexpression in human cancer cells inhibited tumor growth both in vitro and in vivo. A majority of these studies using immunodeficient animal models have focused on demonstrating the direct anticancer properties of IL-24. Very few studies have focused on studying the immunotherapeutic properties of IL-24 despite it being reported to function as a Th1 cytokine. A phase I clinical trial using an adenovirus vector expressing IL-24 (Ad-IL24/INGN241) reported Ad-IL24 treatment of cancer patients resulted in changes in cytokines and T cells. However, well-designed and detailed preclinical studies to support the clinical findings are warranted. Demonstrating immune modulation by IL-24 will provide a rationale for developing IL-24-based immunotherapeutic approaches for cancer treatment.

In the present chapter, we provide experimental details for conducting IL-24-based immunotherapy studies. As it is not possible for the authors to cover all of the information the authors recommend reading other immunology-based literature and procedures for a better understanding of conducting preclinical studies.

Key words: IL-24, mda-7, IL-10, cytokine, cancer, gene therapy, tumor suppressor genes, immunity.

1. Introduction

IL-24/mda-7 is a novel cytokine/tumor suppressor gene that was initially identified in terminally differentiated human melanoma cells (1). IL-24 is a member of the IL-10 family located on

P. Yotnda (ed.), *Immunotherapy of Cancer*, Methods in Molecular Biology 651,
DOI 10.1007/978-1-60761-786-0_14, © Springer Science+Business Media, LLC 2010

chromosome 1q 32 (2). Other members of IL-1-0 cytokine family that are also located at the same locus include IL-10, IL-19, and IL-20 (3). The IL-10 cytokine family comprises six members: IL-10, IL-19, IL-20, IL-22, IL-24, and IL-26. More recently, IL-28 and IL-29 have been included in the IL-10 superfamily (4).

IL-24 gene has limited sequence homology with IL-10 with IL-24 protein having ~19% amino acid identity with other IL-10 family members. Because of its physical location within the IL-10 family locus, its limited homology with IL-10, and its cytokine activity, IL-24 is included in the IL-10 cytokine family (3, 5, 6). Thus a combination of structural data, homology to known cytokines, chromosomal localization, a predicted N-terminus secretion signal peptide, and evidence of its regulation of cytokine secretion, all support IL-24 as an IL-10 family cytokine (2, 7, 8). Furthermore, IL-24-specific receptors have been identified defining IL-24 as a cytokine.

IL-24 unlike IL-10 and its family members is a novel cytokine with unique tumor-specific apoptotic, antiangiogenic, and cytokine properties that make it especially attractive for use in cancer therapy applications (2, 8–10). Studies from our laboratory and others have demonstrated virus and non-viral mediated IL-24 overexpression results in tumor growth inhibition and cell death both in vitro and in vivo (11). The tumor suppressor function of IL-24 is independent of other tumor suppressor gene mutations and selective for tumor cells with no toxicity to normal cells (2, 11).

The fact IL-24 is a cytokine has lead to preclinical studies focused on characterizing the cytokine and immune properties of IL-24. Initial in vitro studies demonstrated IL-24 is expressed at low levels in human peripheral blood mononuclear cells (PBMC) (12). Furthermore, phytohemagglutinin (PHA) or bacterial lipopolysaccharide (LPS)-mediated nonspecific stimulation of PBMCs resulted in increased IL-24 expression in natural killer (NK) and B-cell subpopulations of PBMCs (12–14). Additionally, activation of signal transducer and transcriptional activator (STAT)-3 with induction of IFN-gamma, TNF-alpha, IL-6, IL-12, and GM-CSF secretion in IL-24-treated PBMCs was demonstrated, suggesting IL-24 functions as a pro-Th1 cytokine. Keratinocytes has also been shown to express IL-24 (15).

Subsequent studies by other investigators have reported IL-24 induction and its ability to modulate other cytokines under different pathological conditions. Regulation of IL-24 and its receptor expression by type I interferons (IFN) and LPS in the liver has been reported (16). IL-24-mediated induction of IFN-γ expression in tuberculosis patients has been demonstrated suggesting IL-24 and IFN-γ function in an autoregulatory mechanism (17). Regulation of T-cells and cytokines by IL-24 and other IL-10 family members was also reported (18). Expression of IL-24 has been observed in inflammatory diseases such as psoriasis, rheumatoid arthritis, spondyloarthropathy, palmoplantar pustulosis, and bacteria-associated infections (19–22). Studies from our laboratory demonstrated human melanoma cells when treated with IL-24 protein, induced secretion of IFN-γ and IL-6, but not of IL-4 or IL-5 (11).

All of the studies described above establish IL-24 as a cytokine. However, all of these results were obtained from in vitro studies. Till date there have not been many in vivo studies to demonstrate the immune functions of IL-24. Furthermore, the potential of IL-24 being used as an immunotherapeutic for cancer therapy have not been investigated in detail. We have recently demonstrated IL-24 has immunotherapeutic properties by performing in vivo studies (23). In this study, we showed treatment of tumor-bearing mice with Ad-IL24 resulted in tumor suppression. Molecular and cellular analysis showed T-cell proliferation and induction of TNF-α and IFN-γ in vivo (23). Additionally, T-cell memory response in rejecting tumor challenge was demonstrated in this study. These results established IL-24 as a potential cancer immunotherapeutic agent. Combining the proapoptotic and antiangiogenic activity with its recently identified immunotherapeutic function makes IL-24 a potent anticancer drug.

In this chapter, we provide a step by step procedure for testing the immunotherapeutic properties of IL-24 for cancer therapy. Experimental procedures and assays for testing IL-24 for cancer immunotherapy both in vitro and in vivo are provided. It is anticipated that by following the described steps the reader will easily be able to conduct tests in his/her laboratory.

It is however to be noted that the methods provided in this article are primarily for development and testing of IL-24 in preclinical studies. However, several additional assays that are required to fully characterize IL-24 as an immunotherapeutic may not be covered as it is not possible for the authors to cover all of the information in the present article. The procedures described below are therefore recommended as a guideline for development and testing of IL-24 as a cytokine for cancer immunotherapy.

2. Materials

2.1. In Vitro Studies

2.1.1. Cell Culture

1. Bright-field inverted microscope (Nikon, Melville, NY).

2. BCA Protein Assay Reagent Kit (Pierce, Rockford, IL).

3. Cell lysis buffer: 0.125 M Tris–HCl (pH 6.8), 2% (w/v) sodium dodecyl sulfate (SDS), 10% (w/v) Glycerol, 6 M

Urea, 5% (w/v) 2-β-mercaptoethanol (2-ME), 0.1 ml of 5% (w/v) bromophenol blue. Store at −20°C.

4. Cold calcium-free phosphate buffered saline (PBS).

5. Adenovirus-type 5 containing IL-24 gene (Ad-IL24; Introgen Therapeutics Inc., Houston, TX).

6. Adenovirus-type 5 containing luciferase gene (Ad-luc; Introgen Therapeutics Inc.).

7. Falcon® 6-well tissue culture plates (Becton Dickinson, Franklin Lakes, NJ).

8. Fetal bovine serum (FBS; GIBCO/BRL, Invitrogen Corporation, Grand Island, NY).

9. Murine cancer (MCA16; UV2237m) and fibroblast (10T1/2) cell lines (American Type Culture Collection, Rockville, MD).

10. Tissue culture medium: Dulbecco's modified Eagle's medium (DMEM; GIBCO-BRL, Invitrogen Corporation, Grand Island, NY).

11. Non-essential amino acids (NEAA; GIBCO-BRL).

12. L-glutamine (GIBCO-BRL).

13. Trypsin-containing EDTA (1×; GIBCO/BRL).

14. Trypan-blue (Sigma Chemicals, St. Louis, MO).

15. Eppendorf pipettes (P-1000, P-200, and P-20).

16. Sterile disposable pipette tips (1–200 μl and 1 ml; USA Scientific Inc.).

17. Sterile disposable serological pipettes (1, 5, and 1 ml; Corning Inc., Corning, NY).

18. Biological safety cabinet (BL-2).

19. Tissue culture room for handling adenovirus.

20. Latex-free gloves.

21. Eye glasses.

22. Biohazard disposable bags.

23. Bleach (10%).

2.1.2. Western Blotting Analysis for Transgene Expression

2.1.2.1. Sodium Dodecyl Sulfate (SDS)-Polyacrylamide Gel Electrophoresis (PAGE)

1. Ammonium persulfate (APS): Prepare 10% (w/v) APS solution and aliquot in 0.5 ml volume and store at −20°C.

2. Bis-acrylamide: Prepare 30% bis-acrylamide solution in water and store at +4° C.

3. Prestained molecular weight markers: The markers can be purchased from several commercial vendors (e.g., Bio-Rad, Hercules, CA; Santa Cruz Biotechnology, Santa Cruz, CA).

4. Power/Pac 200 (BioRad, Hercules, CA).

5. Running buffer: Prepare a 10× stock by mixing 0.025 M Tris, 0.192 M glycine, and 0.1% SDS solution. Store the solution at room temperature.

6. Sample loading buffer: Mix 5 ml of cell lysis buffer with 0.5 ml of 2-mercaptoethanol (2-ME) and adjust the final volume to 1 ml with water.

7. Separating buffer: 3.0 M Tris–HCl (pH 8.8). Store the solution at room temperature.

8. Stacking buffer: 0.5 M Tris–HCl (pH 6.8). Store the solution at room temperature.

9. Sodium dodecyl sulfate (SDS): 10% (w/v). Store the SDS solution at room temperature.

10. N, N, N, N'-tetramethyl-ethylenediamine (TEMED; Bio-Rad, Hercules, CA).

11. Water-saturated isobutanol: Mix distilled water with isobutanol in 1:1 ratio (v/v) and allow the two phases to separate. Use the upper phase of the water saturated isobutanol.

12. Western blot apparatus with transfer system (BioRad, Hercules, CA).

2.1.3. Protein Transfer and Detection

1. Bio-Max ML film (Kodak, Rochester, NY).

2. Enhanced chemiluminescent (ECL) reagent (Amersham Biosciences).

3. Horse-radish peroxidase (HRP)-conjugated secondary antibody (Jackson Immunoresearch, West Grove, PA).

4. Nitrocellulose membrane (Millipore, Bedford, MA).

5. PBS-T Blocking buffer: Add 25 g of fat-free milk powder to 450 ml of phosphate-buffered saline (PBS) and mix thoroughly using a magnetic stirrer. Add 0.5 ml of Tween-20, continue to mix, and adjust the final volume to 500 ml. Store the solution at +4°C.

6. Primary antibody – anti-human IL24 antibody (Introgen Therapeutics Inc., Houston, TX). For other antibodies that are commercially (e.g., Santa Cruz Biotechnology, Santa Cruz, CA; Cell Signaling, Worcester, MA) available, the investigator can purchase the antibodies as per his/her preference.

7. Stripping buffer: Mix equal volumes of H_2O_2 and PBS in 1:1 ratio. Always prepare the solution fresh and store at room temperature until use.

8. TBS-T blocking buffer: Add 25 g of fat-free milk powder to 450 ml of Tris–buffered saline (TBS) and mix thoroughly using a magnetic stirrer. Add 0.5 ml of Tween-20, continue to mix and adjust the final volume to 500 ml. Store the solution at +4°C.

9. Transfer buffer: 25 mM Tris, 0.192 mM glycine, and 20% (v/v) methanol. Store the buffer solution at room temperature.

10. Whatmann chromatography paper (3 M; Whatmann, Maidstone, UK).

2.1.4. Flow Cytometry

1. Fluorescein isothiocyanate (FITC) conjugated antibodies to major histocompatibility complex (MHC) class I (anti-H-2K^k and anti-H-2D^k (Becton and Dickinson-Pharmingen).

2. Fluorescein isothiocyanate (FITC) conjugated mouse anti-CD3e antibody; phycoerythrin-conjugated mouse anti-CD4 (L3T4) antibody; allophycocyanine-conjugated anti-CD8a (Ly-2) antibody (eBiosceince, San Diego, CA).

3. Phosphate buffered saline (PBS) containing 0.2% bovine serum albumin and 0.1% sodium azide (flow cytometry buffer).

4. 15-ml centrifuge tubes (Falcon).

5. Table-top high-speed centrifuge (Beckman Coulter, Fullerton, CA).

6. 1% paraformaldehyde.

7. Tumor (UV2237) cell line.

8. Splenocytes.

9. Ad-IL24.

10. Ad-Luc.

11. Vybrant carboxyfluorescein acetate succinimidyl ester (CFDA SE) cell tracer kit (Molecular Probes, Eugene, OR).

12. FACSCalibur flow cytometer (BD Biosciences, Mountain View, CA).

13. Cell Quest software (BD Biosciences).

2.1.5. Cytokine Measurement

1. Splenocytes from the spleens of mice used in the study

2. UV2237m tumor cells

3. Dissecting scissors (Fisher Scientific, Pittsburgh, PA)

4. Glass slides

5. Cell strainer (70 μm nylon; Becton-Dickinson, Franklin Lakes, NJ)

6. Histopaque-1077 (Sigma-Aldrich, St. Louis, MO)

7. Hank's balanced salt solution (GIBCO-BRL)

8. Centriplus YM-10 concentrator (Millipore Co., Bedford, MA)

9. Mouse cytokine 10-Plex (Biosource, Camarillo, CA)

10. Luminex 100 (Luminex Co., Austin, TX)

11. RPMI-1640 (GIBCO-BRL)

12. 2-Mercaptoethanol (Sigma Chemicals)

13. 1% sodium pyruvate (GIBCO-BRL)

14. 1% non-essential amino acids (NEAA)

15. Antibiotics (100 units/ml penicillin and 100 mg/ml streptomycin; GIBCO-BRL)

16. Tissue culture plates

17. Eppendorf pipettes (P-1000, P-200, and P-20)

18. Sterile disposable pipette tips (1–200 μl and 1 ml; USA Scientific Inc.)

19. Sterile disposable serological pipettes (10, 5, and 1 ml; Corning Inc., Corning, NY)

20. Biological safety cabinet (BL-2)

21. Tissue culture room

22. Latex hypoallergenic gloves (Fisher Scientific, Pittsburgh, PA)

23. Biohazard disposable bags

24. Bleach (10%)

2.1.6.
Immunohistochemistry

1. Organ (e.g., spleen, subcutaneous tumor)

2. Positively charged glass slides (Fisher Scientific)

3. Cover slips (Fisher Scientific)

4. Buffered formalin (Fisher Scientific)

5. Ethanol (Fisher Scientific)

6. Xylene (Fisher Scientific)

7. Non-sterile PBS

8. Primary antibodies against target of interest (e.g., CD3, CD4, CD8, NK)

9. Vectastain kit (Vector Laboratories)

10. Fume hood

11. Dark slide incubating box

12. Slide box (Fisher Scientific)

13. Slide holder (Fisher Scientific)

14. Tissue sectioning instrument

15. Hematoxylin (Fisher Scientific)

16. Diaminobenzidine (DAB; Sigma Chemicals)

17. Incubator set to 37°C

18. Oven set to 60°C

19. Steamer (available in general electrical stores)

20. Citrate buffer – 6.3 g of citric acid made to 3 l with water and pH set to 6.0

21. Endogenous blocking solution - 5 ml of 30% hydrogen peroxide (H_2O_2) and 95 ml of methanol

22. Substrate solution – 100 mg of diaminobenzidine tetrahydrochloride (DAB) dissolved in 16.6 ml of PBS. Aliquot and store at –20°C

23. Blocking solution – 10 drops of normal serum (e.g., goat, rabbit, mouse; provided in commercially available staining kits) added to 10 ml of PBS

24. Secondary antibody – 1 drop of biotinylated antibody (provided in commercially available staining kits) added to 10 ml of blocking solution

25. ABC reagent (provided in kit) – 1 drop of solution "A" and 1 drop of solution "B" mixed with 5 ml of blocking solution

26. Bright field microscope (Nikon; Single or double head) with CCD camera attached to a computer for image capturing

2.2. In Vivo Adenovirus Delivery and Therapy

1. 1-cc disposable syringe (Becton Dickinson, Franklin Lakes, NJ)

2. 150-mm CellStar® tissue culture plates (Greiner Bio-One GmBH, Frickenhausen, Germany)

3. Blunt and pointed end forceps (Fisher Scientific, Pittsburgh, PA)

4. Calipers Formalin (Sigma Chemicals, St. Louis, MO)

5. Cold calcium free phosphate buffered saline (PBS)

6. Dissection board (Fisher Scientific, Pittsburgh, PA)

7. Dissection scissors (Fisher Scientific, Pittsburgh, PA)

8. Ad-IL24 (Introgen Therapeutics Inc.)

9. Ad-Luc (Introgen Therapeutics Inc.)

10. Face mask (Fisher Scientific, Pittsburgh, PA)

11. Female C3H/HeN mice (4–6 weeks old; National Cancer Institute-Frederick Cancer Research Facility, Frederick, MD)

12. Female athymic nude mice (4–6 weeks old; Charles River Laboratories, Wilmington, DE)

13. Fetal bovine serum (FBS; GIBCO/BRL, Invitrogen Corporation, Grand Island, NY)

14. UV2237m cancer cells (American Type Culture Collection, Rockville, MD)

15. Latex hypoallergenic gloves (Fisher Scientific)

16. Needles ($25G^{5/8}$ and $27G^{1/2}$; Becton Dickinson, Franklin Lakes, NJ)

17. Rib-Back Carbon Steel Scalpel blade (Becton Dickinson Acute Care, NJ)

18. Tissue culture medium: DMEM (GIBCO-BRL, Invitrogen Corporation, Grand Island, NY)

19. Trypsin containing EDTA ($1\times$; GIBCO/BRL, Invitrogen Corporation, Grand Island, NY)

20. Tyvek suit (Fisher Scientific, Pittsburgh, PA)

3. Methods

3.1. Preparation of Ad-IL24 and Ad-Luc

1. Take out the adenovirus (Ad-IL24, Ad-Luc) stock solution (10^{11}–10^{12} viral particles (v.p.)/ml) that is required for preparing the working viral concentrations from its storage area (–80°C).

2. Allow the reagents to sit inside the BL-2 level biological safety culture hood for few minutes to reach room temperature.

3. While the reagents are thawing, take two 1.5-ml microcentrifuge tubes and label the tubes appropriately to distinguish between Ad-IL24 and Ad-Luc.

4. Wipe the outside of the reagent vials with rubbing alcohol.

5. With a pipettor take the appropriate volume of Ad-IL24 and Ad-Luc that is equivalent to the virus concentration needed to conduct the studies and add to the 1.5-ml microcentrifuge tube.

6. Make the final volume as desired with serum free tissue culture medium.

7. Gently mix by pipetting up and down five times using a 1-ml Eppendorf pipette.

8. The resulting adenovirus solution is ready for use during in vitro and in vivo studies.

3.2. In Vitro Transfection

1. From a tissue culture incubator take out a tissue culture plate (100 mm^2) actively growing a monolayer of cells that is approximately 70–80% confluent.

2. Trypsinize cells by adding 0.5 ml of 1% trypsin containing 0.1% EDTA and incubating at room temperature for 1–2 min.

3. Neutralize the trypsin activity by adding 0.5 ml of serum-free culture medium and gently tap the culture plate to loosen all of the attached cells.

4. Collect the detached cells using a 1-ml pipette and transfer into a 2-ml culture grade sterile polystyrene tube.

5. Gently pipette ten times to make a single cell suspension.

6. Take 100 μl of the cell suspension and add to the tube containing 100 μl of trypan blue. Gently mix by pipetting three times.

7. Transfer 10 μl of the cell suspension in 90 μl of trypan blue into the chambers of a micrometer that is routinely used for cell counting.

8. Place the micrometer under an inverted bright-field microscope and adjust the focus to see the center of the micrometer that contains the "box." The box contains four equal squares.

9. Count the number of cells present in each of the four squares and add the total number of cells present in the four squares.

10. Divide the total number of cells by 4 to get the average number of cells.

11. Calculate the total number of cells per milliliter using the formula:

    Average number of cells × dilution in trypan blue × 10^4 = number of cells/ml.

    For example, if the number of cells counted were 40, then the average number of cells is $40/4 = 10$.

    Then the total number of cells present is 10 × dilution factor =10 (10 μl of cell suspension diluted in 90 μl of trypan blue) × $10^4 = 100 \times 10^4 = 1 \times 10^6$ cells/ml.

12. Seed cells (5×10^5/well) in 2 ml of culture medium in a six-well tissue culture plate (*see* **Note 1**).

13. Incubate the culture plate in a tissue culture incubator set at 37°C temperature and 5% CO_2 for 18–24 h.

14. The next day remove the plate, aspirate the medium with a 5-ml sterile pipette and replace with 1 ml of sterile PBS. Gently swirl the plate to remove traces of the culture medium.

15. Remove the PBS and add 1 ml of serum-free culture medium to the wells and leave the plate inside the biological safety hood for 10 min.

16. Take out a freshly prepared Ad-IL24 or Ad-Luc (described in **Section 3.1**) and using a 20-μl pipette take different volumes (1, 2.5, 5, and 10 μl) equivalent to different concentrations of the viral particles (e.g., 1000, 2500, 5000, and 10,000) and add to each well. Gently swirl the plate for the virus to infect the monolayer of attached cells.

17. Return the culture plate to the incubator and incubate the plate for 3 h.

18. After incubation is complete, take out the plate from the incubator and place inside the biological safety hood. Add 2 ml of 10% serum containing culture medium and return the plate to the incubator.

19. Incubate the plate at 37°C, 5% CO_2.

20. At different time points (24, 48, and 72 h) after virus treatment, remove the plate from the incubator and analyze for cell viability, transgene expression, or flow cytometry as described below.

3.2.1. Cell Viability

1. At different time points after Ad-IL24 and Ad-Luc treatment, take out the tissue culture plates from the incubator.

2. Analyze the cell morphology under a bright-field microscope.

3. Place the plates inside the biosafety (BL2) hood and aspirate the tissue culture medium from each plate.

4. To each plate add 1 ml of sterile PBS and gently rotate the plates to remove traces of serum.

5. Aspirate the PBS into a discard container containing 10% bleach.

6. Trypsinize the cells attached to the bottom of the culture plate by adding 0.5 ml of 1% trypsin containing 0.1% EDTA and incubating at room temperature for 1–2 min.

7. Neutralize the trypsin activity by adding 0.5 ml of serum-free culture medium and gently tap the culture plate to loosen all of the attached cells.

8. Follow steps 5–11 described above in **Section 3.2.**

9. Determine the number of viable cells in each treatment group including untreated control group.

10. Calculate the differences in cell viability among different groups for statistical significance.

3.2.2. Transgene Expression

1. To the wells containing cells that were untreated, or treated with Ad-Luc or Ad-IL24, follow the steps 1–7 described in **Section 3.2.1.**

2. Collect the trypsinized cells into 1.5-ml Eppendorf tubes appropriately labeled as control, Ad-IL24, or Ad-Luc.

3. Place the Eppendorf tubes in a table-top microcentrifuge and spin for 10 min at 13,000 rpm, room temperature.

4. Cells will appear as a pellet at the bottom of the tube with a clear supernatant at the top.

5. Carefully aspirate the upper supernatant without disturbing the pellet.

6. To the cell pellet, add 0.5 ml of cell lysis buffer and gently pipette up and down ten times.

7. Place the tube in a microcentrifuge and spin for 10 min at 13,000 rpm, room temperature.

8. Collect the upper layer of supernatant that contains the total cellular protein using a 1-ml pipette and transfer into a new 1.5-ml Eppendorf tube. Be careful not to collect the cell debris present at the bottom of the tube.

9. The collected supernatant can be stored at –80°C until use. Prior to storing, an aliquot of the supernatant is used to determine the protein concentration.

10. Protein concentration is determined using the bicinchoninic acid (BCA) method (Pierce) and expressed as microgram (μg) of protein per microliter (μl).

11. When ready for use, appropriate volume of the supernatant that contains 50 μg of protein is mixed with a gel loading dye and subjected to gel electrophoresis and Western blotting analyses as described below.

3.2.3. Sodium Dodecyl Sulfate-Poly Acrylamide Gel Electrophoresis (SDS – PAGE)

1. Wipe the glass slides with ethanol and mount them into the stand.

2. Add dH$_2$O to check for leakage.

3. Drain the dH$_2$O and dry using a Whatmann 3 M blotting paper.

4. Prepare the resolving gel according to the molecular weight of the protein to be investigated. For example, to detect

low molecular weight proteins prepare a 12.5% gel; for high molecular weight protein prepare 7. 5% gel.

	7.5%	10%	12.5%
Acrylamide-bis (30%)	3.75 ml	5 ml	6.25 ml
3 M Tris–Hcl (pH 8.8)	3.75 ml	3.75 ml	3.75 ml
dH₂O	7.25 ml	6.0 ml	4.75 ml
TEMED	12.0 μl	12.0 μl	12.0 μl
10% SDS	150 μl	150 μl	150 μl
10% APS	150 μl	150 μl	150 μl

5. Mix the gel by pipetting and then add 7.4 ml of the gel between the slides.

6. Add 300 μl water-saturated isobutanol to remove the bubbles.

7. Let stand for 45 min to 1 h until the gel polymerizes.

8. Prepare the Stacking gel:

Acrylamide-bis (30%)	1.3 ml
0.5 M Tris–HCl (pH 6.8)	2.5 ml
dH₂O	6.1 ml
TEMED	15.0 μl
10% SDS	100 μl
10% APS	150 μl

9. After 1 h drain the isobutanol and wash with dH₂O to remove the remaining isobutanol.

10. Carefully remove excess dH₂O using a blotting paper, so as not to touch the gel.

11. Mix the stacking gel and add on top of the separating gel.

12. Put the comb to make the wells (1.5 mm 10 well comb or 15 well comb can be used depending on the number of wells required).

13. Let stand for 45 min to 1 h until the gel polymerizes.

14. After 1 h remove the combs carefully and gently wash with dH₂O to remove excess gel.

15. Suction out the dH₂O carefully, remembering not to touch the gel.

16. Remove the glass slides from the gel stand and put it into the electrophoresis stand.

17. Pour 1× running buffer between the slides.

18. Centrifuge the proteins needed for loading at 13,000 RPM for 5–10 min.

19. Mix the loading buffer and proteins according to the prepared chart to get equal loading concentration of the proteins.

20. Using a sampler comb load 2 µl of the prepared proteins to each well.

21. Add 1 µl of protein ladder to one of the wells.

22. Run the gel at 100 V, monitoring the blue sample buffer line.

23. Stop the gel once the blue line reaches at the bottom of the gel.

24. Drain off the running buffer and remove the slides from the stand.

25. Carefully open the two slides and remove the gel for transfer.

26. Transfer the proteins from the polyacrylamide gel to the nitrocellulose membrane.

3.2.3.1. Western Blotting

1. Add 1× transfer buffer in a dish and place the transfer case in the buffer.

2. Place a sponge on the case followed by blotting paper, nitrocellulose paper, polyacrylamide gel, 3 M Whatmann blotting paper, and another sponge (so-called "sandwiching" between two electrodes).

3. Put the transfer case into the transfer stand with the black side of the case toward the red side of the transfer kit/stand (depending on the direction you are running the current).

4. Put the kit in a plastic container and pour 1× transfer buffer.

5. Put in a magnetic stirrer and an ice pack to keep the gel cool.

6. Transfer the gel at 100 V for 1–2 h (depending on the molecular weight of the proteins you want to check – longer transfer may be required for high molecular weight proteins) and replacing the ice pack whenever needed.

7. Following transfer, remove the stand and cut the nitrocellulose membrane at the gel marks with a scalpel.

8. Place this membrane in a blocking dish and block with PBS-T or TBS-T blocking buffer depending on the antibody to be used for 1 h to block non-specific binding sites.

9. After 1 h drain the blocking buffer.

10. Add appropriate primary antibody (e.g., mouse anti-human IL-24 antibody) diluted 1:500–1:1000 in PBS-T or TBS-T blocking buffer.

11. Leave the membrane on a shaker set at slow speed (500 rpm) overnight at +4°C.

12. The next morning remove the PBS-T containing the primary antibody.

13. Add PBS-T blocking buffer to the membrane and wash the membrane for 15 min by placing it on a rotary shaker set at a speed of 1000 rpm.

14. Repeat step "13" two more times with washing time of 5 min for each wash.

15. Drain the washing buffer.

16. Add appropriate secondary antibody (e.g., goat anti-mouse antibody) at a dilution of 1:5000 in PBS-T blocking buffer.

17. Place on a rotary shaker set a speed of 500 rpm and allow shaking for 1 h.

18. Wash the membrane as indicated in steps "14" and "15."

19. Wash the membrane with PBS twice. Each wash includes shaking for 5 min on a rotary shaker set at 1000 rpm.

20. Drain the PBS.

21. Add 10 ml of Amersham chemiluminescence ECL Reagent (Detection Reagent 1: Detection Reagent 2 mixed in a ratio of 1:1) and shake for 1 min on the rotary shaker.

22. Drain the ECL reagent and blot dry the membrane using a Whatmann blotting paper.

23. Place the membrane in the X-ray film cassette and expose the membrane using Biomax ML film or any other appropriate film in a dark room.

24. Develop the film in the dark room after exposing for a few minutes or as appropriate. Exposure times vary depending on the signal obtained. If the signal is too weak, expose the film overnight.

25. Protein at the expected molecular size can be detected that can be imaged and quantitated (**Fig. 14.1**).

3.2.3.2. Stripping and Reprobing

1. After obtaining the appropriate result, take out the membrane from the X-ray film cassette.

2. Place the membrane in the dish previously used for washing the membrane.

3. Add 10 ml of stripping buffer to the membrane contained in the dish.

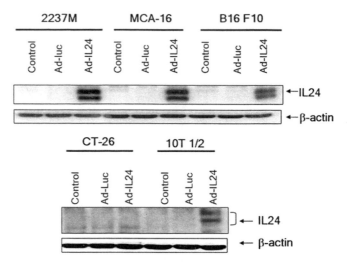

Fig. 14.1. Determination of transgene expression. Murine tumor (UV2237M, MCA-16, B16/F10, CT-26) and normal fibroblast (10T1/2) cells treated with Ad-luc or Ad-IL24 were harvested at 72 h after transfection, lysed, and subjected to Western blotting. Cells that were untreated served as controls. Cells expressing the exogenous IL-24 protein were detected using anti-human IL24 antibody. Beta-actin was used as an internal loading control.

4. Place the dish on a rotary shaker set at 1000 rpm and shake for 30 min.

5. Drain the stripping buffer.

6. Add PBS-T buffer solution containing antibody to beta-actin (1:1000).

7. Repeat steps 11–24 described in **Section 3.2.3.1** and step 2.

8. Detection of a signal on the X-ray film corresponding to the expected protein size for beta-actin will allow the investigator to determine equal loading of protein samples and serve as an internal control. Detection of the equal levels of beta-actin will reflect true changes in the protein of interest that was investigated in **Section 3.2.3.1** and step 2.

3.2.4. Flow Cytometry

3.2.4.1. Tumor Cell
Analysis

1. Seed UV2237m tumor cells (3×10^5) in 10 cm tissue culture dishes and incubate in an incubator at 37°C, 5% CO_2.

2. The next day, take out the culture dish from the incubator and place inside a BL2 safety cabinet.

3. Prepare Ad-IL24 and Ad-Luc working solution (concentration of viral particles to be used depends on the investigator and studies) as described in **Section 3.1** and steps 1–8 inside a BL2 safety cabinet.

4. Aspirate the medium from the culture dishes and infect the cells with Ad-IL24 or Ad-Luc as described in **Section 3.2**. Cells that are not treated with the virus will serve as controls.

5. Follow steps 16–20 described in **Section 3.2**.

6. At different time points after the Ad-IL24 and Ad-Luc treatment, take out the tissue culture plates from the incubator.

7. Follow steps 1–7 described in **Section 3.2.1**.

8. Collect the trypsinized cells into 15-ml Falcon centrifuge tubes and make the final volume to 10 ml with sterile PBS or serum-free tissue culture medium.

9. Place the Falcon tubes in a table-top high-speed centrifuge and spin for 10 min at 1500 rpm at +4°C.

10. After centrifugation, take the tubes back to the culture room and place inside the biosafety cabinet.

11. Carefully aspirate the upper supernatant layer and the cell pellet should be visible at the bottom of the tube.

12. Add 10 ml of sterile PBS to the cell pellet and gently break the cell aggregates by pipetting ten times with a 5-ml pipette.

13. Repeat steps 9–11.

14. Resuspend the cell pellet in 1 ml of PBS and make sure the pellet is disaggregated into single cell suspension by gentle pipetting.

15. Add the appropriate concentration of FITC-conjugated anti-H-2K^k or anti-H-2D^k antibody (1:100–1:1000 dilution) to the cells.

16. Incubate the cells in the dark for 30 min at room temperature.

17. After incubation is complete, take out the tubes and aspirate the antibody.

18. Add 10 ml of flow cytometry buffer and perform steps 9–12.

19. Repeat step 18.

20. To the cell pellet add 1 ml of 1% paraformaldehyde and resuspend into single cell suspension.

21. Analyze the fixed cells with an EPICS XL-MCL flow cytometer for the number of H-2K^k and H-2D^k cells.

22. Analyze at least 5000 cells per sample to obtain relevant information.

23. Collect the data and subject it to statistical significance using appropriate statistical program.

3.2.4.2. Splenocyte
Analysis

**3.2.4.2.1. Cell
Proliferation**

1. Splenocytes prepared from the spleen of mice receiving different treatments (*see* **Section 3.3.1** step 5 below) are actively grown in culture for 7 days.

2. Actively growing splenocytes are harvested by trypsinization and washed as described in steps 8–14 in **Section 3.2.4.1**.

3. Label the splenocytes with carboxyfluorescein acetate succinimidyl ester (CFSE) using the Vybrant CFDA SE cell tracer kit as per manufacturer's recommendation (24, 25).

4. Seed the CFSE-labeled splenocytes (2×10^6) in 48-well tissue culture plates and incubate for 6 days in an incubator at 37°C, 5% CO_2.

5. After incubation is complete, take out the culture plate from the incubator and place inside a BL2 safety cabinet.

6. Collect the cells into a 15-ml Falcon tube and make the final volume 10 ml with PBS or serum-free culture medium.

7. Place the Falcon tubes in a table-top high-speed centrifuge and spin for 10 min at 1500 rpm at +4°C.

8. After centrifugation, take the tubes back to the culture room and place inside the biosafety cabinet.

9. Aspirate the upper layer of supernatant with the cell pellet at the bottom of the tube.

10. Repeat steps 6–9 one more time.

11. Resuspend the CFSE-labeled splenocytes in 1 ml of PBS and analyze with an EPICS XL-MCL flow cytometer for determining the kinetics of proliferating lymphocyte population.

12. Collect the data and analyze using Cell Quest software.

**3.2.4.2.2. Cell Surface
Immune Marker
Analysis**

1. Splenocytes freshly prepared from the spleen of mice receiving different treatments (*see* **Section 3.3.1** and step 5. below) are used in this assay.

2. Follow steps 9–14 in **Section 3.2.4.1**.

3. Add appropriate concentration of FITC-conjugated anti-CD3e, phycoerythrin-conjugated anti-CD4 (L3T4), or allophycocyanine-conjugated anti-CD8a (Ly-2) (1:100 – 1:1000 dilution) to the splenocytes.

4. Incubate the cells in the dark for 60 min at room temperature.

5. After incubation is complete, take out the tubes and aspirate the antibody.

6. Follow steps 18–23 described in **Section 3.2.4.1**.

3.2.5. Cytokine Measurement

1. Grow UV2237m cells to 70% confluency in a 10-cm tissue culture dish.

2. Aspirate tissue culture medium and wash once with sterile PBS to remove traces of serum.

3. Trypsinize tumor cells and follow steps 8–14 as described in **Section 3.2.4.1**.

4. Irradiate the tumor cells to a cobalt source (5 Gray).

5. Seed irradiated tumor cells (1×10^5 cells/well) in a 48-well tissue culture plate.

6. Incubate overnight at 37°C, 5% CO_2.

7. The next day, aspirate the culture medium.

8. To the wells, add splenocytes (2×10^6 cells/well) harvested from the spleens of mice receiving various treatments. The splenocyte (effector) to tumor (target) cell ratio is 20:1.

9. Incubate the plate for 6 days at 37°C, 5% CO_2.

10. Collect the tissue culture medium every other day and replenish with fresh culture medium.

11. Pool the collected supernatant (2 ml/sample) and concentrate to a 200 μl volume using a Centriplus YM-10 concentrator.

12. Mix the concentrated sample with mouse cytokine 10-plex (TNF-alpha, IL-1beta, IL-2, IL-4, IL-5, IL-6, IL-10, IL-12, GM-CSF, and IFN-gamma) beads and follow the manufacturer's instructions.

13. Analyze the cytokine levels in each of the samples using the Luminex-100 instrument according to the manufacturer's recommendations.

14. Analyze the samples in triplicate and determine the results.

15. Express the cytokine levels as the mean of triplicate for each treatment group and determine the statistical significance.

3.3. In Vivo Adenovirus Delivery

3.3.1. Subcutaneous Tumor Model in Mice

1. Seed UV2237m tumor cells (1×10^6) suspended in appropriate tissue culture medium in 150-mm^2 tissue culture plates (*see* **Note 2**).

2. Incubate the plates in an incubator set at 37°C, 5% CO_2.

3. Monitor the plates every day for cell growth and confluency.

4. When the cells are at 70–80% confluency, remove the plates from the incubator and take it to the biological safety hood.

5. Harvest cells by trypsinization (*see* **Section 3.2**), transfer to a 50-ml Falcon tube, and suspend in 5 ml of serum-free medium for cell counting.

6. Perform cell counting by trypan-blue assay method (*see* **Section 3.2**).

7. Place the 15-ml Falcon tube containing the cells in a table-top clinical centrifuge and spin at 1200 rpm for 10 min at 4°C.

8. Take out the 50-ml Falcon tube and place it inside the culture hood.

9. Aspirate the upper layer of culture medium and retain the cell pellet visible at the bottom of the tube.

10. Add 10 ml of sterile cold PBS to the cell pellet and gently pipette ten times using a 5-ml pipette to disassociate the cell pellet.

11. Centrifuge as indicated in step 7.

12. Repeat steps 8–10 two times.

13. Resuspend the cell pellet in an appropriate volume of cold PBS to give a final cell concentration of 5×10^6 cells per 200 μl of PBS.

14. Place the Falcon tube on ice and take it to the animal room where the mice are housed and are to be injected with the tumor cells.

3.3.2. Preparation of Mice

3.3.2.1. Immunocompetent Mice

1. Place the request for appropriate number of female C3H/HeN mice (4–6 weeks old) to be used for the experiment 1-week prior to start of the experiment (*see* **Note 3**).

2. One day prior to injection of tumor cells, check the number of mice required for the study and their health.

3. The number of mice per cage should not be more than 5.

3.3.2.2. Immunodeficient Mice

1. When using immunodeficient nude mice, steps 1–3 are the same as described for immunocompetent mice. However, additional steps are involved when using nude mice as described below.

2. Take the nude mice to a source of cesium irradiation available in the institute.

3. Subject individual mice to total body cesium radiation at 350 rads (*see* **Note 4**).

4. After irradiation, return the mice to the cages and return the cages to the assigned animal room in the veterinary department.

5. Allow the mice to recover from the radiation induced stress for 24 h.

6. The nude mice are now ready to be injected with the tumor cells.

3.3.3. Injection of Tumor Cells to Mice

1. Before entering the animal room, wear shoe covers, tyvek body suit, cap to cover the head, mask, and gloves.

2. In the animal room, clean the biological safety hood with alcohol (70%) thoroughly.

3. Spread a disposable diaper on the floor of the safety hood and arrange all of the materials needed (e.g., 25-gauge needle, 1-ml tuberculin syringe, vials containing the cells, etc.).

4. Take out the vial containing tumor cells and mix the suspension by gently flushing with a pipette or with a syringe.

5. Take 1 ml of the cell suspension into a tuberculin syringe and keep it aside.

6. Take one cage containing five mice and place it inside the biological safety hood.

7. Open the cage and take out one mouse and sedate the mouse by anesthesia (Isoflurane 2–5% by inhalation) until the respiration slows down.

8. Gently place the mouse on the floor of the hood and monitor for respiration and pedal reflexes.

9. Identify the lower right flank.

10. Wipe the flank with cotton gauze dipped in rubbing alcohol.

11. For C3H mice, shave the area where the tumor cells need to be injected using a commercially available clipper. Removal of hair facilitates easy injection of tumor cells.

12. Slightly stretch the flank of the mice with your non-dominant hand, take the syringe containing the tumor cells (step 5) with your dominant hand and slowly insert the needle underneath the skin of the flank.

13. Slowly inject 200 μl (1×10^6) of the cell suspension.

14. Retain the needle inside the skin for a few seconds after injection to minimize reverse flow and leakage.

15. Return the mouse to the cage and monitor for recovery. The mouse will recover from the sedation in a few minutes.

16. Repeat steps 7–13 for injecting cells into the remaining mice.

17. Monitor the mice every day for their health and tumor growth.

18. Measure the tumor size with a caliper.

19. Palpable tumors (5–6 mm^2) should be observed in 10–14 days and are ready for treatment (**Fig. 14.2**).

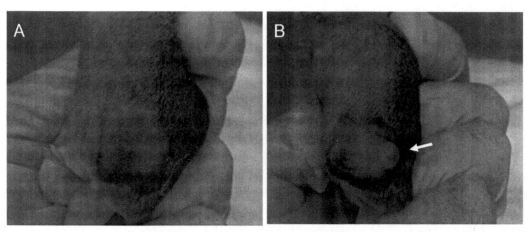

Fig. 14.2. Establishment of subcutaneous tumor. Murine UV2237m fibrosarcoma were established in female C3H/HeN mice by injecting 1 × 10^6 cells on the lower right flank. **A**, Mice were prepared by shaving the lower right flank and injecting tumor cells. **B**, subcutaneous tumors were established 10–14 days after tumor cell injection.

3.3.4. Treatment of Subcutaneous Tumor

1. When the tumor in mice (C3H or nude) is palpable, tag the mice with ear tags to allow easy identification of the individual mice.

2. Determine the tumor size in all of the mice injected with tumor cells using a caliper by measuring the longest (a) and the shortest length (b) of the tumor.

3. Calculate the tumor volume using the formula:

$$a \times b^2/2 = mm^3.$$

4. The tumor volume of each mouse should be between 50–100 mm^3.

5. The tumor–bearing mice are now ready to receive the treatment.

6. Transport the mice to a biohazard room in the veterinary medicine department.

7. Randomize the mice to the different treatment groups.

8. Label the cage cards with the tumor type injected, treatment received, and the ear tag numbers.

9. Freshly prepared Ad-luc or Ad-IL24, as described in **Section 3.1**, is aspirated into a 1 ml tuberculin syringe and kept ready for injection into the tumor.

10. Anesthetize the mice using 2–5% isoflurane as described in step 7 (**Section 3.3.3**).

11. Gently hold the edges of the tumor between the thumb and forefinger of your non-dominant hand.

12. Take the syringe containing Ad-Luc or Ad-IL24 in your dominant hand and slowly insert the needle on one side of the tumor and pass to the middle of the tumor.

13. Slowly inject the viral particles (50–100 µl) into the tumor.

14. Retain the needle inside the tumor after completing the injection for 1 min to prevent reverse flow of the material and leakage.

15. Gently withdraw the needle from the tumor and wipe the injection site with rubbing alcohol.

16. Note the ear tag number in the record book and return the mouse to its cage.

17. Repeat steps 7–13 for injecting virus particles to other tumor-bearing mice.

18. For repeated treatment per experimental design, repeat steps 8–13.

19. Discard used needles and syringes in a Sharps biohazard container; discard used plastic vials and tubes in biohazard bags that are placed in the animal room.

20. Remove all of the protective clothing (gloves, shoe covers, tyvek body suit, etc.) and discard in the designated trash bins.

21. Wash hands with soap.

3.3.5. Analysis of Subcutaneous Tumors for Therapeutic Effect

1. During and after completion of the treatment, measure tumor growth in each mouse using calipers as described in steps 2 and 3 of **Section 3.3.4** and step 2.

2. Measurement of tumor growth can be performed once, twice, or thrice a week and is a choice of the investigator and the experimental design.

3. Record the tumor measurements for each individual mouse in a record book.

4. Calculate the average tumor volume for each treatment group per time point.

5. Enter the values of the average tumor volume for each treatment group per time point in Microsoft Excel spread sheet or other statistical software spreadsheets.

6. Calculate the difference in the tumor volume among the treatment groups for significance using the appropriate statistical method.

7. Statistical analysis can also be performed with the help of a statistician if available in the department or institute.

8. Euthanize the animals by CO_2 inhalation or by any other procedure as recommended and approved by the investigators Institutional Animal Care and Use Committee (IACUC) and by the American Association of Animal Welfare.

9. Place the euthanized mice in biohazard bags and discard in appropriate containers designated by the department of veterinary medicine at the investigators institute.

3.3.6. Rechallenge Studies

1. C3H mice in which the tumors completely regress after Ad-IL24 treatment are separated and monitored for 2–3 weeks after complete tumor regression.

2. Group all of the mice that received Ad-IL24 and demonstrated complete tumor regression.

3. Regroup the mice from step 2 into three groups (groups 3–5).

4. Include two additional groups that comprise naïve C3H mice (groups 1–2).

5. Inject tumor cells (as injected in step 12, **Section 3.3.3**) into the mice as follows:
   Group 1 – naïve C3H mice (1×10^6 tumor cells).

   Group 2 – naïve C3H mice (0.5×10^6; half the original tumor cell number).

   Group 3 – C3H mice cured of tumor (1×10^6 tumor cells).

   Group 4 – C3H mice cured of tumor (0.5×10^6 cells; half the original tumor cell number).

   Group 5 – C3H mice cured of tumor.

6. Follow steps 1–9 described in **Section 3.3.5**.

7. The anticipated result is that tumors in groups 1 and 2 will form and grow progressively. Tumors in groups 3 and 4 will either not form or will form but grow slower when compared to the tumor growth in groups 1 and 2. In group 5, tumor formation should not occur.

8. Demonstration of the anticipated results will provide evidence the contribution of IL-24-mediated immune memory to reject secondary tumor challenge.

9. The splenocytes from these mice can be used for immune marker and cytokine analysis as described in **Sections 3.2.4.2.2.** and **3.2.5.**

3.3.7. Splenocytes

1. Splenocytes is prepared by obtaining the spleen from mice used in therapy studies (**Sections 3.3.1** and step 3 and **3.3.1** and step 4) after euthanization by CO_2 inhalation.

2. The procedure followed is based on the previously described report (26).

3. The freshly isolated spleen is placed in a 10-cm petri dish containing 1 ml of sterile PBS.

4. Mince the spleen into small tissue size with sterile scissors.

5. The tissue is then gently ground between two glass slides for 3–5 min. Grinding results in a separation of splenic cells from the extracellular matrix resulting in single-cell suspension.

6. Pass the 1 ml of PBS containing cell suspension through a 70-μm cell strainer one time with a sterile 15-ml Falcon tube for collecting the cells. Straining the cell suspension eliminates most of the tissue material.

7. Collect the PBS-containing cells with a pipette and layer on the top of a 50-ml Falcon centrifuge tube containing 15 ml of Histopaque-1077.

8. Centrifuge the tube at 15,000 rpm for 10 min at +4°C.

9. Mononuclear cell fraction constituting the splenocytes will appear as a white layer in the Histopaque-1077. Cell debris including RBCs will settle at the bottom of the tube.

10. Carefully, using a sterile glass pipette aspirate the splenocytes into a new sterile 15-ml Falcon centrifuge tube containing 10 ml of Hank's balanced salt solution (HBSS).

11. Wash the cells by centrifugation as described in step 7.

12. Aspirate and discard the upper HBSS solution leaving the cell pellet at the bottom.

13. Repeat steps 10–11 one more time.

14. Resuspend the cell pellet in 2 ml of RPMI-1640 containing 10% FBS 5×10^{-5} M 2-mercaptoethanol, 1% sodium pyruvate, 1% NEAA, 2 mM L-glutamine, 100 units/ml penicillin, and 100 mg/ml of streptomycin.

15. Take an aliquot of the cell suspension and count the number of viable cells by trypan-blue assay as described in **Section 3.2.1** and steps 6–11.

16. The cells are now ready for use in the experiments designed by the investigator.

1. To determine the infiltration and proliferation of immune cells (e.g., CD3, CD4, CD8, or NK cells), tumors, and spleens from mice receiving different treatments are harvested and tissue sections prepared.

2. Cut a part of the tumor or other organ of interest harvested from mice and place the tissue in buffered formalin in appropriately labeled tubes for –24 h.

3. Submit the tissue to the histology laboratory and request for preparation of formalin-fixed paraffin embedded tissue sections. Most institutes and hospitals have a histology laboratory as a core service facility.

4. Prepare 4- to 5-μm-thick tissue sections of the organs harvested from the mice. Tissue sections can be cut as "step-sections" or "serial sections" (see **Note 5**).

5. The tissue sections can be stored in a slide box at room temperature.

6. When ready to stain the tissues follow the below described procedure.
   Take out the slides from the slide box, and label the slides appropriately with a water proof pen.

7. Deparaffinize the tissue sections by placing the slides in an oven set to 60°C for 30 min.

8. Remove the slides and place in a glass slide holder containing xylene for 10 min (see **Note 6**).

9. Rehydrate the slides by serial incubation in different grades of ethanol:
   100% ethanol (EtOH) for 5 min,
   85% EtOH for 5 min,
   60% EtOH for 5 min.
   Distilled water for 2 min.

10. Based on the marker to be stained, the tissue sections may need to be subjected to antigen retrieval (see **Note 7**).

11. Antigen retrieval involves preheating a water-containing steamer for 10 min followed by the following steps:
    (a) Place slides in a plastic slide mailer filled with citrate buffer (5–10 ml).
    (b) Steam for 25 min.
    (c) Remove mailer from steamer and let stand for 2–3 min.
    (d) Remove slides and place them in a glass slide container filled with distilled water for 2–3 min.
    (e) Transfer the slides to another glass container filled with PBS for 2 min.

12. Place the slides in freshly prepared blocking solution for 5–10 min.

13. Wash the slides by placing in PBS for 2 min.

14. Repeat step 13 one more time.

15. Add 100–200 μl of blocking solution and incubate for 30 min at room temperature.

16. Wash slides by incubating in PBS for 2 min.

17. Repeat step 16.

18. Add 100–200 μl of primary antibody diluted (1:100–1:1000) in blocking solution and incubate for 60 min at room temperature.

19. Repeat steps 16 and 17.

20. Add 100–200 μl of secondary antibody diluted (1:100–1:1000) in blocking solution and incubate for 30 min at room temperature.

21. Repeat steps 16 and 17.

22. Add 100–200 μl of ABC reagent (provided in staining kit) and incubate for 45 min.

23. Repeat steps 16 and 17.

24. Add freshly prepared 100–200 μl of DAB solution (500 μl of stock DAB solution mixed with 4.5 ml of blocking solution and 100 μl of 3% H_2O_2) (*see* **Note 8**).

25. Incubate the slides in the dark for 1–5 min at room temperature.

26. Place slides in a glass container and rinse under slow running tap water.

27. Transfer the slides to a container having Mayer hematoxylin for 2 min.

28. Wash slides with water three times to remove excess .hematoxylin.

29. Rehydrate slides by serial transfer into 80, 95 and 100% ethanol with 2 min incubation per each ethanol concentration.

30. Remove slides and air dry.

31. When completely dry, mount the slides with plastic cover slip using water-based or organic solvent based mounting medium (*see* **Notes 8**).

32. Slide is ready for microscopic examination and evaluation of the appropriately stained markers.

4. Notes

1. The number of cells to be seeded for in vitro transfection depends on the cell type and their growth rate. Prior titration using different cell numbers is recommended. Very low cell numbers, however, will lead to toxicity as well as low transfection. Optimization is strongly recommended.

2. Prior to seeding the cells, make sure the cells are healthy and have around 70% confluency. Check for presence of mycoplasma and bacterial contamination as this will interfere with tumor formation when implanted in mice.

3. Mice can be purchased from different vendors. Female mice are relatively easy to handle. Male mice are aggressive and often result in fighting and inflicting wounds on mice within a cage. This will result in isolating mice into separate cages and also the elimination of mice from a study.

4. Nude mice, although indicated as immunodeficient (T- and B-cell deficient), have natural killer (NK) cells. Additionally, some B-cell activity exists. To eliminate the contribution of these cells in IL–24-mediated antitumor-immunity in nude mice, we prefer whole body sub-lethal radiation (350 rads of cesium).

5. The thickness of the tissue section cut can be as thick as 8 μm depending on the antibody and the marker to be stained. "Step section" refers cutting through the tissue and taking the first section followed by taking the fourth or fifth cut section. The sections in-between are discarded. "Serial section" refers to cutting through the tissue and taking a consecutive section for the study. Selection of one procedure over the other is an investigator's decision.

6. Xylene fumes are harmful to human health. It is strongly recommended to handle xylene inside a fume hood. Wear a respiratory mask if necessary.

7. Antigen retrieval is recommended for those markers that are not easy to detect. Antigen retrieval unmasks the antigen and enhances the staining and detection. Paraffin has been shown to mask the antigen during the tissue embedding process.

8. DAB is a carcinogen and the handling of DAB should be performed while wearing gloves. Precautionary measures are recommended. Also, disposal of DAB should be per institutional environmental safety and health (EH&S) guidelines.

Acknowledgments

The authors would like to thank Drs. Ryo Miyahara, Yasuko Miyahara, Kouichiro Kawano, and Sanjeev Banerjee for their immense contribution to the IL-24 immunotherapy studies, and Ms. Jennifer Parker for editorial assistance. This work was supported in part by a sponsored research agreement with Introgen Therapeutics, Inc.

References

1. Jiang, H., Lin, J. J., Su, Z. Z., Goldstein, N. I., and Fisher, P. B. (1995) Subtraction hybridization identifies a novel melanoma differentiation associated gene, mda-7, modulated during human melanoma differentiation, growth and progression. *Oncogene 11*, 2477–2486.

2. Chada, S., Sutton, R. B., Ekmekcioglu, S., Ellerhorst, J., Mumm, J. B., Leitner, W. W., Yang, H. Y., Sahin, A. A., Hunt, K. K., Fuson, K. L., Poindexter, N., Roth, J. A., Ramesh, R., Grimm, E. A., and Mhashilkar, A. M. (2004) MDA-7/IL-24 is a unique cytokine-tumor suppressor in the IL-10 family. *Int Immunopharmacol 4*, 649–667.

3. Huang, E. Y., Madireddi, M. T., Gopalkrishnan, R. V., Leszczyniecka, M., Su, Z., Lebedeva, I. V., Kang, D., Jiang, H., Lin, J. J., Alexandre, D., Chen, Y., Vozhilla, N., Mei, M. X., Christiansen, K. A., Sivo, F., Goldstein, N. I., Mhashilkar, A. B., Chada, S., Huberman, E., Pestka, S., and Fisher, P. B. (2001) Genomic structure, chromosomal localization and expression profile of a novel melanoma differentiation associated (mda-7) gene with cancer specific growth suppressing and apoptosis inducing properties. *Oncogene 20*, 7051–7063.

4. Commins, S., Steinke, J. W., and Borish, L. (2008) The extended IL-10 superfamily: IL-10, IL-19, IL-20, IL-22, IL-24, IL-26, IL-28, and IL-29. *J Allergy Clin Immunol 121*, 1108–1111.

5. Wang, M., Tan, Z., Zhang, R., Kotenko, S. V., and Liang, P. (2002) Interleukin 24 (MDA-7/MOB-5) signals through two heterodimeric receptors, IL-22R1/IL-20R2 and IL-20R1/IL-20R2. *J Biol Chem 277*, 7341–7347.

6. Dumoutier, L., Leemans, C., Lejeune, D., Kotenko, S. V., and Renauld, J. C. (2001) Cutting edge: STAT activation by IL-19, IL-20 and mda-7 through IL-20 receptor complexes of two types. *J Immunol 167*, 3545–3549.

7. Sauane, M., Gopalkrishnan, R. V., Sarkar, D., Su, Z. Z., Lebedeva, I.V., Dent, P., Pestka, S., and Fisher, P. B. (2003) MDA-7/IL-24: novel cancer growth suppressing and apoptosis inducing cytokine. *Cytokine Growth Factor Rev 14*, 35–51.

8. Inoue, S., Shanker, M., Miyahara, R., Gopalan, B., Patel, S., Oida, Y., Branch, C. D., Munshi, A., Meyn, R. E., Andreeff, M., Tanaka, F., Mhashilkar, A. M., Chada, S., and Ramesh, R. (2006) MDA-7/IL-24-based cancer gene therapy: translation from the laboratory to the clinic. *Curr Gene Ther 6*, 73–91.

9. Lebedeva, I. V., Emdad, L., Su, Z. Z., Gupta, P., Sauane, M., Sarkar, D., Staudt, M. R., Liu, S. J., Taher, M. M., Xiao, R., Barral, P., Lee, S. G., Wang, D., Vozhilla, N., Park, E. S., Chatman, L., Boukerche, H., Ramesh, R., Inoue, S., Chada, S., Li, R., De Pass, A. L., Mahasreshti, P. J., Dmitriev, I. P., Curiel, D. T., Yacoub, A., Grant, S., Dent, P., Senzer, N., Nemunaitis, J. J., and Fisher, P. B. (2007) mda-7/IL-24, novel anticancer cytokine: focus on bystander antitumor, radiosensitization and antiangiogenic properties and overview of the phase I clinical experience. *Int J Oncol 31*, 985–1007.

10. Ramesh, R., Mhashilkar, A. M., Tanaka, F., Saito, Y., Branch, C. D., Sieger, K., Mumm, J. B., Stewart, A. L., Boquoi, A., Dumoutier, L., Grimm, E. A., Renauld, J. C., Kotenko, S., and Chada, S. (2003) Melanoma differentiation-associated gene 7/interleukin (IL)-24 is a novel ligand that regulates angiogenesis via the IL-22 receptor. Cancer Res 63, 5105–5113.

11. Chada, S., Bocangel, D., Zheng, M., Mhashilkar, A. M., and Ramesh, R. (2007) MDA-7/IL-24 is a tumor-targeting apoptotic cytokine (apokine). A. Zdanov, (Ed.),

Class II Cytokines. Transworld Research Network, India, 177–191.

12. Poindexter, N. J., Walch, E. T., Chada, S., and Grimm, E. A. (2005) Cytokine induction of interleukin-24 in human peripheral blood mononuclear cells. *J Leukoc Biol 78*, 745–752.

13. Caudell, E. G., Mumm, J. B., Poindexter, N., Ekmekcioglu, S., Mhashilkar, A. N., Yang, X. H., Retter, M. W., Hill, P., Chada, S., and Grimm, E. A. (2002) The protein product of the tumor suppressor gene, melanoma differentiation-associated gene 7, exhibits immunostimulatory activity and is designated IL-24. *J Immunol 168*, 6041–6046.

14. Mumm, J. B., Ekmekcioglu, S., Poindexter, N. J., Chada, S., and Grimm, E. A. (2006) Soluble human MDA-7/IL-24: characterization of the molecular form(s) inhibiting tumor growth and stimulating monocytes. *J Interferon Cytokine Res 26*, 877–886.

15. Kunz, S., Wolk, K., Witte, E., Witte, K., Doecke, W. D., Volk, H. D., Sterry, W., Asadullah, K., and Sabat, R. (2006) Interleukin (IL)-19, IL-20 and IL-24 are produced by and act on keratinocytes and are distinct from classical ILs. *Exp Dermatol 15*, 991–1004.

16. Wegenka, U. M., Dikopoulos, N., Reimann, J., Adler, G., and Wahl, C. (2007) The murine liver is a potential target organ for IL-19, IL-20 and IL-24: Type I Interferons and LPS regulate the expression of IL-20R2. *J Hepatol 46*, 257–265.

17. Wu, B., Huang, C., Kato-Maeda, M., Hopewell, P. C., Daley, C. L., Krensky, A. M., and Clayberger, C. (2008) IL-24 modulates IFN-gamma expression in patients with tuberculosis. *Immunol Lett 117*, 57–62.

18. Oral, H. B., Kotenko, S. V., Yilmaz, M., Mani, O., Zumkehr, J., Blaser, K., Akdis, C. A., and Akdis, M. (2006) Regulation of T cells and cytokines by the interleukin-10 (IL-10)-family cytokines IL-19, IL-20, IL-22, IL-24 and IL-26. *Eur J Immunol 36*, 380–388.

19. Kõks, S., Kingo, K., Vabrit, K., Rätsep, R., Karelson, M., Silm, H., and Vasar, E. (2005) Possible relations between the polymorphisms of the cytokines IL-19, IL-20 and IL-24 and plaque-type psoriasis. *Genes Immun 6*, 407–415.

20. Kragstrup, T. W., Otkjaer, K., Holm, C., Jørgensen, A., Hokland, M., Iversen, L., and Deleuran, B. (2008) The expression of IL-20 and IL-24 and their shared receptors are increased in rheumatoid arthritis and spondyloarthropathy. *Cytokine 41*, 16–23.

21. Kingo, K., Mössner, R., Kõks, S., Rätsep, R., Krüger, U., Vasar, E., Reich, K., and Silm, H. (2007) Association analysis of IL19, IL20 and IL24 genes in palmoplantar pustulosis. *Br J Dermatol 156*, 646–652.

22. Buzas, K., and Megyeri, K. (2006) Staphylococci induce the production of melanoma differentiation-associated protein-7/IL-24. *Acta Microbiol Immunol Hung 53*, 431–440.

23. Miyahara, R., Banerjee, S., Kawano, K., Efferson, C., Tsuda, N., Miyahara, Y., Ioannides, C. G., Chada, S., and Ramesh, R. (2006) Melanoma differentiation-associated gene-7 (mda-7) /interleukin (IL)-24 induces anticancer immunity in a syngeneic murine model. *Cancer Gene Ther 13*, 753–761.

24. Lyons, A. B., and Parish, C. R. (1994) Determination of lymphocyte division by flow cytometry. *J Immunol Meth 171*, 131–137.

25. Kurts, C., Carbone, F. R., Barnden, M., Blanas, E., Allison, J., Heath, W. R., and Miller, J. F. (1997) CD4+ T cells help impairs CD+ T cells deletion induced by cross-presentation of self antigens and favors autoimmunity. *J Exp Med 186*, 2057–2062.

26. Love-Schimenti, C. D., and Kripke, M. L. (1994) Dendritic epidermal T cells inhibit T cell proliferation and may induce tolerance by cytotoxicity. *J Immunol 53*, 3450–3456.

Chapter 15

Liposomes for Gene Transfer in Cancer Therapy

Nancy Smyth Templeton

Abstract

We developed improved liposomes that produce efficacy for the treatment of cancer, cardiovascular diseases, and HIV-1-related diseases in small and large animal models. Because our processes are reproducible, we have standard operating procedures (SOPs) for the cGMP manufacture of these reagents that have been approved by the Food and Drug Administration for use in phase I/II clinical trials.

Key words: Liposomes, nanotechnology, clinical trials, cGMP, gene therapy, non-viral.

1. Introduction

We developed improved liposomes that produce efficacy for the treatment of cancer (1–3), cardiovascular diseases, and HIV-1 related diseases in small and large animal models. These liposomes condense nucleic acids, mixtures of nucleic acids and proteins, and viruses (4) on the interior of bilamellar invaginated vesicles (BIVs) produced by a novel extrusion procedure (5). These nucleic acid:liposome complexes have extended half-life in the circulation, are stable in physiological concentrations of serum, have broad biodistribution, efficiently encapsulate various sizes of nucleic acids and other molecules, are targetable to specific organs and cell types, penetrate through tight barriers in several organs, are fusogenic with cell membranes, are optimized for nucleic acid:lipid ratio and colloidal suspension in vivo, can be size fractionated to produce a totally homogenous population of complexes prior to injection, and can be repeatedly administered. We can add specific ligands either by ionic interactions or by

P. Yotnda (ed.), *Immunotherapy of Cancer*, Methods in Molecular Biology 651,
DOI 10.1007/978-1-60761-786-0_15, © Springer Science+Business Media, LLC 2010

covalent attachments to the surface of these nucleic acid-liposome complexes to accomplish targeted delivery to specific cell surface receptors. The ligands include monoclonal antibodies, Fab fragments, peptides, peptide mimetics, small molecules and drugs, proteins, and parts of proteins. In addition, the charge on the surface of these complexes can be modified in order to avoid uptake by non-target cells using our novel technology called "reversible masking." We have also achieved high dose systemic delivery of these complexes without toxicity in vivo by further purification of plasmid DNA. We have developed proprietary technologies for the detection and removal of contaminants found at high levels in clinical grade plasmid DNA preparations produced by several different companies. For instance, these DNA contaminants preclude high dose delivery of complexes that may be required for the treatment of metastatic cancer. Our "Super Clean DNA" also provides for elevated levels of gene expression and prolonged transient expression in vitro and in vivo. Our complexes have been injected into mice, rats, rabbits, pigs, nonhuman primates, and humans. Currently, these complexes are injected intravenously into patients in clinical trials to treat lung cancer and will be used in upcoming trials to treat breast, pancreatic, head and neck cancers; Hepatitis B and C, and restenosis (*see* **Note 1**). This liposomal delivery system has been used successfully in a phase I clinical trial to treat end-stage non-small cell lung carcinoma patients who have failed to respond to chemotherapy (6). These patients have prolonged life spans and have demonstrated objective responses including tumor regression. This chapter focuses on the production of these BIV liposomes (*see* **Note 2**) and on mixing nucleic acid-liposome complexes (*see* **Notes 3** and **4**). Because our processes are reproducible, we have standard operating procedures (SOPs) for the cGMP manufacture of these reagents that have been approved by the Food and Drug Administration for use in phase I/II clinical trials.

2. Materials

The following materials are necessary:
1. ethanol,
2. paper towels,
3. gloves,
4. spatulas,
5. 1-l round-bottomed flask,
6. cork ring to hold the round-bottomed flask,

7. timer,

8. small weigh boats,

9. sterile 5% dextrose in water (D5W; Abbott Laboratories Inc. Part No. 1522-02),

10. cGMP grade (Cat. No. 770890) or GLP grade (Cat. No. 890890) 18:1 dimethyldioctadecylammonium bromide (DOTAP) powder form (Avanti Polar Lipids),

11. cGMP grade synthetic cholesterol (Sigma Cat. No. C1231),

12. ACS grade chloroform (Fisher Cat. No. C298-1),

13. 0-grade argon gas, RBS pF detergent concentrate (Pierce Cat. No. 27960),

14. sterile glass vials with screw tops,

15. sterile 50-ml polypropylene conical tubes (Falcon Cat. No. 352098, Becton Dickinson Labware),

16. sterile 15-ml polypropylene conical tubes (Falcon Cat. No. 352097),

17. sterile polysulfone syringe filters 1.0-μm pore size 13 mm dia (Whatman Cat. No. 6780-1310),

18. sterile polysulfone syringe filters 0.45-μm pore size 13 mm dia (Whatman Cat. No. 6780-1304), sterile ANOTOP syringe filters 0.2-μm pore size 10 mm dia (Whatman Cat. No. 6809-1122),

19. sterile ANOTOP syringe filters 0.1-μm pore size 10 mm dia (Whatman Cat. No. 6809-1112),

20. glass pipettes,

21. sterile polystyrene pipettes,

22. lens paper,

23. parafilm

24. sterile 10-cc syringes (Becton Dickinson Cat. No. 309604),

25. sterile water (Baxter Cat. No. 2F7114), sterile microfuge tubes,

26. sterile pipette tips with no barriers,

27. latex control particles (Beckman-Coulter Part No. 6602336),

28. plastic cuvettes with caps (Beckman-Coulter Part No. 7800091),

29. conductivity calibration standard (Beckman-Coulter Part No. 8301355),

30. EMPSL7 mobility standard (Beckman-Coulter Part No. 8304073),

31. Class II Type A/B3 laminar flow biological safety cabinet (hood),

32. vortex,

33. analytical balance,

34. rotary evaporator (Buchi model R-114, Brinkmann Instruments),

35. vacuum aspirator (Brinkmann model B-169),

36. water baths,

37. circulating water bath (Lauda model E100),

38. freeze dryer (Labconco model Freezone 4.5),

39. low frequency sonicator (Lab-Line TansSonic model 820/H,

40. pipette aid,

41. pipetmen,

42. spectrophotometer (Beckman model DU640B, Beckman-Coulter),

43. spectrophotometer turbidity cell holder (Beckman Part No. 517151),

44. UV-Silica masked semi-microcell (Beckman Part No. 533041),

45. submicron particle size analyzer with computer (Coulter model N4 Plus, Beckman-Coulter),

46. zeta potential analyzer (Coulter model Delsa 440SX).

3. Methods

3.1. Liposome Preparation

This procedure prepares 30 ml of BIV liposomes. The final yield is about 95%, and therefore, approximately 28.5 ml of 5X stock liposomes are produced.

1. Clean all work surfaces and the hood with 70% ethanol.

2. Allow lipids, DOTAP, and synthetic cholesterol to come to room temperature (RT).

3. Weigh 420 mg of DOTAP and place into a 1-l round-bottomed flask.

4. Weigh 208 mg of synthetic cholesterol and place into the 1-l round-bottomed flask.

5. Dissolve the lipids in 30 ml of chloroform.

6. Rotate on the rotary evaporator at 30°C for 30 min to make a thin film.

7. Dry the film in the flask under vacuum for 15 min.

8. Under the hood, add 30 ml of D5W to the film, cover with parafilm, and make small holes in the parafilm with a syringe needle.

9. Rotate the flask in a 50°C water bath for 45 min, rotating and swirling the flask until the film is in solution.

10. Place the flask in a 37°C water bath and continue to swirl for 10 min.

11. Cover the flask with more parafilm (over the parafilm with holes) and allow the flask to sit overnight at RT.

12. The next day, remove the parafilm with no holes and sonicate the flask at low frequency (35 kHz) for 5 min at 50°C.

13. Under the hood, place the contents from the flask into a sterile 50-ml tube, and aliquot liposomes evenly into three sterile 15-ml tubes.

14. Place one 15-ml tube into a circulating water bath at 50°C (nearby the hood) for 10 min.

15. Under the hood, remove the plungers from four sterile 10-cc syringes and attach one of each pore size sterile filter (1.0, 0.45, 0.2, and 0.1 μm) to the syringes.

16. Under the hood, rapidly filter the liposomes through all four filters, starting with the largest pore size (1.0 μm) and ending with the smallest pore size (0.1 μm).

17. Under the hood, collect liposomes in a sterile 50-ml tube.

18. Repeat steps 14–16 for the remaining two 15-ml tubes and collect all liposomes in the same sterile 50-ml tube (listed in step 17) under the hood.

19. Under the hood, aliquot the liposomes into sterile glass tubes with screw caps, flush with argon or nitrogen gas through a 0.2-μm filter, and store at 4°C.

20. Rinse the round-bottomed flask with hot water, then with ethanol, and fill with 1X RBS and allow to sit overnight. The next day, rinse out the flask, then rinse with hot water, then with distilled water, and finally with ethanol. Seal the flask with parafilm after it is dry.

3.2. Quality Assurance/Quality Control Testing for the Liposome Stock

1. Place 10 μl of liposomes into 190 μl of sterile water. Read the sample on the spectrophotometer at OD400 using the turbidity holder and corresponding cuvette. The reading should be about 4.0, and the acceptable range is any reading lower than 4.5 OD400.

2. Determine the size for the L100 and L200 standards using the particle size analyzer. If the standards are within range, proceed to assess the liposome stock. Place 12 μl of

liposomes into 4 ml of sterile water in the plastic cuvette. Determine the particle size that should be about 200 nm, and the acceptable range is between 50 and 250 nm.

3. Access the mobility for the conductivity calibration standard and the mobility standard using the zeta potential analyzer. If the standard is within range, proceed to assess the liposome stock. Place 120 μl of liposomes into 1880 μl of sterile water. Determine the zeta potential that should be about 65 mV, and the acceptable range is between 50 and 80 mV.

4. Assays for residual chloroform in the liposome stock should not detect any chloroform. All sterility tests should show no observable growth or no contamination.

3.3. Complex Preparation

Using pipetmen and microfuge tubes, final volumes ranging from 50 to 1200 μl of complexes can be prepared.

1. Bring all reagents to RT.

2. Under the hood, dilute the 5X stock liposomes to 2X in D5W in a microfuge tube. For example, to mix a 300 μl final volume of complexes, dilute 60 μl of 5X stock liposomes in 90 μl of D5W.

3. Under the hood in a second microfuge tube, dilute the stock nucleic acid in D5W to 1 μg/μl. The volume of diluted nucleic acid must be identical to the volume of diluted stock liposomes in step 2. The final mixed complexes have a concentration of 0.5 μg of nucleic acid/μl. Note: the stock nucleic acid should be vortexed well prior to removing any aliquot for mixing complexes.

4. Under the hood, pipette the diluted nucleic acid into the diluted liposomes by rapid mixing at the surface of the liposomes. Rinse up and down about twice using the pipetman.

5. Read the sample (10 μl of the complexes in 190 μl of sterile water) on the spectrophotometer at OD400 using the turbidity holder and corresponding cuvette. The OD400 should be about 0.8, and the acceptable range is between 0.65 and 0.95 OD400. If the complexes fall out of this range, then the amount of nucleic acid used for mixing must be adjusted. Specifically, if the OD400 is too low, then more nucleic acid must be used for mixing. If the OD400 is too high, then less nucleic acid must be used for mixing. If the nucleic acid is not adequately pure, then the appropriate OD400 of the complexes will not be obtained. Note: to avoid wasting material in order to establish the proper mixing conditions, we mix final volumes of complexes at 50 μl

first before we begin large scale mixing using new lots of nucleic acids.

6. When the proper mixing volumes have been established, more complexes can be mixed if needed following the steps above. All complexes can be pooled after mixing, and the OD400 of the pooled complexes should be measured and should fall between 0.65 and 0.95 OD400.

7. The particle size of the complexes can also be measured. Determine the size for the L300 and L500 standards using the particle size analyzer. If the standards are within range, proceed to assess the complexes. Place 12 μl of complexes into 4 ml of sterile water in the plastic cuvette. Determine the particle size that should be about 400 nm, and the acceptable range is between 200 and 500 nm.

8. Because the encapsulation of nucleic acids is spontaneous, the complexes can be administered after mixing. Complexes can also be stored in glass vials at 4°C and administered the following day.

4. Notes

1. The complexes can be administered and re-administered into animals and humans by any delivery route. The dose and administration schedule will be determined by the specific nucleic acid therapeutic and disease model of the investigator, and therefore, must be optimized.

2. Many investigators are not set up to produce liposomes in their laboratories. Therefore, the BIV liposomes and other custom services can be purchased from our non-viral core facility at the Baylor College of Medicine (contact Nancy Smyth Templeton at **ntempleton@gradalisinc.com** to place orders).

3. Using the optimal liposomes for transfection is not necessarily enough to ensure success. Other reagents must be optimized such as the expression plasmid design (6) and the plasmid DNA preparation (7) for applications that use plasmid DNA.

4. We have found that BIV DOTAP is best for transfection of cells in culture (4, Templeton, unpublished data). The same protocol is used to produce these liposomes; however, cholesterol is not added. Complexes made with BIV DOTAP are mixed using the same procedure above.

References

1. Ramesh, R., Saeki, T., Templeton, N. S., Ji, L., Stephens, L. C., Ito, I., Wilson, D. R., Wu, Z., Branch, C. D., Minna, J. D., and Roth, J. A. (2001) Successful treatment of primary and disseminated human lung cancers by systemic delivery of tumor suppressor genes using an improved liposome vector. *Mol Ther* 3, 337–350.

2. Shi, H. Y., Liang, R., Templeton, N. S., and Zhang, M. (2002) Inhibition of breast tumor progression by systemic delivery of the maspin gene in a syngeneic tumor model. *Mol Ther* 5, 755–761.

3. Tirone, T. A., Fagan, S. P., Templeton, N. S., Wang, X. P., and Brunicardi, F. C. (2001) Insulinoma induced hypoglycemic death in mice is prevented with beta cell specific gene therapy. Ann Surg *233*, 603–611.

4. Yotnda, P., Chen, D.-H., Chiu, W., Piedra, P. A., Davis, A., Templeton, N. S., and Brenner, M. K. (2002) Bilamellar cationic liposomes protect adenovectors from preexisting humoral immune responses. *Mol Ther* 5, 233–241.

5. Templeton, N. S., Lasic, D. D., Frederik, P. M., Strey, H. H., Roberts, D. D., and Pavlakis, G. N. (1997) Improved DNA: liposome complexes for increased systemic delivery and gene expression. *Nature Biotech 15*, 647–652.

6. Lu, H., Zhang, Y., Roberts, D. D., Osborne, C. K., and Templeton, N. S. (2002) Enhanced gene expression in breast cancer cells in vitro and tumors in vivo. *Mol Ther 6*, 783–792.

7. Templeton, N. S. (2002) Liposomal delivery of nucleic acids in vivo. *DNA Cell Biol 21*, 857–867.

Chapter 16

Oncolytic HSV as a Vector in Cancer Immunotherapy

Hongtao Li and Xiaoliu Zhang

Abstract

It is well documented that immunotherapy has a great potential for cancer treatment. The ideal cancer immunotherapeutic strategies should be relatively simple, but able to trick the host's immune system to elicit a robust immune response to the tumor target. Herpes Simplex Virus (HSV) has been engineered for the purpose of oncolysis. These so-called oncolytic HSVs can selectively replicate within tumor cells, resulting in their destruction and in the production of progeny virions that can spread to adjacent tumor cells. In addition to their direct oncolytic effect, tumor lysis by oncolytic viruses releases tumor antigens in their native form and configuration in an individualized way. Immune responses thus generated would be more likely to recognize the original tumor than would tumor vaccines produced by other methods, most of which require extensive in vitro modification and manipulation. Several recently published studies have shown that HSV-elicited antitumor immune responses are an essential part of the overall antitumor effect produced by oncolytic HSVs, not only for controlling primary tumor growth, but also for preventing long distance metastases. In this chapter several key methods will be illustrated to monitor the immune response elicited by oncolytic HSVs.

Key words: Oncolytic HSV, immunotherapy, CTL, virotherapy, cancer.

1. Introduction

Despite the steady improvements in standard treatment of cancer by surgery, radiation, and chemotherapy, cancer is still the second leading cause of death in the US. The main reason is the failure of these standard cares to eradicate the established tumors that reside either in the orthotopic organ or at the distant metastatic sites. There is ample evidence to suggest that the host's immune system, if harnessed effectively, can not only combat infectious diseases caused by bacteria and viruses, but also protect the body against cancer occurrence or treat the established tumors (1).

P. Yotnda (ed.), *Immunotherapy of Cancer*, Methods in Molecular Biology 651,
DOI 10.1007/978-1-60761-786-0_16, © Springer Science+Business Media, LLC 2010

Cancer immunotherapy has been frequently designed with the purpose to increase the potential of either tumor-specific antibodies or cellular immune responses against the targeted tumor. Several drugs based on cytokines and antibodies have been approved for clinical use in treating cancer patients (2).

Oncolytic viruses are genetically modified to replicate in tumor cells but not in normal cells (3). Tumor destruction in situ by an oncolytic virus should release large quantities of tumor antigens in their native forms and configurations, thus affording an attractive means to produce a whole tumor vaccine (4). Tumor antigens released after virotherapy can be presented to T cells either directly by tumor cells or indirectly via cross-presentation by professional antigen-presenting cells, such as dendritic cells. Several mechanisms can facilitate the access of antigenic materials from malignant cells to the exogenous pathway of antigen-presenting cells for class I and class II presentation (5). Chief among them is the inflammatory milieu, which can be created during virotherapy in the tumor site in situ. The inflammatory microenvironment can attract migration as well as stimulate maturation of antigen presentation cells. The direct oncolytic effect and subsequent induction of antitumor immunity during virotherapy may provide a unique combination that can potentially eradicate locally invasive or metastatic tumors that are difficult to manage with conventional agents and thus represents a highly promising strategy of cancer treatment.

Replication selective oncolytic viruses have shown great promise as antitumor agents for solid tumors and are currently in clinical trials for treating several malignant diseases (6). Oncolytic HSV has several attractive features to make it a good candidate for cancer immunotherapy study. First, HSV can infect a wide variety of tumor cells with relatively low infection particles. Second, HSVs have evolved several molecular mechanisms to escape host immune clearance. Third, HSV is well characterized and can be easily controlled by the anti-virus drugs such as acyclovir and gancyclovir. Finally, the mouse and monkey animal model are readily available for the immune study of oncolytic HSV (7–12). Several commonly used methods that have been used in studying the immune responses elicited by oncolytic HSVs will be discussed and illustrated on this chapter.

2. Materials

2.1. Cell Lines and Mouse Splenocytes Suspension

1. Dulbecco's modified Eagle medium (DMEM), high-glucose formulation, containing 5, 10, or 20% FBS, heat-inactivated 1 h at 56°C, 2 mM L-glutamine, 50 µM 2-ME, 100 U/ml penicillin, and 100 µg/ml streptomycin sulfate.

2. RPMI 1640 medium containing 2, 5, 10, 15, or 20% FBS, heat-inactivated 1 h at 56°C, 2 mM L-glutamine, 50 μM 2-ME, 100 U/ml penicillin, and 100 μg/ml streptomycin sulfate.

3. For splenocytes preparation, 60 × 15-mm petri dishes, scissors and forceps, kept in sterile beaker with 70% ethanol, 6-ml syringe with 19-G needle, 200-μm mesh nylon screen.

4. Red blood cell lysing buffer: 8.29 g NH_4Cl (0.15 M), 1 g $KHCO_3$ (10.0 mM), and 37.2 mg Na_2EDTA (0.1 mM). Add 800 ml H_2O and adjust pH to 7.2–7.4 with 1 N HCl. Add H_2O to 1 l. Filter sterilize through a 0.2-μm filter. Store at room temperature.

5. High-density solution: Ficoll-Paque (Ficoll and sodium diatrizoate; Pharmacia LKB) or Lympholyte-M (Cedarlane) 12- or 50-ml polypropylene centrifuge tubes.

2.2. Virus Propagation and Titration

1. Overlay medium: DMEM containing 1% FBS and 1.2% carboxylmethylcellulose. Store at room temperature.

2. Crystal violet stock solution: 1 % crystal violet in 20% ethanol. Crystal violet working solution: stock solution 4 ml; ethanol 8 ml; water 30 ml (This is approximately 0.1% crystal violet in 20% ethanol).

3. Carboxylmethylcellulose stock solution: 12% carboxylmethylcellulose in PBS, autoclaved. Carboxylmethylcellulose working solution: 1:10 dilution into EMEM containing 1% FBS.

2.3. Immunohistochemistry

1. 10% neutral-buffered formalin: prepare a 10% (w/v) solution in PBS fresh for each experiment. The solution may need to be carefully dissolved, and then cool to room temperature for use.

2. Mayer's hematoxylin buffer: aluminium ammonium sulfate 200 g, hematoxylin 20 g, ethanol 40 ml, sodium iodate 4 g, acetic acid 80 ml, glycerol 1200 ml, and distilled water 2800 ml. Mix well and store (see Note 1).

3. Scott's tap water substitute: sodium hydrogen carbonate 10 gm, magnesium sulfate 100 gm, and distilled water 5 L. Dissolve the salts in the water. Store stock solutions at room temperature.

4. Eosin buffer: 1% eosin 400 ml, 1% phloxine 40 ml, 95% alcohol 3100 ml, and acetic acid 16 ml. Mix and stir well.

5. Mounting medium: Antifade (Molecular Probes, Eugene, OR).

2.4. Elispot

1. 96-well PVDF-backed microplate (Millipore plate, Cat. No. S2EM004M99), and two antibodies for mouse interferon-γ (BD Bioscience, Cat. No.551881).

2. Coating buffer (PBS): 8 g NaCl; 0.2 g KCl; 1.44 g Na_2HPO_4-$7H_2O$, 0.24 g KH_2PO_4; dissolved in H_2O to a final volume of 1 liter. Adjust pH to 7.2, filter sterilize (0.2 μm), and store at 4°C.

3. Blocking Solution: complete tissue culture medium (e.g., RPMI 1640 containing 10% FBS and 1% penicillin–streptomycin, L-glutamine).

4. Wash Buffer I: 1× PBS containing 0.05% Tween-20 (0.5 ml Tween-20 per 1 L PBS).

5. Wash Buffer II: 1× PBS.

6. Dilution Buffer: 1× PBS containing 10% FBS.

7. ELISPOT AEC Substrate.

   (a) Prepare AEC (3-Amino-9-ethyl-carbazole; Sigma A-5754) stock solution: mix 100 mg AEC in 10 ml DMF (N,N dimethylformamide; Sigma D-4551). Caution: dispense DMF in fume hood. Store solution in glassware.

   (b) Prepare 0.1 M acetate solution: add 148 ml of 0.2 M acetic acid/glacial acidic acid to 352 ml of 0.2 M sodium acetate. Adjust volume to 1 L DI water; adjust pH to 5.0.

   (c) For final substrate solution, add 333.3 μl of AEC stock solution to 10 ml 0.1 M acetate solution. Filter through 0.45-μm filter. Add 5 μl of H 202 (30%) and use immediately.

3. Method

The antitumor immune responses during virotherapy are routinely investigated using syngeneic murine tumor models. Several cell lines and oncolytic HSVs have been used (*see* **Note 2**). Tumors are established either in the orthotopic site or on the flank through tumor cell implantation into syngeneic mouse strain (*see* **Note 3**). For subcutaneous tumors, animals will receive an intratumoral injection of either PBS or oncolytic HSV when the local tumors become palpable in all mice after tumor cell inoculation. Injections are given slowly at two to three different sites across the tumor to prevent leakage. For orthotopic tumors implanted in internal organs, virotherapy will usually be given at 7–10 days after tumor implantation, either intratumorally or intraperitoneally (e.g., for ovarian or pancreatic cancers). To examine the innate immune response, the lymphocyte infiltration into the tumor site will be detected by flowcytometry and immunohistochemistry (*see* **Note 3**). The adaptive immune response is usually monitored by analyzing the harvested splenocytes, as detailed in the following sections.

3.1. Viral Preparation

3.1.1. Preparation of Stocks of HSV on VERO or BHK Cells

1. Grow cells to 90% confluency.
2. Remove medium.
3. Infect with 0.1 pfu/cell.
4. Leave 2 days until CPE is achieved.
5. Shake or scrape cells off flask into medium and keep on ice from this point onwards.
6. Spin cells for 5 mins at 2500 rpm at 4°C.
7. Remove supernatant.
8. Resuspend pellet in 1 ml DMEM medium.
9. Sonicate for 1 min – see notes below.
10. Aliquot in 0.1-ml volumes.
11. Label aliquots as "stock" with batch no. "H-", and the date.
12. Freeze at –80°C.

3.1.2. Titration of HSV

1. Sonicate virus stock for 1 min on full power or repeatedly freeing/thawing 3×.
2. Make initial virus dilutions in 1× EMEM (without additions) as follows, depending on the estimated concentration of virus in the stock:
   - 100× 10.1 µl to 1 ml → 10–2
   - 100× 10.1 µl to 1 ml → 10–4
3. Make 10× virus dilutions from these dilutions as follows:
   - 10× 111.1 µl to 1 ml → 10–5
   - 10× 111.1 µl to 1 ml → 10–6
   - 10× 111.1 µl to 1 ml → 10–7
   - 10× 111.1 µl to 1 ml → 10–8
4. Remove the medium from the cells (Vero cells in 6-well dishes) and add 500 µl of each virus dilution to each of two wells. (If you start at the lowest virus dilution you can use the same tip for all the dilutions.)

5. Incubate at 37°C for 1 h, rocking the plates every 15 min to spread the virus inoculum.

6. Prepare overlay medium.

7. Remove medium containing virus from plates, starting at dilution with least virus, and add overlay medium to plates (2 ml per well of 6-well dish, 3 ml per 5-cm dish).

8. After 2 days stain plaques with crystal violet (*see* **Note 4**).

3.1.3. Staining Plaques
with Crystal Violet

1. First remove the agarose overlay if any.

2. Put on enough Crystal violet working solution to cover the cells without drying out (1 ml).

3. Leave for 15 min.

4. Remove stain. Wash cells by dunking in a beaker of water.

5. Blot plates dry on tissues and leave to dry in the hood for 15–30 min.

6. Count plaques.

3.2. Harvest of Mouse Splenocytes

3.2.1. Harvest of Freshly
Removed Spleen from
Mice

1. Place freshly removed organs in 60 × 15-mm petri dishes (one for each type of organ to be removed) containing 3 ml complete RPMI-5 or DMEM-5. With scissors, cut the organs in several places.

2. Using a circular motion, press the pieces against bottom of the petri dish with the plunger of a 6-ml syringe until mostly fibrous tissue remains.

3. Further disperse clumps in the suspension by drawing up and expelling the suspension several times through a 6-ml syringe equipped with a 19-G needle.

4. Expel suspension into a centrifuge tube through a 200-μm mesh nylon screen. Wash petri dish with ~4 ml complete medium. Repeat if necessary and add wash to tube.
About 5 ml of complete medium (containing 5% FCS) is used during the processing of each spleen, thymus, and set of lymph nodes from one mouse.

5. Centrifuge 10 min in Sorvall H-1000B rotor at 1000 rpm ($200 \times g$) and discard supernatant (see support protocols if removal of red blood cells or dead cells is required). Resuspend pellet in 20 ml complete medium, centrifuge again, and resuspend in a volume suitable for counting.

3.2.2. Removal of Red
Blood Cells from Spleen
Cell Suspensions

Before counting the total number of lymphocytes in suspensions of spleen cells, it is desirable to remove the red blood cells (RBC), as the inexperienced eye will often have trouble distinguishing those from the white blood cells.

1. Resuspend pellet of spleen cells in lysing buffer, using ~5 ml per spleen; use a 12-ml test tube for one or two spleens, or a 50-ml tube for more spleens.

2. Incubate 5 min at room temperature with occasional shaking.

3. Add wash medium to fill the tube, spin 10 min at $200 \times g$ in a low-speed centrifuge and discard supernatant. Wash pellet again and resuspend in appropriate medium and volume for next procedure (e.g., dead cell removal, cell counting, or fractionation).

3.2.3. Removal of Dead Cells Using the One-Step Gradient Method

1. Resuspend cells in complete RPMI-5 and distribute into centrifuge tubes at $0.5–1 \times 10^8$ cells/2 ml (12-ml tube) or $1–5 \times 10^8$ cells/5 ml (50-ml tube) (*see* **Note 5**).

2. Layer 3 ml (for 12-ml tubes) or 5 ml (for 50-ml tube) high-density solution under the cell suspension by drawing the high-density solution into a pipette, placing tip of pipette at bottom of tube, and slowly letting the solution flow under the cell suspension.

3. Centrifuge 15 min in Sorvall H-1000B rotor at 2000 rpm ($800 \times g$), room temperature (*see* **Note 6**).

4. Isolate live cells floating on top of the high-density solution by slowly moving tip of pipette over surface of high-density layer and drawing cells up in a 5-ml pipette (try to collect as little high-density solution as possible). Transfer live cells to another tube.

5. Add complete RPMI-5 (10 ml for the small volume, 40 ml for the larger volume) and centrifuge 10 min at $200 \times g$, room temperature. Repeat this washing procedure.

6. Resuspend cells in appropriate medium and volume for subsequent procedure.

3.3. Immunohisto-chemistry

For histologic examination of tumor specimens, mice were euthanized at different times after treatment and sections of tumor were fixed in 10% neutral-buffered formalin for 24 h, dehydrated in serial ethanol, and embedded in paraffin. Sections (5-μm thick) were prepared, mounted on slides, and stained with Hematoxylin and Eosin (13).

1. Hydrate the tissue section: put the slide into the 100% ethanol after issue section. Rinse the rack with tap water to remove ethanol for 5 min.

2. Stain nucleus with Hematoxylin: Put the rack into a container filled with Hematoxylin for 10 min. Rinse the rack

with tap water for 10 min to remove Hematoxylin. Dip the rack into a jar containing 0.1% HCl 3 times and into tap water 3–4 times. Dip the rack into a jar containing 0.1% NH₄OH three times and into tap water 3–4 times.

3. Stain cytoplasm with Eosin and dehydrate: dip the rack into the following solutions for 5 min.
AcetoneEosin ethanol (100%); ethanol (100%); ethanol (100%) with 0.1% acetic acid; acetone; xylene; xylene.

4. Mounting: drop 2–3 drops of mountantonto the slide and, then, put a cover glass onto the slide.
An example of the results produced is shown in **Fig. 16.1**.

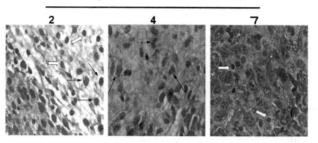

Days after FusOn-H2 treatment

Fig. 16.1. Tumor histology after HSV therapy. Tumor nodules were explanted on days 2, 4, and 7 after the start of therapeutic injections of oncolytic HSV (FusOn-H2). One typical field within H&E-stained tumor sections from mice treated with FusOn-H2 alone is presented at each time point. The infiltrating lymphoid cells (⇨), monocytic cells (➔) , and LLC cells (➡) are labeled. Some of the indicated tumor cells show degeneration and/or necrosis with prominent vacuolar cytoplasm. Original magnification, 400×.

3.4. Chromium51 Release Assay

For quantifying CTL activity, mice were sacrificed 14 days after intratumoral injection of oncolytic HSV into immune-competent Balb/c mice bearing 4T1 tumor. Splenocytes were isolated from mice in each treatment group. Effector cells were obtained by coculturing splenocytes with irradiated tumor cells, supplemented with recombinant human interleukin-2. After 5 days of restimulation, the effector cells to lyse target cells were quantified by using the standard 4-h chromium release assay (14).

1. Select the appropriate targets (tumor cell lines *see* **Note 7**) expressing the restricting HLA class I allele and transfer the required number of cells into a 15-ml conical tube (*see* **Note 8**).

2. Spin cells down for 10 min at 1500 rpm. Aspirate supernatant to about 200 μl. Add 50 uCi of Cr^{51} per target, then resuspend cells with the same pipette tip you used to add the chromium. Incubate cells for 1 h at 37° C.

3. Purified splenocytes were added as effector cells to the 96-well plate; count the effectors and resuspend them at the proper concentration (*see* **Note 9**).

4. After the hour is up, wash the targets three times with 12 ml cold R10 at 1000 rpm for 7 min in a cold centrifuge. Count cells and resuspend. Add 100 μl target tumor cells to each 96 well. Incubate plates for 4 h in the incubator.

5. After 4 h, harvest 30 μl of supernatant were harvested and Cr^{51} release was measured with a scintillation counter (*see* **Note 10**).
    An example result is shown in **Fig. 16.2**.

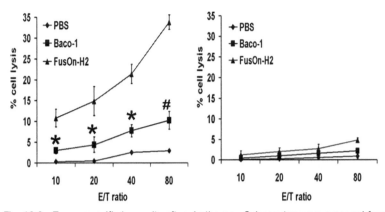

Fig. 16.2. Tumor-specific immunity after virotherapy. Splenocytes were prepared from spleens collected from Balb/c mice bearing 4T1 tumor and treated with the indicated agents. In vitro stimulated effector cells were then assayed for CTL activity against (**A**) 4T1 tumor cells or (**B**) syngeneic MethA sarcoma cells. All results were means ± SD of triplicate assays. *$p<0.05$, comparing FusOn-H2 with PBS and Baco-1; #$p<0.01$, comparing FusOn-H2 with PBS and Baco-1.

3.5. ELISPOT Assay

The splenocytes prepared for Fig. 2 were also quantitated by ELISPOT assays. The chromogenic alkaline phosphatase substrate was added. The colorimetric reaction was terminated within 5–20 min by washing with tap water. After drying, the spots were counted (15).

1. Dilute capture antibody in coating buffer. Add 100 μl of diluted antibody solution to each well of an ELISPOT plate; Store plates at 4°C overnight.

2. Discard coating antibody. Wash wells 1× with 200 μl/well blocking solution. Add 200 μl/well blocking solution and incubate for 2 h at room temperature.

3. Discard blocking solution. Prepare antigen (*see* **Note 7**), diluted in complete tissue culture medium. Add 100 μl/well to ELISPOT plate. Prepare cell suspensions at different densities, (e.g., 1×10^5/ml to 2×10^6 cells/ml) Add 100 μl/well of each cell suspension to ELISPOT plate wells. Replace ELISPOT plate lid. Incubate ELISPOT plate at 37°C, 5% CO_2 and 99% humidity (*see* **Note 11**).

4. Aspirate cell suspension. Wash wells 2× with deionized (DI) water. Allow wells to soak for 3–5 min at each wash step. Wash wells 3× with 200 μl/well wash buffer I. Discard wash buffer. Dilute detection antibody in dilution buffer. Replace lid and incubate for 2 h at room temperature.

5. Discard detection antibody solution. Wash wells 3× with 200 μl/well wash buffer I. Dilute Streptavidin-Horseradish Peroxidase (HRP) in dilution buffer. Add 100 μl/well diluted Streptavidin-HRP. Replace lid; incubate for 1 h at room temperature.

6. Discard Streptavidin-HRP solution. Wash wells 4× with 200 μl/well wash buffer I. Wash wells 2× with 200 μl/well wash buffer II. Add 100 μl of final substrate solution (AEC) to each well. Monitor spot development from 5 to 60 min (*see* **Note 12**).

7. Enumerate spots manually using a dissecting microscope or automatically using an ELISPOT Analyzer.
   An example result is shown in **Fig. 16.3**.

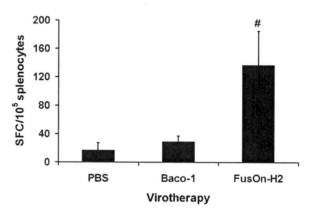

Fig. 16.3. ELISPOT assay after virotherapy. Splenocytes were prepared from spleens collected from the experiment 3. All results were means ± SD of triplicate assays. #$p <$ 0.01, comparing FusOn-H2 with PBS and Baco-1.

4. Notes

1. Add the hematoxylin powder to the alcohol. Pour the strong alcoholic solution of hematoxylin into the cooled alum solution stir to dissolve. Add the sodium iodate, acetic acid, and finally the glycerol.

2. Cell lines and oncolytic HSV viruses developed by this study that have been used for studying antitumor immune responses are listed here.

Cell lines: African green kidney (Vero) cells; 4T1 cells, a 6-thioguanine-resistant cell line derived from a BALB/c spontaneous mammary carcinoma; Meth-A, a methylcholanthrene-induced sarcoma cell line of BALB/c origin; Murine neuroblastoma Neuro-2A and Sa-I murine sarcoma cell lines (ATCC) (*see* **Note 1**).

Viruses: HSV type 1 oncolytic viruses: Baco-1 and Synco-2D (16); HSV type 2 oncolytic virus: FusOn-H2 was derived from the wild-type HSV-2 strain 186 (17) (*see* **Note 2**).

3. For the mouse neuroblastoma Neuro-2A inoculation in this study, 6- to 8-week-old immunocompetent A/J mice were used. For the mouse mammary 4T1, 6- to 8-week-old female Balb/c mice were used.

4. Vortex each dilution for at least 5 seconds before making next dilution. Use a fresh yellow tip for each dilution.

5. The efficacy of the separation procedures is dependent on the interface diameter; therefore, 50-ml tubes are used when separation of higher numbers of cells is desired, while 12-ml tubes can be used for lower cell numbers. For minimum cell loss due to adherence, polypropylene tubes are recommended over polystyrene tubes.

6. Best separations are obtained when rapid acceleration and slow deceleration (no brake) are used. A slightly higher centrifugation speed than normally used is recommended because the Ficoll solution is of higher density.

7. Using MethA cells as the control for 4T1 cells, Sa-I as the control for Neuro2A cells.

8. Transfer 1–1.5 million cells per target into a 15 ml conical tube, depending on how many targets you will need for the assay; plan the assay in advance so that you will know how many cells you need.

9. Different effector/target ratios were employed in a series of studies. The commonly used ratio is 80:1, 40:1, 20:1, and 10:1. It is critical to include the syngeneic tumor cell line as a control to show the specificity of the immune response.

10. RPMI medium served as a negative control. Supernatants Spontaneous release was measured in wells containing target cells alone. Triton X-100 was used to lyse the target cells maximally. The percentage of specific lysis was calculated by the following formula: percent of specific lysis = [(experimental release cpm – spontaneous release cpm)/(maximum release cpm – spontaneous release cpm)] × 100 (14).

11. The duration of the incubation time can be varied (e.g., 2 –24 h) depending on the nature of the stimulatory cell

culture system. Specific activation conditions and incubation times will vary, depending on cell type, kinetics, and cytokine of interest. After step 3, aseptic conditions are no longer needed.

12. Stop substrate reaction by washing wells with DI water. Air-dry plate for 2 h – overnight at room temperature in the dark, until the plate is completely dry. Store plate in the dark, prior to analysis.

References

1. Weiner, L. M. (2008) Cancer immunotherapy – the endgame begins. *N Engl J Med 358*, 2664–2665.

2. Waldmann, T. A. (2003) Immunotherapy: past, present and future. *Nat Med 9*, 269–277.

3. Russell, S. J., and Peng, K. W. (2007) Viruses as anticancer drugs. *Trends Pharmacol Sci 28*, 326–333.

4. Heath, W. R., Belz, G. T., Behrens, G. M., Smith, C. M., Forehan, S. P., Parish, I. A., Davey, G. M., Wilson, N. S., Carbone, F. R., and Villadangos, J. A. (2004) Cross-presentation, dendritic cell subsets, and the generation of immunity to cellular antigens. *Immunol Rev 199*, 9–26.

5. Wolfers, J., Lozier, A., Raposo, G., Regnault, A., Thery, C., Masurier, C., Flament, C., Pouzieux, S., Faure, F., Tursz, T., Angevin, E., Amigorena, S., and Zitvogel, L. (2001) Tumor-derived exosomes are a source of shared tumor rejection antigens for CTL cross-priming. *Nat Med 7*, 297–303.

6. Todo, T. (2008) Oncolytic virus therapy using genetically engineered herpes simplex viruses. *Front Biosci 13*, 2060–2064.

7. Varghese, S., and Rabkin, S. D. (2002) Oncolytic herpes simplex virus vectors for cancer virotherapy. *Cancer Gene Ther 9*, 967–978.

8. Randazzo, B. P., Kesari, S., Gesser, R. M., Alsop, D., Ford, J. C., Brown, S. M., Maclean, A., and Fraser, N. W. (1995) Treatment of experimental intracranial murine melanoma with a neuroattenuated herpes simplex virus 1 mutant. *Virology 211*, 94–101.

9. Wong, R. J., Kim, S. H., Joe, J. K., Shah, J. P., Johnson, P. A., and Fong, Y. (2001) Effective treatment of head and neck squamous cell carcinoma by an oncolytic herpes simplex virus. *J Am Coll Surg 193*, 12–21.

10. Mineta, T., Rabkin, S. D., Yazaki, T., Hunter, W. D., and Martuza, R. L. (1995) Attenuated multi-mutated herpes simplex virus-1 for the treatment of malignant gliomas. *Nat Med 1*, 938–943.

11. Wong, R. J., Patel, S. G., Kim, S., DeMatteo, R. P., Malhotra, S., Bennett, J. J., St-Louis, M., Shah, J. P., Johnson, P. A., and Fong, Y. (2001) Cytokine gene transfer enhances herpes oncolytic therapy in murine squamous cell carcinoma. *Hum Gene Ther 12*, 253–265.

12. Ino, Y., Saeki, Y., Fukuhara, H., and Todo, T. (2006) Triple combination of oncolytic herpes simplex virus-1 vectors armed with interleukin-12, interleukin-18, or soluble B7-1 results in enhanced antitumor efficacy. *Clin Cancer Res 12*, 643–652.

13. Li, H., Zeng, Z., Fu, X., and Zhang, X. (2007) Coadministration of a herpes simplex virus-2 based oncolytic virus and cyclophosphamide produces a synergistic antitumor effect and enhances tumor-specific immune responses. *Cancer Res 67*, 7850–7855.

14. Li, H., Dutuor, A., Fu, X., and Zhang, X. (2007) Induction of strong antitumor immunity by an HSV-2-based oncolytic virus in a murine mammary tumor model. *J Gene Med 9*, 161–169.

15. Li, H., Dutuor, A., Tao, L., Fu, X., and Zhang, X. (2007) Virotherapy with a type 2 herpes simplex virus-derived oncolytic virus induces potent antitumor immunity against neuroblastoma. *Clin Cancer Res 13*, 316–322.

16. Fu, X., Tao, L., Jin, A., Vile, R., Brenner, M. K., and Zhang, X. (2003) Expression of a fusogenic membrane glycoprotein by an oncolytic herpes simplex virus potentiates the viral antitumor effect. *Mol Ther 7*, 748–754.

17. Fu, X., Tao, L., Cai, R., Prigge, J., and Zhang, X. (2006) A mutant type 2 herpes simplex virus deleted for the protein kinase domain of the ICP10 gene is a potent oncolytic virus. *Mol Ther 13*, 882–890.

Chapter 17

Generation of Chimeric T-Cell Receptor Transgenes and Their Efficient Transfer in Primary Mouse T Lymphocytes

Linda J. Howland, Nicole M. Haynes, and Phillip K. Darcy

Abstract

Gene modification of T cells with chimeric T-cell receptor (TCR) transgenes offers a novel way to generate tumor-specific T cells for cancer immunotherapy. Retroviruses have been utilized as the most common means of efficiently transducing primary T lymphocytes with these transgenes. In this section we describe methods for generation of chimeric TCR's and utilization of retroviral vectors for efficient transduction of these transgenes in primary mouse T lymphocytes.

Key words: Retrovirus, murine, T lymphocytes, chimeric T-cell receptor, transfection, transduction, retronectin, packaging cells, enrichment.

1. Introduction

Adoptive immunotherapy, involving transfer of tumor-reactive T cells into patients, is an emerging new approach for the treatment of cancer. Studies involving the transfer of tumor-infiltrating lymphocytes, expanded with IL-2, into patients with advanced melanoma disease has resulted in some remarkable anti-cancer responses and regression of disease (1). The inclusion of lymphoablative conditioning has led to enhanced persistence of transferred T cells and increased anti-tumor effects (2). Nevertheless, the broad application of this approach has been limited by the difficulty of isolating tumor-specific T cells for all tumor types.

P. Yotnda (ed.), *Immunotherapy of Cancer*, Methods in Molecular Biology 651,
DOI 10.1007/978-1-60761-786-0_17, © Springer Science+Business Media, LLC 2010

An alternative strategy to address this problem involves the genetic modification of T cells with chimeric single-chain (scFv) receptors that can specifically recognize tumor-associated antigen (TAA). One advantage of this approach is that T cells gene-modified with these receptors can be specifically directed toward a variety of TAAs on different tumor types in patients of any HLA type. A number of studies have demonstrated enhanced tumor recognition by primary T cells using this approach (3, 4). More recently, chimeric scFv receptors incorporating both co-stimulatory and primary signaling domains linked in tandem (scFv-CD28-ζ) have been shown to optimally activate T cells following specific-antigen stimulation in vitro (3, 4) and in adoptive transfer experiments in mice (5).

Retroviral vectors have been the most commonly used vehicles to gene modify human peripheral blood lymphocytes (PBL) with scFv and/or T-cell receptor (TCR) transgenes for adoptive transfer into patients (6–8). Transduction of human PBL using RetroNectin® and incorporation of centrifugation steps into the protocol have been reported to enhance the level of gene transfer. Despite these advances for increasing transgene expression in human T cells, only a few studies have reported efficient transduction of mouse T lymphocytes for reasons that are not entirely clear (9). The ability to achieve good levels of transduction of primary mouse T lymphocytes is particularly important for adoptive immunotherapy approaches that involve optimization of specific chimeric receptor transgenes in a compatible in vivo system.

Investigations in our laboratory have found that the level of transgene expression in primary mouse splenic T cells can be increased by two to three levels of magnitude over that obtained by spin infection methods, by co-culturing mouse T lymphocytes with high titer retrovirus-producing packaging cells in the presence of phytohemagglutinin (PHA) and recombinant human IL-2 (rh-IL-2). The enhanced transduction efficiency, achieved by co-cultivation, is most likely due to optimal infection by the virus due to cell–cell contact and high local virus concentration. The incorporation of a c-*myc* tag recognition epitope within the extracellular region of our scFv gene constructs has allowed for direct detection of transgenes on the surface of transduced mouse T cells. This transduction protocol results in the rapid, reproducible and high level expression of chimeric TCR receptors in both primary mouse CD8$^+$ T cells (40–50%) and CD4$^+$ T cells (20–30%) without the need for antibiotic selection. This is an important advantage over conventional strategies, that generally involve the selection of transduced T cells by treatment with Geneticin (G418), as this avoids prolonged culture times and any negative effect that this may have on their biological activity following adoptive transfer. This is particularly important considering recent evidence demonstrating that persistence of adoptively transferred

T cells and their anti-tumor effects correlated well with cells being in an early state of effector T-cell differentiation (10). In this report, we describe methods for construction of chimeric TCR and a new transduction protocol for expressing these transgenes in primary mouse T cells.

2. Materials

1. MFE-23 vector (contains the scFv anti-CEA antibody)
2. pRSV-scFv-R vector (*see* **Note 1**)
3. pSW50-5 vector (contains the scFv anti-erbB2 antibody)
4. pGEM3Z-ζ (contains human TCR-ζ signaling domain)
5. LXSN retroviral vector (11) (*see* **Note 2**)
6. Restriction enzymes: *Xba* I, *BstE* II, *Xho* I, *Sna* B1, *Hpa* I
7. Murine ecotropic GP+E86 packaging cell line (12)
8. PA317 amphotropic packaging cell line (12)
9. NIH3T3 cells (mouse fibroblast cell line)
10. Human peripheral blood mononuclear cells (PBMC)
11. COS-7 cells
12. Jurkat E6-1 cells
13. 9E10 cells (hybridoma for anti-c-*myc* antibody)
14. Dulbecco's Modified Eagle's Medium (DMEM) (Gibco-BRL, Grand Island, NY)
15. Complete medium: DMEM supplemented with 10% (vol/vol) heat-inactivated fetal calf serum (FCS), 2 mM L-glutamine (Gibco-BRL), 100 U/ml penicillin (Gibco-BRL), and 100 μg/ml streptomycin (Gibco-BRL)
16. Selection medium: Geneticin (G418; Gibco-BRL, Grand Island, NY) 100 μL of 50 mg/ml stock in 10 ml DMEM (final concentration of 500 μg/ml)
17. Recombinant human IL-2 (rh-IL-2; Biological Resources Branch Preclinical Repository, National Cancer Institute); stock at 10^6 U/ml
18. Polybrene (Sigma, St. Louis, MO): 4 mg/ml stock
19. Phytohemagglutinin (PHA; Sigma, St. Louis, MO): 1 mg/ml stock
20. 1x Phosphate buffered saline (PBS)
21. 0.9% saline solution

22. Trypsin

23. 2x HEPES buffered saline (HBS): 50 mM HEPES, pH 7.05 (5.0 g), 10 mM KCl (0.37 g), 12 mM Dextrose (1.0 g), 28 mM NaCl (8.0 g), 1.5 mM Na_2HPO_4 (0.1065 g), and make up to 500 ml with distilled water (*see* **Note 3**)

24. Calcium Chloride Solution: 2 M $CaCl_2$ (29.4 g) in 100 ml in distilled water

25. Polyethylene glycol 8000 (Fisher Scientific, Fairlawn, NJ)

26. May-Grunwald stain: May-Grunwald stain (Sigma, St Louis, MO) 0.3 g/100 ml of 100% methanol. Following 24 h settling time, sterilize by passing through a 0.2 μM filter

27. Nylon wool (Polysciences Inc, Warrington, PA)

28. 10 ml syringe (Becton Dickinson, San Jose, CA)

29. Stop-cock (Becton Dickinson, San Jose, CA)

30. ACK lysis buffer: 0.15 M NH_4Cl (8.29 g), 1.0 mM $KHCO_3$ (1.0 g), 0.1 mM Na_2EDTA (37.2 mg) made up to 800 ml with distilled water and pH adjusted to 7.2–7.4 with 1 M HCL, then top up to 1 l with more distilled water. Sterilize through a 0.2-μM filter and store at room temperature

31. 2x Lysis Buffer: 1% SDS, 0.6 M NaCl, 20 mM EDTA and 20 mM Tris–HCL (pH 7.4)

32. Formaldehyde solution: 7.5% formaldehyde, 1.5 M NaCl and 150 mM sodium citrate (pH 7.0)

33. 10 mm tissue culture dishes (Corning)

34. 60 mm tissue culture dishes (Corning)

35. T25 tissue culture flasks

36. 0.45 μM filter for syringes

37. 70 μM nylon sieve (Becton Dickinson, San Jose, CA, USA)

38. Dissection equipment (scissors and forceps sterilized)

39. MACs buffer: 1x PBS with 0.5% bovine serum albumin (BSA; Sigma)

40. MACs Dynabeads: anti-mouse CD8 monoclonal antibody (mAb) conjugated beads, and anti-mouse CD4 mAb conjugated beads (Miltenyi Biotec, Bergisch Gladbach, Germany)

41. Dynal MPC-50 magnet (Invitrogen, Mount Waverley, VIC, Australia)

42. Falcon 50 ml polypropylene tubes (Becton Dickinson, San Jose, CA)

43. Nylon membrane–Hybond-N$^+$ (Amersham, Cleveland, OH)

44. ^{32}P-αCTP radiolabel (PerkinElmer Life and Analytical Sciences, Shelton, CA)

45. ^{32}P-αCTP radiolabeled Neomycin probe

46. Neomycin specific gene primers:
5′-ATGATTGAACAAGATGGATTGCA-3′ and
5′-AGGCATCGCCATGGGTCACGACGAGAT-3′

47. Mouse anti-*c-myc* tag monoclonal antibody

48. FITC-labeled anti-mouse IgG monoclonal antibody (Becton Dickinson, San Jose, CA)

49. PE-labeled anti-mouse monoclonal antibodies against: CD4, CD8, CD44, and CD62L (Becton Dickinson, San Jose, CA)

50. FACs fix solution: 1% formaldehyde, 2% glucose in 500 ml of 1x PBS

51. Vanadyl ribonuclease complex (Gibco BRL)

52. Tris–EDTA buffer (pH 7.4) (Sigma, St. Louis, MO)

53. Yeast tRNA (Gibco BRL)

54. QIAGEN RNA extraction kit (QIAGEN Pty Ltd, Doncaster, Australia)

55. 24-well tissue culture plate

56. Mouse anti-CD3 and anti-CD28 purified antibodies

57. NUNC Maxisorp Immuno Plate

58. Binding buffer: 0.1 M Na$_2$HPO$_4$, pH to 9 with HCL

59. Wash solution: 5 ml Tween-20 in 1 L PBS

60. Blocking solution: PBS with 10% FCS, or 10% NCS or 1% BSA

61. Hydrogen peroxide (H$_2$O$_2$)

62. IFNγ standards of known quantity (5×10^6 pg/ml)

63. Biotin-labeled anti-IFNγ capture antibody

64. Streptavidin–Horseradish peroxidase (SA-HRP)

65. 3,3′,5,5′-Tetramethylbenzidine (TMB) tablets

66. Citrate phosphate buffer (CPB) (10x stock): Add 18.24 g Na$_2$HPO$_4$ to 12.77 g citric acid and make up to 250 ml with distilled water and pH adjust to 5. Make a (1x) working stock by diluting 1:10

3. Methods

Detailed procedures are described for (1) chimeric single chain (scFv) receptor gene construction, (2) generation of stable retrovirus vector expressing cells, (3) transduction of mouse T cells, and (4) functional characterization of transduced T cells.

3.1. Chimeric Single Chain (scFv) Gene Construction

We have generated in our laboratory several chimeric scFv receptor gene constructs containing different signaling domains reactive with either carcinoembryonic antigen (CEA) or the human epidermal growth factor receptor antigen (erbB2) by standard molecular biological techniques. The following section describes detailed methods for the construction of scFv transgenes composed of the V_H and V_L regions of the anti-CEA mAb or anti-erbB2 mAb, joined via a flexible human CD8 hinge to signaling domains comprising a human CD28 co-stimulatory domain, and the human TCR-ζ signaling domain. The expression cassettes used in these studies include the Rous Sarcoma Viral vector (pRSV-scFv-R) (*see* **Note 1**) and the retroviral vector pLXSN (*see* **Note 2**).

3.1.1. Cloning Anti-CEA or Anti-erbB2 scFv into the pRSV-scFv-R Vector

1. For cloning of the anti-CEA gene construct, first amplify a 767-bp fragment of DNA coding for the scFv of anti-CEA from the vector MFE-23 (13) and a c-*myc* tag marker epitope by PCR using the primers designated:
   Sense 5'-ATAATG<u>TCTAGA</u>CAGGTGAAACTGCAG-3'
   Antisense 5'-AGAGAC<u>GGTGACC</u>CCATTCAGATCCTCT TCTGAGATGAGTTTTTGTTCTGCGGCCGCCCGTTT CAGCTCCAGCTT-3'.
   The primers incorporate an *Xba* I site and *BstE* II site, respectively (denoted by the underline).

2. For the anti-erbB2 gene construct, amplify a 767-bp fragment of DNA coding for the scFv of anti-erbB2 from the pSW50-5 vector (a kind gift from Dr. Winfried Wels, Institute of Experimental Cancer Research, Germany) (14) and a c-*myc* tag marker epitope by PCR using the primers designated:
   Sense 5'-ATAATG<u>TCTAGA</u>CAGGTACAACTGCAG-3'
   Antisense 5'-AGAGAC<u>GGTGACC</u>CCATTCAGATCCTCT TCTGAGA TGAGTTTTTGTTCGATCTCCAATTTTGT-3'
   The primers incorporate a *Xba* I site and a *BstE* II site respectively (denoted by the underline).

3. Digest the anti-CEA or anti-erbB2 scFv fragments containing the c-*myc* tag epitope with *Xba* I and *BstE* II restriction enzymes, and clone into the *Xba* I/*BstE* II digested pRSV-scFv-R vector.

4. Identify positive clones by restriction digest and sequence verify.

*3.1.2. Cloning the
Human CD28 Signaling
Domain into the
pRSV-anti-erbB2 or
pRSV-anti-CEA Vectors*

1. Amplify the transmembrane (TM) and cytoplasmic (CYT) domains of human CD28 by PCR from cDNA derived from activated human peripheral blood mononuclear cells (PBMC) using the primers designated:
   Sense: 5′-GAGAGGATCCTCTTTTGGGTGCTG-3′
   Antisense: 5′-GAGACTCGAGTCAGGAGCGATAGGC-TG-3′
   The primers incorporate *Bam* HI and *Xho* I restriction sites, respectively (denoted by the underline).

2. Digest the human CD28 PCR product with *Bam* HI and *Xho* I restriction enzymes and clone into the *Bam* HI/*Xho* I digested pRSV-scFv-R vector (either pRSV-scFv-anti-CEA or pRSV-scFv-anti-erbB2) to generate a gene construct that consists of either scFv-anti-CEA or scFv-anti-erbB2 containing a c-*myc* tag epitope, a CD8 hinge region, and the TM and CYT regions of human CD28.

3. Identify positive clones by restriction digest and sequence verify.

*3.1.3. Cloning the
Human TCR-ζ Signaling
Domain into the
pRSV-scFv-R Vector*

1. Amplify the human TCR-ζ cytoplasmic (CYT) domain containing *Xho* I and *Sal* I restriction sites by PCR from the vector pGEM3Z-ζ (15) using the primers designated:
   Sense 5′-GAGAGACTCGAGAGAGTGAAGTTCAGC-3′
   Antisense 5′-CTAGCTCGAGTTAGCGAGGGGGCAGG-3′ (restriction sites denoted by the underline).

2. Digest the TCR-ζ PCR product with *Xho* I restriction enzyme and clone into calf intestinal phosphatase (CIP) treated *Xho* I digested pRSV-scFv-anti-CEA-hCD28 or pRSV-scFv-anti-erbB2-hCD28 vectors. The gene construct now consists of scFv-anti-CEA or scFv-anti-erbB2 and a c-*myc* tag epitope linked to a CD8 hinge region, a TM and CYT human CD28 domain, and a CYT human TCR-ζ signaling domain.

3. Sequence-verify the entire gene construct cloned into the pRSV-scFv-R vector and to confirm the orientation of the TCR-ζ domain.

4. The complete scFv transgene can be excised using appropriate restriction enzymes and cloned into the retrovirus vector pLXSN as described below.

*3.1.4. Cloning of
Chimeric T-Cell
Receptors into the
Retrovirus pLXSN Vector*

1. Partially digest the pRSV-scFv-R vector containing the chimeric T-cell receptor genes (scFv-anti-CEA-hCD28-hTCRζ or scFv-anti-erbB2-hCD28-hTCRζ) with *Sna* BI and *Xho* I and clone into the *Hpa* I/*Xho* I digested retroviral vector (pLXSN).

2. Identify positive clones by restriction digest and sequence verify entire scFv receptor gene construct.

3.2. Generation of Stable Retroviral Vector Producing Cell Lines

3.2.1. Preparation of PA317 Amphotropic Packaging Cells for Transfection (Day –1)

1. Plate 1×10^6 PA317 cells into a 10 cm tissue culture dish with 10 ml of complete medium (*see* **Note 4**). Incubate the plate in a humidified 37°C, 5% CO_2 incubator.

2. Cells should be 60–70% confluent the following day.

3.2.2. Calcium Phosphate Transfection of PA317 Cells (Day 0)

1. Transfect PA317 cells by combining 6–10 µg of plasmid LXSN retroviral vector containing the scFv gene construct or vector alone for a negative control, with calcium chloride solution in a volume of 500 µl (*see* **Notes 5**). Then add 500 µl of 2x HBS (pH 7.05) dropwise while gently bubbling air through the solution so that it mixes well. Immediately (within 1–2 min) overlay 1 ml of this solution onto plates containing PA317 cells and medium.

2. After 10 h incubation at 37°C and 5% CO_2 remove the medium and replace with 10 ml of fresh complete medium, and incubate overnight at 37°C and 5% CO_2.

3.2.3. Preparation of GP+E86 Ecotropic Packaging Cells for Transduction (Day 1)

1. The PA317 cells should be approximately 80–90% confluent after 24 h transfection.

2. Seed five plates of the parental GP+E86 ecotropic packaging cells in complete medium at 2×10^6 cells/10 cm plate.

3.2.4. Transduction of GP+E86 Packaging Cells (Days 2–4)

1. Harvest supernatant from transfected PA317 cells that are producing retrovirus progeny expressing the transgene and pass through a 0.45 µM Millipore filter (maintaining supernatant on ice throughout procedure).

2. Aspirate the medium off the previously prepared plates of GP+E86 cells and overlay the cells with PA317 retrovirus as follows

Plate number	1	2	3	4	5
Complete medium (ml)	8	9	10	10	10
PA317 retrovirus supernatant (ml)	2	1	0.4	0.2	0.1
Polybrene 4 mg/ml (µl)	10	10	10	10	10

3. After 24 h incubation (day 3) at 37°C and 5% CO_2 replace the medium with 10 ml complete medium and continue to incubate for a further 24 h.

4. Once GP+E86 cells have reached confluency (day 4), harvest the GP+E86 cells from all five plates separately by treatment with trypsin, centrifuge to pellet the cells then resuspend each cell pellet (five in total) in 10 ml of complete medium. For each of the five cell suspensions generated above, plate out a further 5×10 cm plates as follows:

Plate number	1	2	3	4	5
Complete medium (ml)	18	19	20	20	20
GP+E86 cells (ml)	2	1	0.5	0.25	0.125

5. Leave plates (total 25 new plates) overnight at 37°C in a 5% CO_2 incubator.

3.2.5. Antibiotic Selection of Transduced GP+E86 Clones (Day 5)

1. Aspirate supernatant and replace medium with 10 ml complete medium containing the selection antibiotic geneticin (G418; 500 μg/ml).

2. Replace the selection medium every 3–4 days.

3. Incubate the cells at 37°C and 5% CO_2 for 10–14 days before isolating colonies.

3.2.6. RNA Slot-Blot Analysis for Isolation of High Viral Titer Clones (Days 10–14)

1. Collect supernatants from the plates of selected retroviral producing cells and filter through a 0.45-μM Millipore filter.

2. Precipitate the retroviral RNA from 1 ml of each supernatant with 30% polyethylene glycol 8000 and 1.5 M NaCl and leave on ice for 30 min. Centrifuge the precipitate to generate a pellet, discard the supernatant then resuspend the pellets in 200 μl of Tris–EDTA buffer (pH 7.4) containing 10% (vol/vol) vanadyl ribonuclease complex and 100 μg/ml of yeast tRNA.

3. Lyse the solution by adding 200 μl of 2x lysis buffer and extract the retroviral RNA from the lysed solution using a QIAGEN RNA extraction kit.

4. Reconstitute RNA with 500 μl of a formaldehyde solution. Subsequently, load 100 and 400 μl of each RNA sample into adjacent wells of a slot-blot apparatus Minifold II (Schleicher and Schuell, Keene, NH) and transfer onto a nylon membrane Hybond-N$^+$ (Amersham, Cleveland, OH).

5. After transfer, hybridize filters firstly with a ^{32}Pα-CTP radiolabeled Neomycin probe and then a probe recognizing the gene of interest to select for high expressing clones.

6. Upon analysis of gene expression in the separate clones, the positive GP+E86 clones are frozen at –70°C in liquid nitrogen (*see* **Note 6**).

**3.3. Determination
of Virus Titer by
Infection of NIH3T3
Cells (Days 0–14)**

1. Plate the GP+E86 retroviral-producing cells (high virus titer clones selected in **Section 3.2.6**) at 1×10^6 per T25 flask in 5 ml of complete medium. Incubate the cells at 37°C and 5% CO_2 for 24 h until 90–100% confluent.

2. Discard medium by aspiration (day 1) and replace with 4 ml of fresh complete medium.

3. Seed 14×60 mm culture dishes with 2×10^5 NIH3T3 cells for each of the GP+E86 clones plated above. The plates are required for duplicate analysis of each of the six ten-fold virus dilutions (12 plates) generated of each GP+E86 clone and control plates (2 plates) containing no virus in the following analysis.

4. Collect viral supernatant from GP+E86 retrovirus-producing clones after 18 h ($\sim$ 4 ml volume) (day 2), filter through a 0.45 µM Millipore filter and chill on ice for immediate use. The supernatants can also be stored at –70°C for further analysis at another time if required.

5. Prepare virus dilutions (10^{-1} to 10^{-6}) in 0.8–1 ml volume of complete medium and keep everything on ice (*see* **Note 6**). Add polybrene at 4 µg/ml to each virus dilution.

6. Remove medium from NIH3T3 cells and immediately add 0.5 ml of virus/polybrene mixture dropwise to the NIH3T3 cells. Duplicate plates are required for each virus dilution (in particular 10^{-3}, 10^{-4}, and 10^{-5} dilutions). Cultivate for 2 h at 37°C and 5% CO_2 with gentle rocking of each plate every 15–30 min; then gently add 3 ml of complete medium, pre-warmed to 37°C, to the edge of tilted plates.

7. Culture the infected NIH3T3 cells for further 72 h in a 37°C and 5% CO_2 incubator.

8. Harvest the infected NIH3T3 cells (day 5) by treatment with trypsin, centrifuge to pellet the cells and resuspend the pellet in 2.5 ml complete medium.

9. Seed 0.125 ml of NIH3T3 cell suspension onto two 60-mm culture dishes and add 3 ml of selection medium containing G418 (500 µg/ml final concentration) to each culture dish.

10. Incubate the plates for a further 10–14 days and replace the G418 selection medium every 3–4 days to isolate positively transduced clones.

11. Aspirate medium from plates, cover dish with May-Grunwald stain, and leave for 5 min at room temperature. Following removal of the stain, wash plates with distilled water and count colonies of G418-resistant NIH3T3

clones. Viral titer in colony-forming units per ml (cfu/ml) is determined by dividing the number of colonies by the volume (in 1 ml) of virus used for the infection and multiplying by 5 to correct for the 1:5 cell dilution.

3.4. Retroviral-Mediated Transduction of Mouse Lymphocytes

3.4.1. Enrichment of Splenic Mouse T lymphocytes

1. To isolate mouse splenocytes dissect the spleen(s) from syngeneic donor mice, transfer to a sterile 10-cm culture dish and homogenize under manual force.

2. Resuspend the cells in 5–8 ml of hypotonic ACK lysis buffer to deplete the red blood cells present in the suspension, and then neutralize by the addition of 8 ml of complete medium.

3. Strain the cell suspension through a 70 μM nylon sieve to produce a single cell suspension, centrifuge at 1250 rpm for 7–10 min, wash once with PBS, then resuspend in 4 ml of fresh DMEM.

4. Enrich primary mouse T lymphocytes by passing the splenocyte culture through a nylon wool column. Prepare a nylon-wool column by weighing 1.26 g of nylon wool (Polysciences Inc, Warrington, PA). Rinse the nylon wool three times in distilled water, and load tightly into the barrel of a 10 ml syringe using forceps. Sterilize nylon wool columns by autoclaving.

5. Attach a stop-cock to the end of the column, which has been pre-warmed and maintained at 37°C, and equilibrate the column with 20 ml of warmed 0.9% saline solution, 20 ml of warmed DMEM (no FCS or supplements) and finally 20 ml of warmed complete medium. Load the splenocyte suspension onto the column and incubate at 37°C and 5% CO_2 for 45 min before harvesting T cells in 15–20 ml of warmed complete medium into a sterile 50-ml polypropylene tube. This procedure generally results in >90% enrichment of primary mouse T cells.

3.4.2. Immunomagnetic Separation (Negative Selection) for Isolation of Mouse CD8+ and CD4+ T-Lymphocyte Populations

1. For some experiments it may be necessary to further enrich mouse T lymphocyte subsets by magnetically activated cell sorting (MACS). To generate enriched mouse CD8+ or CD4+ T cells, wash nylon-wool column-enriched T cells with MACS buffer (×2) and incubate with either anti-mouse CD8 antibody-conjugated beads (10 μg/ml) or anti-mouse CD4 antibody-conjugated beads (10 μg/ml) for 15 min on ice. Following incubation, wash cells with cold MACS buffer

($\times 2$) and separate on magnetic depletion columns in a Vario MACs separator (Miltenyi, Germany).

2. Verify efficiency of isolating separate T-cell subsets by flow cytometry.

3.4.3. Retroviral Transduction of Enriched Mouse T-lymphocyte Population (Co-cultivation Method)

1. Plate out 1×10^6 GP+E86 retroviral-producing packaging cells into 10 cm dishes containing 10 ml of complete medium without G418 selection (*see* **Note 7**) (day 0).

2. On day 1, add enriched primary mouse T lymphocytes (1×10^7) to retroviral-producing packaging cells together with PHA (5 μg/ml), rh-IL-2 (100 U/ml) and polybrene (4 μg/ml) and co-cultivate at 37°C in a 5% CO_2 incubator for 72 h.

3. On day 4, remove T lymphocytes from packaging cells and transfer to a 10 cm plastic dish for 3 h to allow any remaining GP+E86 packaging cells to adhere to the surface.

4. Remove supernatant containing only the non-adherent transduced T lymphocytes, pellet by centrifugation at 1250 rpm for 5–10 min and wash with complete medium.

5. Subsequently, culture the transduced T lymphocytes (1×10^6/ml) into six-well plates containing complete medium supplemented with rh-IL-2 at 100 U/ml.

6. The efficiency of retrovirus transduction can then be determined immediately by flow cytometry.

3.5. Analysis of Transduction Efficiency by Flow Cytometry

Cell surface expression of the transgene can be determined by staining the transduced mouse T lymphocytes with a mAb directed against a tag epitope that has been incorporated in the extracellular region (3′ end) of the retrovirus insert.

1. We use a c-*myc* tag antibody purified from supernatants of mouse 9E10 cells (16) to determine the level of transgene expression, followed by staining with a FITC-labeled anti-mouse IgG mAb for detection by flow cytometry. The transduced population can then be sorted and enriched further, eliminating the requirement for selection with G418 treatment (*see* **Note 7**).

2. Cell surface phenotyping of transduced cells can then be determined by flow cytometry using phycoerythrin (PE)-conjugated anti-mouse CD4, CD8, CD44, and CD62L antibodies. This involves staining 5×10^5 of transduced T lymphocytes with 100 μl of appropriately diluted antibody at 4°C for 30 min, washing twice in PBS, and resuspending cells in 0.5 ml of FACS fix solution. The phenotype of the cell population can then be determined by flow cytometry.

3.6. Determining Antigen-Specific Cytokine Secretion by Transduced T Cells

3.6.1. Co-culture of T cells with Antigen Positive and Negative Target Cells

1. Culture tumor cells (antigen positive or negative) in 24-well tissue culture plates at 5×10^5 cells/well. Incubate for 2–3 h to allow cells to adhere to the plate.

2. For positive controls, include anti-CD3/anti-CD28 antibody coated wells by diluting each of the purified antibodies 1/1000 in 1 ml PBS and add to a single well of the 24-well plate. Also, coat a single well with purified anti-c-*myc* tag antibody (diluted 1/1000 in 1 ml of PBS) as a positive control for T cells transduced with the chimeric T-cell receptor. Incubate at 37°C 5% CO_2 for 2–3 h.

3. Following the 2–3 h incubation, aspirate the supernatant from all the wells.

4. Add gene-modified or control T cells (5×10^5 cells/well) onto the target cells (1:1 ratio) or antibody coated wells (1 ml total volume/well). Add T cells alone to a well as a negative control.

5. Co-culture T cells and target cells overnight at 37°C 5% CO_2.

6. The following day, spin the 24-well plates at 1250 rpm for 10 min at room temperature. Collect the supernatants from the wells using a 1 ml pipette and filter tips, and transfer the supernatants to another 24- or 48-well tissue culture plate in preparation for analysis by ELISA (*see* **Note 8**).

3.6.2. Enzyme Linked Immunosorbent Assay (ELISA) for Assessing IFNγ Secretion

1. Coat an ELISA 96-well plate (NUNC F96 Maxisorp Immuno Plate) with purified anti-IFNγ mAb diluted 1/1000 in binding buffer and incubate at 4°C overnight. Wash the plate (x 4) with wash solution.

2. Block the plate with 200 μL/well of blocking solution and incubate at room temperature for 1 h. Wash the plate ($\times$ 4) with wash solution.

3. Serially dilute IFNγ standards (two-fold) in PBS and add 100 μL/well in duplicate wells to the plate. For blank wells add 100 μL/well of PBS in duplicate.

4. Add T-cell supernatant samples (derived in **Section 3.6.1**) to appropriate wells of the plate in duplicate at the following dilutions; neat, diluted 1:10 in PBS, or using a further dilution if required (*see* **Note 9**).

5. Incubate the plate with IFN-γ standards and T-cell supernatant samples loaded, at room temperature for 2 h. Wash the plate ($\times$ 6) with wash solution and gently tap the plate dry onto a paper towel.

6. Dilute the biotin labeled capture anti-IFNγ mAb 1/1000 in PBS and add 100 μL/well to the plate. Incubate at room temperature for 1 h. Wash the plate ($\times$ 6) with wash solution and gently tap the plate dry onto a paper towel.

7. Dilute the streptavidin-HRP conjugate 1/500 in PBS, and add 100 μL/well to the plate. Incubate at room temperature for 45 min to 1 h. Wash plate ($\times$ 8) with wash solution and gently tap the plate dry onto a paper towel.

8. Dilute a single TMB substrate tablet in 10 ml of citrate phosphate buffer and wait until completely dissolved before adding 2 μL hydrogen peroxide solution (*see* **Note 10**). Add 50 μL/well TMB substrate solution and incubate at room temperature until blue color develops.

9. Stop the reaction with 1 M H_2SO_4 50 μL/well (turns the color of the reaction yellow). Read the optical density (OD) of the wells using a plate reader at 450 nm wavelength.

10. Analyze and calculate the IFNγ levels using the equation generated from the linear portion of the standard curve.

4. Notes

1. The pRSV-scFv-R vector obtained from Zelig Eshhar (Weizmann Institute, Rehovot, Israel) contains a scFv receptor linked to a CD8 hinge region and gamma. This vector is used as a template to excise the existing scFv construct and insert the scFv of interest. Further additions of TCR or co-stimulatory signaling domains can be added to the construct. The complete chimeric scFv construct can then be cloned into a retrovirus vector (i.e., pLXSN) to enable stable transduction of primary T cells.

2. Retroviral vectors utilizing the Moloney Murine Leukemia Virus (MoMLV) long terminal repeat (LTR) promoter for expression are efficient in directing high levels of gene expression in all T-lymphocyte subpopulations. The pLXSN vector also contains a neomycin resistance (neo[r]) gene.

3. Stock solutions may be prepared and frozen at $-20°C$. The HBS solution required for $CaPO_4$ transfection should be prepared every 6–12 months.

4. Prior to splitting the cells for transfection it is important that the cells are not overgrown. It is important to passage the cells 1:3 to 1:4 to prevent cell clumping which occurs when the cells are passaged at low density or when they are allowed to become over confluent. The key for successful transfection and for achieving high viral titers is to have a large number of single cells evenly spread on the dish. Mycoplasma infection of cell lines can also inhibit efficient transfection/transduction.

5. Plasmid DNA should be prepared either by double spun caesium chloride gradients or by QIAGEN columns. Both methods result in similar transfection efficiencies.

6. With regard to freeze/thawing of retroviral stocks: Freeze stocks immediately at $-70°C$ or keep chilled on ice to maintain viral titer. Do not freeze/thaw more than once as it destroys the integrity of the virus DNA. Once thawed, discard remainder.

7. It is possible to detect and select transduced cells by treatment with G418; however, the potential for this treatment to negatively affect the biological activity of T cells and reduce the already limited lifespan of T cells makes G418 selection unfavorable.

8. Supernatants may be frozen at $-20°C$ and analyzed at a later time point.

9. Absolute values should not be extrapolated outside of the standard curve if the OD values for samples lie outside the limits of the standards.

10. TMB substrate solution is best made fresh, no more than 20 mins prior to use. The addition of hydrogen peroxide is essential for the color reaction to occur.

References

1. Rosenberg, S. A. (1990) Adoptive immunotherapy for cancer. *Sci Am 262*, 62–69.
2. Dudley, M. E., Wunderlich, J. R., Robbins, P. F., Yang, J. C., Hwu, P., Schwartzentruber, D. J., Topalian, S. L., Sherry, R., Restifo, N. P., Hubicki, A. M., Robinson, M. R., Raffeld, M., Duray, P., Seipp, C. A., Rogers-Freezer, L., Morton, K. E., Mavroukakis, S. A., White, D. E., and Rosenberg, S. A. (2002) Cancer regression and autoimmunity in patients after clonal repopulation with antitumor lymphocytes. *Science 298*, 850–854.
3. Finney, H. M., Lawson, A. D., Bebbington, C. R., and Weir, A. N. (1998) Chimeric receptors providing both primary and costimulatory signaling in T cells from a single gene product. *J Immunol 161*, 2791–2797.
4. Maher, J., Brentjens, R. J., Gunset, G., Rivière, I., and Sadelain, M. (2002) Human

T-lymphocyte cytotoxicity and proliferation directed by a single chimeric TCRzeta /CD28 receptor. *Nat Biotechnol 20*, 70–75.

5. Moeller, M., Haynes, N. M., Kershaw, M. H., Jackson, J. T., Teng, M. W., Street, S. E., Cerutti, L., Jane, S. M., Trapani, J. A., Smyth, M. J., and Darcy, P. K. (2005) Adoptive transfer of gene-engineered CD4+ helper T cells induces potent primary and secondary tumor rejection. *Blood 106*, 2995–3003.

6. Morgan, R. A., Dudley, M. E., Wunderlich, J. R., Hughes, M. S., Yang, J. C., Sherry, R. M., Royal, R. E., Topalian, S. L., Kammula, U. S., Restifo, N. P., Zheng, Z., Nahvi, A., de Vries, C. R., Rogers-Freezer, L. J., Mavroukakis, S. A., and Rosenberg, S. A. (2006) Cancer regression in patients after transfer of genetically engineered lymphocytes. *Science 314*, 126–129.

7. Kershaw, M. H., Westwood, J. A., Parker, L. L., Wang, G., Eshhar, Z., Mavroukakis, S. A., White, D. E., Wunderlich, J. R., Canevari, S., Rogers-Freezer, L., Chen, C. C., Yang, J., Rosenberg, S. A., and Hwu, P. (2006) A phase I study on adoptive immunotherapy using gene-modified T cells for ovarian cancer *Clin Cancer Res. 12*, 6106–6115.

8. Lamers, C. H., van Elzakker, P., Luider, B. A., van Steenbergen, S. C., Sleijfer, S., Debets, R., and Gratama, J. W. (2008) Retroviral vectors for clinical immunogene therapy are stable for up to 9 years. *Cancer Gene Ther 15*, 268–274.

9. Lee, J., Sadelain, M., and Brentjens, R. (2009) Retroviral transduction of murine primary T lymphocytes. *Methods Mol Biol 506*, 83–96.

10. Zhou, J., Shen, X., Huang, J., Hodes, R. J., Rosenberg, S. A., and Robbins, P. F. (2005) Telomere length of transferred lymphocytes correlates with in vivo persistence and tumor regression in melanoma patients receiving cell transfer therapy. *J Immunol 175*, 7046–7052.

11. Miller, A. D., and Rosman, G. J. (1989) Improved retroviral vectors for gene transfer and expression *BioTechniques 7*, 980–982, 84–86, 89–90.

12. Miller, A. D., and Buttimore, C. (1986) Redesign of retrovirus packaging cell lines to avoid recombination leading to helper virus production. *Mol Cell Biol 6*, 2895–2902.

13. Chester, K. A., Robson, L., Keep, P. A., Pedley, R. B., Boden, J. A., Boxer, G. M., Hawkins, R. E., and Begent, R. H. (1994) Production and tumour-binding characterization of a chimeric anti-CEA Fab expressed in Escherichia coli. *Int J Cancer 57*, 67–72.

14. Wels, W., Harwerth, I. M., Mueller, M., Groner, B., and Hynes, N. E. (1992) Selective inhibition of tumor cell growth by a recombinant single-chain antibody-toxin specific for the erbB-2 receptor. *Cancer Research 52*, 6310–6317.

15. Weissman, A. M., Hou, D., Orloff, D. G., Modi, W. S., Seuanez, H., O'Brien, S. J., and Klausner, R. D. (1988) Molecular cloning and chromosomal localization of the human T-cell receptor zeta chain: distinction from the molecular CD3 complex. *Proc Natl Acad Sci USA 85*, 9709–9713.

16. Evan, G. I., Lewis, G. K., Ramsay, G., and Bishop, J. M. (1985) Isolation of monoclonal antibodies specific for human c-myc proto-oncogene product. *Mol Cell Biol 5*, 3610–3616.

Chapter 18

Multi-walled Carbon Nanotube (MWCNT) Synthesis, Preparation, Labeling, and Functionalization

Babak Kateb, Vicky Yamamoto, Darya Alizadeh, Leying Zhang, Harish M. Manohara, Michael J. Bronikowski, and Behnam Badie

Abstract

Nanomedicine is a growing field with a great potential for introducing new generation of targeted and personalized drug. Amongst new generation of nano-vectors are carbon nanotubes (CNTs), which can be produced as single or multi-walled. Multi-walled carbon nanotubes (MWCNTs) can be fabricated as biocompatible nanostructures (cylindrical bulky tubes). These structures are currently under investigation for their application in nanomedicine as viable and safe nanovectors for gene and drug delivery. In this chapter, we will provide you with the necessary information to understand the synthesis of MWCNTs, functionalization, PKH26 labeling, RNAi, and DNA loading for in vitro experimentation and in vivo implantation of labeled MWCNT in mice as well as materials used in this experimentation. We used this technique to manipulate microglia as part of a novel application for the brain cancer immunotherapy. Our published data show this is a promising technique for labeling, and gene and drug delivery into microglia.

Key words: cancer immunotherapy, microglia, macrophage, glioma, nanotechnology, nano-medicine, MWCNT application, brain tumor, nano-vector, carbon nanotube.

1. Introduction

Nanomedicine is a growing field with a great potential for delivering targeted and personalized therapeutic agents. Amongst new generation of nano-vectors are carbon nanotubes (CNTs), which can be produced as single or multi-walled. CNTs are generally considered low- to virtually non-toxic if they are pristine (purity at 99% or more), properly coated or functionalized, used in certain

P. Yotnda (ed.), *Immunotherapy of Cancer*, Methods in Molecular Biology 651,
DOI 10.1007/978-1-60761-786-0_18, © Springer Science+Business Media, LLC 2010

working concentration (1–5), and are used locally (6). While in vitro and in vivo studies show much progress, further studies are needed to resolve long-term safety and toxicity issues (7, 8), should these nano-vectors be considered for clinical trials. Nevertheless, CNTs hold great promise in cancer therapy as there are many reports in the literature about application of CNTs as gene and drug delivery vehicles (9–15) and their potential use for glioma immunotherapy (6, 16).

Malignant glioma is considered to be the most common and fatal brain tumors in adults. Despite advancement in surgical resection techniques, radiotherapy, and chemotherapy, the survival rate and prognosis of glioma patients remain poor with a median survival of 12–15 months (17). Other multimodal approaches have been desperately sought by clinicians and researchers to eradicate gliomas or even improve survival rate. One of the recent promising approaches is the use of immunotherapy.

While the central nervous system (CNS) was considered to be immunologically privileged organ, this is no longer the axiom and researchers have shown that immune cells, such as activated T cells, can cross the blood–brain barrier (18–20). Moreover, there are numerous reports that microglia, a type of glial cells whose function is similar to macrophages and essential for nerve injury repair, are the primary immune effector cells in the CNS and are associated with various neurological disorders (21–23). There is also evidence of tumor-associated antigens (24–27) and the expression of class I and II MHC by brain tumors which could potentially activate the CNS innate immune system (26, 28, 29). However, the role of microglia in brain tumor immunology is still unclear. The current limited literature indicates that microglia, along with tumor-associated macrophages, are recruited by tumor but whether the tumor infiltrating microglia promote or suppress tumor growth has not been determined yet (30–33). Therapeutic potential of microglia activation in brain tumors are maximized if we are able to direct microglial function toward tumor eradication via gene, RNAi, or drug introduction. This approach could increase phagocytotic activity, boost immune response, and prevent the cancer growth-promoting function of microglia. Consequently, having effective genes, drug, and/or RNAi delivery into macrophage is crucial to achieve this goal.

In this chapter we have introduced a method that utilizes MWCNT as a gene/RNAi delivery carrier. This method is potentially useful in immunotherapy application in treating cancer, since we have proven that the MWCNT itself is taken up preferentially by microglia and macrophages without causing significant immune reaction both in vivo and in vitro (6,16). Additionally, siRNA and plasmid DNA can be loaded into MWCNT efficiently. This can pave the way for the use of CNT as a new gene or drug delivery vehicle. The following is the description of methods for synthesis of high-quality, fluorescent-labeled MWCNT and loading of MWCNTs with DNA or siRNA.

2. Materials

2.1. Cell Culture

1. BV2, murine microglia cell line.
2. The complete media. Dulbecco's modified Eagle's media (GIBCO, 11995-073) supplemented with 10% heat-inactivated fetal bovine serum (Omega Scientific, FB-02, batch tested), 100 U/ml penicillin-G, 100 µg/ml streptomycin (Cellgro, MT-30-002-CI), and 0.01 M HEPES (Irvine Scientific, 9319).
3. Trypsin (Irvine Scientific, 9341).
4. Sterile phosphate-buffered saline (PBS).
5. General equipments, such as 37°C water bath, centrifuge, cell counter, sterile plastic or glass pipettes, laminar flow cabinets, and 37°C humidified incubator at 5% CO_2.

2.2. MWCNT PKH26 Labeling

1. Sterile blade or scalpel
2. Level II biosafety cabinet
3. Multi-walled carbon nanotubes(MWCNT)
4. Mini Beadbeater-8 (Biospec Products)
5. VirSonic 300 (The Virus Company)
6. PKH26 Red Fluorescent Cell Linker Kit for General Cell Membrane Labeling (Sigma-Aldrich, PKH26GL-1KT)
7. Pluronic F108 (PF108) (BASF Corporation)
8. Ultracentrifuge machine
9. Ultracentrifuge Ultra-Clear Tubes (Beckman, 344057)
10. Laser or confocal microscope

2.3. In Vivo Application of MWCNT

1. Mice, 7- to 8-week-old (We use C57BL6 mice but other strains can be used)
2. Ketamine/Xylazine or other anesthetics (refer to your institute's recommendation)
3. Buprenex or other analgesia
4. Betadine
5. 70% ethanol
6. Electric hair clipper

7. Electric drilling instrument

8. Stereotactic frame

9. Scalpel

10. Hamilton Syringe (for MWCNT injection)

11. 27-G needle and 1 ml syringe (for injection of anesthetics/analgesia)

12. Sterile gauze or cotton tip

13. Timer

14. Wound glue or clips

15. Warm blanket or heat lamp

16. Eye ointment

3. Methods

3.1. Maintaining BV2 Cells

1. Thaw a frozen vial of BV2 cells in 37°C water bath (*see* **Note 1**).

2. Transfer cells into 15-ml conical tube containing 9 ml pre-warmed complete media. Centrifuge at 450 g (or Relative Centrifugal Force) for 5 min (*see* **Note 2**).

3. Aspirate the supernatant and re-suspend the pellet gently in 5 ml of the complete media. Transfer the cells into a T-75 (total of 13 ml media) or T-25 (5 ml) (*see* **Note 3**). Incubate cells at 37°C, 5% CO_2. The cells should be confluent after 2–4 days depending upon how many cells are plated.

4. Remove the media and wash once with PBS. Coat the cells with a layer of trypsin (1–3 ml) and let it sit for a few seconds. Aspirate the trypsin and place flask in the 37°C incubator for about 5 min. If some cells are still attached on the flask, facilitate detaching by gently tapping the flask). Add the complete media.

5. For maintenance, split cells into 1:4–1:5 dilutions. For in vitro imaging of CNT uptake by BV2, seed 2×10^5 cells in a 6-well dish.

3.2. MWCNT Synthesis

MWCNT is available commercially and should be pristine and sterile enough to be used in cell culture and in vivo study. Our team obtained MWCNT from the NASA- Jet Propulsion Laboratory (JPL) through an institutional collaboration agreement. Due to proprietary agreement with JPL, the detailed protocol cannot be disclosed. However, the following is a brief description and synopsis of how the MWCNTs for the current application were produced by JPL.

MWCNTs were synthesized using the catalytic chemical vapor deposition technique in a tube furnace which contained a pressure-regulated 2-inch-diameter quartz tube. This technique is known to generate high quality MWCNTs with no defects. The MWCNTs were grown on catalyst-coated substrates under a flowing mixture of ethylene and hydrogen. Typical MWCNT growth conditions are as follows: C_2H_4 flow, 380 sccm; H_2 flow, 190 sccm; total pressure, 200 Torr; temperature, 650°C; growth time, 15 min. The substrates consisted of silicon wafers with a 400-nm layer of thermal silicon oxide (SiO_2). These substrates were patterned with a thin film, approximately 10-nm thick, of sputtered iron catalyst using electron beam lithography and lift-off processing, and then inserted into the tube furnace for MWCNT growth. Under these conditions, MWCNTs were grown on the substrates only in the areas patterned with Fe catalyst as bundles. The individual tube diameter was ~20 nm (34–36). (*see* **Fig. 18.1**).

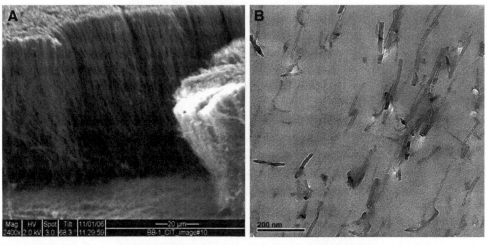

Fig. 18.1. MWCNTs were imaged using scanning electron microscopy (SEM) and transmission electron microscopy (TEM). (**A**) MWCNTs were imaged using SEM before processing to observe homogenous growth and size. (**B**) Processed MWCNTs were imaged using TEM to ascertain the consistency in length of the MWCNTs after processing. MWCNTs were determined to be between 200 and 400 μm for more than 80% of the suspension. (6)

3.3. MWCNT Functionalization

This section describes the protocol to functionalize MWCNT Pluronic F108, a non-ionic, difunctional block copolymer surfactant. This step is extremely important as the functionalization makes the carbon nanotubes soluble and prevents the nanotubes from being cytotoxic and immunogenic. Additionally, this protocol makes the nanotubes biodegradable; this permits nanotubes to release RNAi or genes in an efficient manner.

1. Using a sterile scalpel or blade, scrape and transfer MWCNT into a dish containing 1.5 ml of 1% Pluronic F108 (PF108) in a level II biosafety cabinet. The weight is determined at the beginning where you scrape off the CNTs from the

strips. Measure the length and width of each strip and the weight is determined based on a table provided by a manufacturer (*see* **Note 4**).

2. Transfer the MWCNT in 1% PF108 suspension into an Eppendorf tube on ice and homogenize it using the Mini Beadbeater-8 for 45 min. Alternatively, do high-shear mixing (Polyscience X520) for 1 h.

3. Sonicate the MWCNT-PF108 suspension using a sonicator at 540 W, 4–5 min each time, for 30 min (*see* **Note 5**).

4. Transfer the suspension into an ultracentrifuge tube and spin down at $122,000 \times g$ for 4 h at room temperature.

5. Decant the upper clear layer (typically, upper 50–60%) carefully, leaving micelle-suspended nanotube solution. There should be a light grey layer between the clear top layer and bottom dark grey pellet. Transfer the light-gray middle layer to a new Eppendorf tube (*see* **Note 6**).

6. Re-suspend the pellet to a stock concentration of 80 μg/ml using PF108 (*see* **Note 7**). The processed MWCNT shall be named as pMWCNT afterwards. You may go directly to 3.5 to label pMWCNT with PKH26 if it is not necessary to load pMWCNTs with plasmid and/or siRNA.

3.4. Loading pMWCNTs with Plasmid and/or siRNA

1. Process pMWCNTs as described in **Section 3.3**.

2. Incubate pMWCNT with DNA (any plasmids, shRNA, or siRNA) at a ratio (by weight) of pMWCNT : DNA 4:1 for 4 h in 4°C in 1% PF108. It may be necessary to optimize the ratio and incubation time.

3. Centrifuge the pMWCNT : DNA at $122,000 \times g$ for 4 h at 4°C (*see* **Note 8**). Resuspend the pellet with 1% PF108 (to 80 μg/ml) and centrifuge again at $122,000 \times g$ for 4 h at 4°C. Resuspend the pellet with 1% PF108 and proceed to 3.5 for PKH labeling.

3.5. PKH26 Labeling

1. Prepare the PKH26 stock solution (1×10^{-3} M). Dilute the stock further using Diluent C to 2×10^{-6} M. Refer to the kit's instruction for details.

2. Add 7 μl of 2×10^{-6} M PKH26 per 10 μg of pMWCNT. Mix well, cover the tube to avoid light exposure, and let it stands for 5 min at room temperature. Place the tube on a shaker for about 10 min.

3. Ultracentrifuge the suspension at $122,000 \times g$ for 4 h at 4°C.

4. Resuspend the pellet to 80 μg/ml using 1% PF108 for in vitro experiment. For in vivo experiment, resuspend the pellet

to 400 to 500 μg/ml. Store the pMWCNT-PKH26 in 4°C until use (*see* **Note 9**).

3.6. In Vitro Introduction of MWCNT

This section describes the procedure for introducing the DNA- or RNAi-loaded carbon nanotubes into murine microglia.

1. Add 3 μg of PKH26-labeled pMWCNT to BV2 cells in complete media per well (6-well dish). Incubate the cells overnight at 37°C. 24-h incubation should generate 70–80% uptake rate by the cells without significant cytotoxicity effect to the cells.

2. Observe the cells that uptake the PKH26-labeled pMWCNT using laser or confocal microscope. The HeNe 543 nm lasers should be used to monitor PKH26 (red)-labeled pMWCNT. (*see* **Fig. 18.2**)

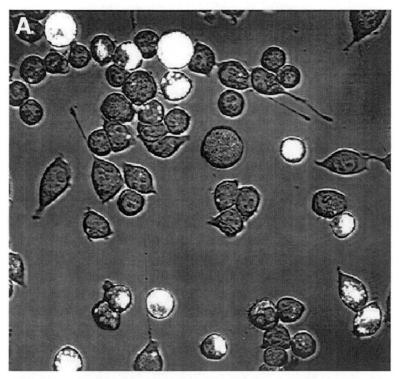

Fig. 18.2. pMWCNTs-PKH positive BV2 cells. The cells were imaged using an LSM 510 Meta confocal microscope at 48 h post-incubation with PKH-labeled MWCNT (×400). (6)

3.7. In Vivo Implantation of MWCNT

1. Sterilize procedure area with 70% ethanol.

2. Anesthetize the mouse with Ketamine (132 mg/kg) and Xylazine (8.8 mg/kg) solution.

3. Clip all hair from scalp and wipe the surgical area with beta-dine solution using sterile cotton tips.

4. Make a small sagital paramedian incision, about 1 cm, with a sterile scalpel blade. Wipe blood from the wound with cotton tips or gauze.

5. Drill an injection site (1 mm right of midline and 1 mm forward of bregma) on the scull carefully. Stop drilling after you make a small burr hole and start to see dura. You may stop drilling just before the drilling instrument punctures the scull completely in order to avoid damaging brain tissues.

6. Mount the mouse on a stereotactic head frame.

7. Load 10 µl of labeled pMWCNT-PKH (4–5 µg) into a Hamilton syringe.

8. Line up the syringe to the top of the hole on the scull straight. Carefully move the needle tip to the injection site. The tip should now touch the dura or on the surface of the injection site on the scull. Move the needle tip down by 3 mm into the brain.

9. Inject the 10 µl of labeled pMWCNT-PKH into the brain slowly over a period of 10 min. Ideally, inject 2 µl every 2 min. In this way, damage to the brain by injection will be minimal.

10. After the injection, let the syringe needle sit for one more minute and then slowly withdraw the needle from the brain.

11. Wipe the injection site with sterile gauze or cotton tip.

12. Close the incision area with wound glue or clips. Apply eye ointment to the mouse's eyes to prevent over-dryness.

13. Place the mouse on an electric warm blanket (heated to 37–38°C) or under the heat lamp in a cage until the mice start to wake up. To alleviate possible post-op pain, inject Buprenex or other analgesia into peritoneum cavity.

14. Move back the mouse to its home cage after the mouse become fully alert.

To assess the uptake of the labeled MWCNT by microglia, fix and harvest the mouse brain on 7 and/or 14 day post-injection. The red dye from PKH can be observed in cryosectioned brain samples. The in vivo study has many applications, such as investigating the efficacy of targeted drug, gene, or siRNA delivery and its potential use in brain tumor treatment. Further in vivo studies will shed light on the important applicability of carbon nanotubes in brain tumor immunotherapy.

4. Notes

1. Thaw and transfer the cells into regular media as quickly as possible. Dimethyl sulfoxide (DMSO) or other cryoprotective additive is often toxic to the cells.

2. All materials, media, reagents, and supplies for cell culture must be sterile. Media and reagents need to be filter-sterilized using 0.2-μM filter. Media need to be pre-warmed to 37°C. All the glassware must be detergent-free.

3. Choosing the flask size depends on how many cells you need to grow. Normally, there will be approximately 8×10^6 cells and 2×10^6 cells for T75 and T25, respectively, at the time of confluence.

4. The table will only apply for a specific MWCNT batch you have and it is not a universal table for any MWCNT batches. The length of MWCNT grown on each strip varies, thus you need to measure it every time you scrape them off.

5. We use a VirSonic 300 from The Virus Company, but any sonicator should work.

6. Check the top supernatant by electron microscope. Increase centrifugation time if there are significant amount of MWCNT in the top layer. The very bottom layer contains large CNT particles that can be removed and be further sonicated to increase yield.

7. The processed MWCNT must be used within 96 h.

8. The amount of DNA loaded to the pMWCNTs can be roughly determined by collecting the supernatant and by calculating the differences in the total added DNA or siRNA to the amount of DNA or siRNA present in the supernatant. Adjust the ratio of pMWCNT: DNA and incubation time as necessary.
   The PKH26-labeled pMWCNT must be used within 48 h.

Acknowledgments

Part of the research described in this publication was carried out at the Jet Propulsion Laboratory, California Institute of Technology, under a contract with the National Aeronautics and Space Administration.

References

1. Vittorio, O., Raffa, V., Cuschieri, A. (2009) Influence of purity and surface oxidation on cytotoxicity of multi-wall carbon nanotubes with human neuroblastoma cells. *Nanomedicine: Nanotechnology*, [Epub ahead of print; PMID: 19341817].

2. Liu, Z., Davis, C., Cai, W., He, L., Chen, X., Dai, H. (2008) Circulation and long-term fate of functionalized, biocompatible single-walled carbon nanotubes in mice probed by Raman spectroscopy. *Proc Natl Acad Sci USA 105*(5), 1410–1415.

3. Yehia, H. N., Draper, R. K., Mikoryak, C., Walker, E. K., Bajaj, P., Musselman, I. H., Daigrepont, M. C., Dieckmann, G. R., Pantano, P. (2007) Single-walled carbon nanotube interactions with HeLa cells. *J Nanobiotechnology 5*, 8.

4. Singh, R., Pantarotto, D., Lacerda, L., Pastorin, G., Klumpp, C., Prato, M., Bianco, A., Kostarelos, K. (2006) Tissue biodistribution and blood clearance rates of intravenously administered carbon nanotube radiotracers. *Proc Natl Acad Sci USA 103*(9), 3357–3362.

5. Prato, M., Kostarelos, K., Bianco, A. (2008) Functionalized carbon nanotubes in drug design and discovery. *Acc Chem Res 41*(1), 60–68.

6. Kateb, B., Van Handel, M., Zhang, L., Bronikowski, M. J., Manohara, H., Badie, B. (2007) Internalization of MWCNTs by microglia: possible application in immunotherapy of brain tumors. *Neuroimage, 37*(1), S9–S17.

7. Poland, C. A., Duffin, R., Kinloch, I., Maynard, A., Wallace, W. A., Seaton, A., Stone, V., Brown, S., Macnee, W., Donaldson, K. (2008) Carbon nanotubes introduced into the abdominal cavity of mice show asbestos-like pathogenicity in a pilot study. *Nature Nanotech Nat Nanotechnol 3*(7), 423–428.

8. Ding, L., Stilwell, J., Zhang, T., Elboudwarej, O., Jiang, H., Selegue, J. P., Cooke, P. A., Gray, J. W., Chen, F. F. (2005) Molecular characterization of the cytotoxic mechanism of multiwall carbon nanotubes and nanoonions on human skin fibroblast. *Nano Lett 5*(12), 2448–2464.

9. Podesta, J. E., Al-Jamal, K. T., Herrero, M. A., Tian, B., Ali-Boucetta, H., Hegde, V., Bianco, A., Prato, M., Kostarelos, K. (2009) Antitumor activity and prolonged survival by carbon-nanotube-mediated therapeutic siRNA silencing in a Human Lung Xenograft Model. *Small* [Epub ahead of print: PMID: 19306454].

10. Liu, Z., Chen, K., Davis, C., Sherlock, S., Cao, Q., Chen, X., Dai, H. (2008) Drug delivery with carbon nanotubes for in vivo cancer treatment. *Cancer Res 68*(16), 6652–6660.

11. Bhirde, A. A., Patel, V., Gavard, J., Zhang, G., Sousa, A. A., Masedunskas, A., Leapman, R. D., Weigert, R., Gutkind, J. S., Rusling, J. F. (2009) Targeted killing of cancer cells in vivo and in vitro with EGF-directed carbon nanotube-based drug delivery. *ACS Nano 3*(2), 307–316.

12. Hampel, S., Kunze, D., Haase, D., Krämer, K., Rauschenbach, M., Ritschel, M., Leonhardt, A., Thomas, J., Oswald, S., Hoffmann, V., Büchner, B. (2008) Carbon nanotubes filled with a chemotherapeutic agent: a nanocarrier mediates inhibition of tumor cell growth. *Nanomed 3*(2): 175–182.

13. Villa, C. H., McDevitt MR, Escorcia, F. E., Rey, D. A., Bergkvist, M., Batt, C. A., Scheinberg, D. A. (2008) Synthesis and biodistribution of oligonucleotide-functionalized, tumor-targetable carbon nanotubes. Nano Lett. 8(12):4221–4228.

14. Chen, J., Chen, S., Zhao, X., Kuznetsova, L. V., Wong, S. S., Ojima, I. (2008) Functionalized Single-Walled Carbon Nanotubes as Rationally Designed Vehicles for Tumor-Targeted Drug Delivery. *J Am Chem Soc 130* (49), 16778–16785.

15. Liu, Z., Cai, W., He, L., Nakayama, N., Chen, K., Sun, X., Chen, X., Dai, H. (2007) In vivo biodistribution and highly efficient tumour targeting of carbon nanotubes in mice. *Nat Nanotechnol 2*(1):47–52.

16. VanHandel M, Alizadeh, D., Zhang, L., Kateb, B., Bronikowski, M., Manohara, H., Badie, B. (2009) Selective uptake of multi-walled carbon nanotubes by tumor macrophages in a murine glioma model. *J Neuroimmunol 31, 208*(1–2), 3–9.

17. Wen, P. Y., Kesari, S. (2008) Malignant gliomas in adults, N Engl J Med. 5:492-507.

18. Sehgal, A., Berger, M. S. (2000) Basic concepts of immunology and neuroimmunology. *Neurosurg Focus 9*(6).

19. Engelhardt, B. (2008) The blood-central nervous system barriers actively control immune cell entry into the central nervous system. *Curr Pharm Des 14*(16), 1555–1565.

20. Stevens, A., Klöter, I., Roggendorf, W. (1988) Inflammatory infiltrates and natural killer cell presence in human brain tumors. *Cancer 61*(4), 738–743.

21. Streit, W. J., Conde, J. R., Fendrick, S. E., Flanary, B. E., Mariani, C. L. (2005) Role of microglia in the central nervous system's immune response. *Neurol Res* 27(7), 685–691.

22. Tambuyzer, B.R., Ponsaerts, P., and Nouwen, E. J. (2009) Microglia: gatekeepers of central nervous system immunology. J Leukoc Biol 85(3), 352–370.

23. Pollard, J. W. (2009) Trophic macrophages in development and disease. *Nat Rev Immunol* 9(4):259–270.

24. Chi, J. H., Panner, A., Cachola, K., Crane, C. A., Murray, J., Pieper, R. O., James, C. D., Parsa, A. T. (2008) Increased expression of the glioma-associated antigen ARF4L after loss of the tumor suppressor PTEN. Laboratory investigation. *J Neurosurg* 108(2), 299–303.

25. Hatano, M., Eguchi, J., Tatsumi, T., Kuwashima, N., Dusak, J. E., Kinch, M. S., Pollack, I. F., Hamilton, R. L., Storkus, W. J., Okada, H. (2005) EphA2 as a glioma-associated antigen: a novel target for glioma vaccines. *Neoplasia* 7(8), 717–722.

26. Mitchell, D. A., Fecci, P. E., Sampson, J. H. (2008) Immunotherapy of malignant brain tumors. *Immunol Rev* 222, 70–100.

27. Ueda, R., Iizuka, Y., Yoshida, K., Kawase, T., Kawakami, Y., Toda, M. (2004) Identification of a human glioma antigen, SOX6, recognized by patients' sera. *Oncogene* 23(7):1420–1427

28. Parney, I. F., Farr-Jones, M. A., Chang, L. J., Petruk, K. C. (2000) Human glioma immunobiology in vitro: implications for immunogene therapy. *Neurosurgery* 46(5):1169–1177; discussion 1177–1178.

29. Takamura, Y., Ikeda, H., Kanaseki, T., Toyota, M., Tokino, T., Imai, K., Houkin, K., Sato, N. (2004) Regulation of MHC class II expression in glioma cells by class II transactivator (CIITA) *Glia* 45(4), 392–405.

30. Galarneau, H., Villeneuve, J., Gowing, G., Julien, J. P., Vallières, L. (2007) Increased glioma growth in mice depleted of macrophages. *Cancer Res* 67(18):8874–8881.

31. Geranmayeh, F., Scheithauer, B. W., Spitzer, C., Meyer, F. B., Svensson-Engwall, A. C., Graeber, M. B. (2007) Microglia in gemistocytic astrocytomas. *Neurosurgery* 60(1), 159–66.

32. Graeber, M. B., Scheithauer, B. W., Kreutzberg, G. W. (2002) Microglia in brain tumors. *Glia* 40(2):252–259.

33. Watters, J. J., Schartner, J. M., Badie, B. (2005) Microglia function in brain tumors. *J Neurosci Res* 81(3), 447–455.

34. Manohara, H. M., Bronikowski, M. J., Hoenk, M., Hunt, B. D. and Siegel, P. H. (2006) High-current-density field emitters based on arrays of carbon nanotubes bundles, *J Vac Sci Technol* B 23(1), 157–161.

35. Bronikowski, M. J. (2006) CVD growth of carbon nanotube bundle arrays, *Carbon*, 44, 2822–2832.

36. Bronikowski, M. J., Manohara, H. M., and Hunt, B. D. (2006) Growth of carbon nanotube bundle arrays on silicon surfaces, J Vac Sci Technol, A 24(4) 1318–1322.

Chapter 19

Cellular Immunotherapy of Cancer

Fatma V. Okur and Malcolm K. Brenner

Abstract

Standard therapies for many common cancers remain toxic and are often ineffective. Cellular immunotherapy has the potential to be a highly targeted alternative, with low toxicity to normal tissues but a high capacity to eradicate tumor. In this chapter we describe approaches that generate cellular therapies using active immunization with cells, proteins, peptides, or nucleic acids, as well as efforts that use adoptive transfer of effector cells that directly target antigens on malignant cells. Many of these approaches are proving successful in hematologic malignancy and in melanoma. In this chapter we discuss the advantages and limitations of each and how over the next decade investigators will attempt to broaden their reach, increase their efficacy, and simplify their application.

Key words: Cancer, immunotherapy, tumor vaccines, adoptive cell therapy and T cells.

1. Introduction

Conventional modalities for treating cancer remain unsatisfactory. Despite the introduction of small molecules that target specific molecular lesions or pathways within the cancer cell, cure rates for many common tumors remain low, while adverse events are still distressingly high. Cancer immunotherapy represents a promising extension of highly targeted cancer therapy with a favorable toxicity profile and excellent pharmaco-economics. Although most attention has been on the development of monoclonal antibodies (*see* **Table 19.1**) (1–5) beneficial results with cellular immunotherapy are now being reported. Although to date these have primarily been obtained in subjects with lymphoma, melanoma, or neuroblastoma, methodologies are being developed to allow us to extend the tumor range.

P. Yotnda (ed.), *Immunotherapy of Cancer*, Methods in Molecular Biology 651,
DOI 10.1007/978-1-60761-786-0_19, © Springer Science+Business Media, LLC 2010

Table 19.1
Monoclonal antibodies approved by the FDA for cancer

Monoclonal antibody	Target	Structure	Indication
Rituximab (Rituxan)	CD20	Chimeric	B-cell NHL
Tositumomab (Bexxar)	CD20	Murine mAb linked to ^{131}I	B-cell NHL
Ibritumomab (Zevalin)	CD20	Murine mAb linked to ^{90}Y	B-cell NHL
Gemtuzumab (Myolotarg)*	CD33	Humanized mAb linked to calicheamicin	AML
Alemtuzumab (Campath)	CD52	Humanized mAb	B-CLL, T-cell lymphoma
Transtuzumab (Herceptin)	Her2/Neu	Humanized mAb	Breast Cancer
Cetuximab (Erbitux)	EGFR	Chimeric	Head, neck and colorectal cancers
Panitumumab(Vectibix)	EGFR	Humanized mAb	Colorectal cancer
Bevacizumab (Avastin)	VEGF	Humanized mAb	NSCLC, colorectal cancer, breast cancer

NHL, non-Hodgkin's lymphoma: AML, acute myelogenous leukemia; NSCLC, nonsmall cell lung cancer; mAb, monoclonal antibody
*Subsequently withdrawn as failed post-approval testing (June 2010)

Many human tumors express tumor-specific (TSA) or tumor-associated antigens (TAA) that can be recognized by the host immune system and induce anti-tumor cell-mediated and humoral immune responses. Although these responses may be transient and are not always associated with clinical responses, they provide evidence for the existence of tumor-directed immunity in humans which may also have anti-tumor activity (6–8). Several barriers block the development of more effective anti-tumor immunity in subjects with cancer. First, many human tumors express few MHC molecules or have poor processing of their potential tumor antigens. Even when TAA/TSA are processed and presented, most tumors lack the co-stimulatory molecules necessary to implement a long lived and effective immune response. In addition to these passive defenses against immunity, many tumors can "edit" the immune system to their advantage, secreting cytokines such as TGF-β that directly inhibit cytotoxic effector T-cell growth, function and survival, or that favor expansion of Th2/Treg rather than effector T cells (9, 10). Finally, intensive chemo and radiotherapies can themselves severely reduce immune function by destroying antigen-presenting cells and dividing T lymphocytes. (**Table 19.2**)

As our understanding of the molecular basis of tumor immune escape has increased, it has been possible to derive

Table 19.2
Causes of immunocompromise in cancer patients

Immunosuppression induced by tumor	References
Antigen-specific CD4$^+$/CD8$^+$ T cell tolerance	(97–100)
Defective proximal TCR signaling (decreased expressions of CD3δ chain, p56^{lck}, p59^{fyn} tyrosine kinases)	(101–103)
Impairment of antigen processing machinery (TAP, LMP2, LMP7) or antigen-presenting ability of APCs (downregulation of MHC molecules and co-stimulatory molecules)	(104, 105)
Activation of negative costimulatory signals (CTLA-4, PD-1, B7-H4, BTLA)	(106–109)
Tumor-derived immunosuppressive cytokines (TGF-β, IL-10, VEGF, PGE$_2$)	(110–114)
Expression of immunomodulatory or proapoptotic molecules by tumor (tryptophan-depleting enzyme IDO, galectin-1, FasL, TRAIL)	(115–120)
Recruitment and expansion of immunosuppressive cell populations (regulatory T cells, MDSCs, IDO$^+$ DCs, myeloid/plasmocytoid DCs)	(121–131)
Immunosuppression induced by therapy	
Neutropenia, depletion and functional impairment of monocytes	(132–135)
Hypogammaglobulinemia (decreased levels of IgA and IgM)	(133)
Defective T-cell-mediated immune response	(136–138)

countermeasures that may allow us to induce more potent anti-tumor immune responses, and that will soon allow us to extend effective anti-tumor immune responses to a broad range of common tumors.

2. Types of Cellular Immunotherapy

Cellular immunotherapy may be *active*, using cell-based vaccines derived from tumor cells themselves or antigen-presenting cells expressing TAA/TSA from proteins or peptides, or *passive*, by direct adoptive transfer of viable effector T cells. The former approach relies on the intact afferent and efferent immune system of the host responding to the stimulus with an effective anti-tumor response, while the latter is the cellular equivalent of antibody serotherapy, in which the transferred effector cells are expected to attack the tumor cells directly, albeit with a phase of in vivo expansion.

2.1. Vaccines

Identification of antigens that are tumor-specific (molecules that are unique to cancer cells) or tumor-associated (molecules that are expressed at different levels by cancer cells and normal cells)

Table 19.3
Methods used to prepare cancer vaccines against TAA/TSA

Vaccination strategy	Method of production	References
Peptide/protein subunit vaccines	Manufacturing peptides from class I/II MHC epitopes of tumor target antigens or protein sub-unit containing multiple epitopes	(139–142)
DNA vaccines	Cloning genes encoding tumor target antigens in to a plasmid and delivering it to host by different methods (injection, electroporation, gene gun)	(143–145)
Whole-cell vaccines	Irradiated unmodified autologous tumor cells Autologous/Allogeneic tumor cells engineered to express costimulatory molecules, cytokines, chemokines	(146–153)
Dendritic cell vaccines	Derivation of immature DCs from CD34+hemato poeitic stem cells or peripheral blood monocytes Loading them with tumor antigens (peptides/whole protein, DNA, mRNA), whole necrotic or apop-totic tumor cells, tumor cell lysates, or transducing with viral vectors or fusing with tumor cells Ex vivo maturation with cytokine cocktails ($\pm$) TLR agonists	(154–165)

has supported the development of cancer vaccines (**Table 19.3**). Unlike conventional vaccines for infectious agents, however, these anti-cancer vaccines are expected to function in a host who already has disease. Devising such "therapeutic" vaccines has proved a significant challenge, even in patients with apparently minimal residual disease, in whom they are intended to prevent relapse rather than induce the host to eradicate bulky tumor.

The sine qua non of an effective tumor vaccine is the establishment of a persistent effector cell immune response in vivo, which requires tumor antigens to be appropriately presented by an appropriate professional antigen-presenting cell (APC) To this end, either the APC or the tumor cell itself may need to be genetically modified if a successful immune response is to be mounted and sustained (**Table 19.3**). Hence, optimal design requires knowledge of the both the target antigens and the immune evasion mechanisms used by that particular cancer, so that maximum stimulus is given in the presence of countermeasures to blocking strategies used by the tumor cells. It should be noted that identification of specific cytotoxic T-cell epitopes within a TSA/TAA has helped in the design of subunit or peptide antigens, but it is always important to ensure that the (malignant) tumor cells themselves process and present the same target epitopes as the (normal) antigen-presenting cell, otherwise any immune response generated will be incapable of recognizing the intended target.

2.1.1. Peptide/Protein Subunit Vaccines

Tumor-selective peptides are usually administered with adjuvants that stimulate monocytes and macrophages through their toll-like receptors (TLRs) to generate the danger signals needed for activation and maturation of professional antigen-presenting cells (APC) such as myeloid dendritic cells (mDC), a necessary precondition for recruiting tumor-specific effector cells (**Table 19.3**). Peptides were initially designed to be presented on APC in association with class I MHC antigens and thereby recruit CD8$^+$ cytotoxic T cells. Subsequently, it became apparent that cellular immune responses that were optimal in magnitude and duration also required immune responses mediated by CD4$^+$ T helper cells. Such cells recognize larger peptides, associated with Class II MHC antigens, leading many investigators to use peptide pools containing both short (e.g., 9-mer) and long (e.g., 20-mer) peptides, or to switch to protein subunit vaccines that contained both CD8 and CD4 epitopes. The latter approach also has the advantage that a single protein can be used for a multiplicity of HLA types, whereas individual peptides (particularly those associating with MHC Class I antigens) are usually restricted to association with just one or two specific HLA polymorphisms. Overall, *single* peptide vaccination has fallen from favor, not only because of the limited nature of the cellular immune responses induced, but also because even when clinical responses occur, they are often short-lived, and terminated by the selection of epitope loss variants of the tumor that can grow unscathed.

2.1.2. DNA Vaccines

In this vaccination method, genes encoding specific tumor antigens are cloned and vaccines composed of this DNA are administered by injection or electroporation directly into skin or muscle (**Table 19.3**). Immune responses to DNA vaccines may result directly from expression of antigen by transduced cells such as muscle or skin fibroblasts, or by cross-presentation of the proteins by professional APCs. DNA vaccines can induce both humoral and cellular immune responses and they are stable and inexpensive. Their efficacy can be improved by simultaneous use of cytokines and synthetic oligodeoxynucleotides containing CpG or other motifs that stimulate TLRs (11–13). Indeed many studies use a prime-boost approach in which patients first receive priming with a recombinant viral construct, followed by boosting with peptide immunization to ensure that the dominant immune response is directed to the TAA/TSA rather than to the viral antigens (14, 15). This approach has had variable success in humans (**Table 19.3**).

2.1.3. Whole-Cell
Vaccines

Instead of immunizing with TSA/TAA themselves (as proteins, peptides, or DNA/RNA), the tumor cell itself may be used as the immunogen. This strategy has the potential to be the most physiological means of eliciting a robust immune response because of the presentation of all possible tumor antigens to the host immune system. To enhance the limited inherent immunogenicity of the tumor cells, they are genetically modified either in vivo or ex vivo using viral or non-viral delivery methods. The transferred genes are intended to increase the immunogenicity of the tumors by attracting and activating professional APCs (e.g., GM-CSF), recruiting T cells to the tumor injection site (e.g., lymphotactin), or by activating and expanding antigen-specific T cells (e.g., CD40L or IL2), and may be used alone or in combination (**Table 19.4**). The tumor cells themselves may be autologous or allogeneic. Each source has reciprocal advantages and disadvantages. Autologous tumor cells present the specific TAA/TSA expressed by the patients' own tumor in the context of the correct HLA antigens (if expressed), but the disadvantage of being harder to obtain and standardize. Allogeneic tumor cells lines are readily obtained and standardized, but may lack crucial antigens, and likely require cross presentation by potentially defective host APC to generate an immune response. Both approaches have been used clinically, and tumor responses reported, including complete sustained remissions (**Table 19.3**).

Table 19.4
Methods for enhancing the immunogenicity of tumor cells

Aim	Method	References
Enhancement of cross-priming of T cells via recruitment and activation of APCs	Genetic modification of tumor cells or bystander cells expressing GM-CSF, CD40L, IL-4	(166–172)
	Viral infection and apoptosis of tumor cells (HSVtk, Newcastle disease virus)	
Attraction of T cells	Genetic modification of tumor cells expressing chemokines	(173, 174)
Enhancement of direct-priming T cells by improving antigen-presenting ability of tumor cells	Genetic modification of tumor cells expressing costimulatory molecules (CD80, CD86, CD40), major histocompatibility complex/peptide	(146, 148, 151, 152)
T-cell activation and expansion	Genetic modification of tumor cells or bystander cells expressing cytokines (IL-2, IL-7, IL-12, IFN-γ)	(175–179)

2.1.4. Dendritic Cell
Vaccines

Many of the immune evasion strategies used by human tumor cells target the processing and presentation of antigen by professional antigen-presenting cells (**Table 19.2**). In these tumors, conventional peptide protein or DNA vaccines will be ineffective since the afferent components of antigen uptake, processing and presentation will remain impaired. To overcome these deficits, investigators have used immunization with professional APCs generated ex vivo and pulsed with tumor antigens. Dendritic cells (DCs) are the most potent APCs and can be prepared from myeloid or monocytoid precursor cells in peripheral blood or bone marrow. To enhance DC maturation and activation, a multiplicity of "cocktails" have been described, usually consisting of cytokines such as IL4, GM-CSF and TNF-α, IL-6, IL-1ß, with or without prostaglandin E2 (**Table 19.5**). With the aid of these agents, myeloid/monocytoid DC become better able to take up and present tumor antigens and to increase their expression of co-stimulatory molecules such as CD80, CD86, CD40, and CD54. Moreover, they are then able to polarize the resulting immune response toward a T effector phenotype, rather than to an undesired Treg or tolerogenic outcome. Most studies have pulsed treated DC with peptides, tumor cell lysates, or tumor cell RNA, or transduced them with viral vectors encoding TSA/TAA (16–20). More recently, hybrids between dendritic cells and tumor cells have been made, combining the antigens of the tumor cells with the antigen-presenting capacity of the DC (21). Recent positive results in a large randomized trial of an APC vaccine for the patients with advanced prostate cancer and subsequent licensing approval by the FDA have rekindled interest in this approach (22, 23).

Table 19.5
Protocols used for DC maturation and activation

Protocol	References
Cytokines (TNF-α alone; TNF-α+IL-1β+IL-6+PGE2)	(180–183)
CD40 Ligand (± IFN-γ)	(184, 185)
Cytokines + Toll-like receptor agonists (IFN-γ+ +LPS, TNF-α+IL-1β+PolyI: C+ IFN-γ +IFN-α)	(186, 187)
In situ maturation	(188, 189)

2.1.5. Optimum Clinical Methods for Cancer Vaccination

Most early phase I clinical trials of cancer vaccines have been in subjects with extensive tumor burden, who have been heavily pre-treated with standard chemotherapy protocols prior to vaccination. As described in **Table 19.2**, this is a challenging setting, since the immune evasion activities of the tumor will be high and the responsiveness of the immune system low. Even in subjects with minimal residual disease, it may be necessary to deplete or functionally inactivate the regulatory T cells that frequently surround human tumors (**Table 19.2**). Many methods of

Treg depletion have been tried, ranging from CD25 monoclonal antibodies to ablative chemotherapy and stem cell transplantation, but as yet we have no good Treg depletion methodology. Other issues that must be assessed in the design of cancer vaccine protocols include vaccine schedule and dose and route of injection. Decisions on which design is optimal may have to depend on questionable surrogate markers, such as levels of the anti-tumor immune response measured in vitro, rather than on a direct knowledge of comparative clinical responses.

2.2. Adoptive Cell Therapy with Lymphocytes

In principle, lymphocytes have the ability to traffic through multiple tissue planes and to be self-renewing. These assets, coupled with their ability to destroy tumor or viral infected target cells through a range of mechanisms makes them an appealing resource for adoptive transfer, and a multiplicity of clinical studies using this approach have now been described. Adoptive lymphocyte therapies may use allogeneic or autologous cells, which range from tightly defined specificity (e.g., T-cell clones) to broad phenotype and activity (e.g., tumor-infiltrating lymphocytes). As we have learned more about the molecular basis of immune recognition and immune regulation, it has become possible to genetically modify the infused lymphocytes to alter their specificity or behavior. In this section we describe examples of each type of adoptive transfer and discuss the relative merits and limitations of each (**Table 19.6**).

2.2.1. Adoptive Transfer of Cells with Incompletely Defined Specificity

2.2.1.1. Natural Killer Cell Therapy

Natural killer (NK) cells are bone-marrow derived lymphocytes that do not express mature B- or T-lymphocyte markers (Ig or CD3). As a component of the innate immune system, they can recognize and destroy virally infected cells and a range of tumor cells in a HLA-unrestricted manner. NK cells also serve to connect the innate and adaptive immune responses via bidirectional interactions with DCs (24). They induce DC maturation and help to polarize T-cell responses toward the Th1 phenotype by producing high levels of IFN-γ (25, 26), thus supporting the development of an effective adaptive anti-tumor immune response. NK cells are activated by exposure to the cytokines IL-2, IL-12, IL-15, or IFN-γ and thus increase their cytotoxic activity (27). In the first clinical studies, autologous NK cells were activated and expanded in vitro with IL-2 (lymphokine-activated killer cells, LAK cells) and used in combination with high doses of IL-2 to treat patients with metastatic melanoma and renal carcinoma (28). Comparison of LAK cell therapy and IL-2 with IL-2 alone showed no significant difference in response rates (29), discouraging further

Table 19.6
Current adoptive cell therapy strategies and their challenges

Strategy	Method of production	Challenges
DLI	Harvesting unsensitized peripheral blood leucocytes from leucopheresis product of stem cell donor	GVHD, pancytopenia, infection
LAK	Activation and expansion of autologous NK cells with IL-2 in vitro	Limited clinical efficacy
Allogeneic NK infusion	Harvesting and purification of haploidentical NK cells from donor leucopheresis product via immunomagentic CD3 depletion and ex vivo activation with cytokines (IL-2, IL-15)	Contamination with alloreactive T cells Heterogenecity of individual NK cell repertoire limiting the number of alloreactive NK cells in product
TIL	Isolation of tumor-reactive T cells from tumor tissue or tumor-infiltrated lymph nodes and ex vivo expansion with cytokines	Limited clinical efficacy due to overgrowing non-specific T cells and tumor-induced T-cell anergy
Antigen-specific CTL	In vitro reactivation and expansion of polyclonal virus- or TAA-specific cytotoxic T lymphocytes by repeatedly stimulating with APCs and cytokines	Complexity and length of process Insufficient in vivo expansion and survival of CTLs except latent virus-specific CTLs Inhibition of CTL function by tumor-induced immune evasion mechanisms T cell escapes mutants of virus or tumor
TCR gene transfer	Genetic modification of CTLs through insertion of class I HLA-restricted TCR genes cloned from tumor-reactive T cells	Hybrid TCRs HLA-restricted antigen recognition and T-cell activation T cell escapes mutants of tumor
CARs	Genetic modification of CTLs through insertion of chimeric TCRs engineered by infusing antigen-reconizing scFv of TAA-specific mAb with signaling domain of CD3 δ chain	Anti-CAR antibody response Inability to proliferate and survive in vivo due to costimulatory signaling defect.

study of the approach. More recently, a better understanding of the molecular targets of NK cells have increased interest in using allogeneic NK cells, for example, after HLA mismatched stem cell transplant, to eradicate residual (recipient derived) malignancy (30). This "antigen specific" application of NK cells is described in **Section 2.2.2.1**.

2.2.1.2. Donor Lymphocyte Infusion

It has long been apparent that the curative effects of allogeneic stem cell transplants for many hematological malignancies can be attributed to a graft-versus-leukemia effect from the incoming T cells within the donor graft. Thus, patients with chronic graft versus host disease were well recognized as having a lower probability of relapse than individuals without this unpleasant complication. Similarly, recipients of syngeneic grafts have the lowest rate of GvHD and the highest risk of relapse (31, 32). In 1990, Kolb and colleagues took advantage of this observation and deliberately infused donor lymphocytes in an attempt to eliminate recurrent disease in patients with chronic myeloid leukemia (CML) (33). Their positive results have been confirmed in multiple studies worldwide, and remission can be induced in more than 50% of CML patients who relapse after transplantation by stopping immunosuppressive treatment or infusing donor lymphocytes (34). Unfortunately, DLI are much less effective at treating other types of relapsed leukemias after transplantation, with a 29% remission rate for AML and only 5% for ALL (35). It is not clear why these differences occur, since all these leukemias present the minor histocompatibility antigens that are likely the targets of this graft versus leukemia effect, although they have yet to be fully defined. DLI therapy may also produce severe adverse effects, since the frequency of broadly alloreactive effector cells is usually much higher than the frequency of lymphocytes targeted exclusively to the relapsed malignancy. As a consequence, patients receiving DLI often develop GvHD, which may be manifest by skin, gut, or liver damage, or by pancytopenia if there is significant residual host hemopoietic chimerism (36). Strategies aimed at retaining the benefits of GvL while preventing GvHD have included the depletion of alloreactive T cells in the donor lymphocyte product (37, 38) and the incorporation of suicide genes into the infused CTLs so that they may be killed if the GvHD activity exceeds the benefits from GvL. Examples of suicide genes include the prodrug metabolizing enzyme HSV-TK (addition of ganciclovir killing the cells) which is now in Phase III clinical trial, and more recently an inducible caspase 9, which can be activated by a small molecule, chemical inducer of dimerization and kill cells expressing the transgenic caspase (39–43). Ultimately, however, investigators may wish to identify leukemia-restricted target antigens on the malignant cells and infuse antigen-specific T cells directed to them.

2.2.2. Antigen-Specific Therapies

2.2.2.1. NK-Cell Therapy after KIR-HLA Mismatched Haploidentical SCT

Induction of NK-cell-induced cytolysis depends on the balance between activating and inhibitory signals coming from their specific ligands on target cells. For T-cell-mediated cytotoxicity, activation occurs when the T-cell receptor (TCR) engages an antigenic epitope presented by a Class I or Class II MHC antigen. In contrast, the presence of MHC class I molecules on target cells actually inhibits NK-cell activation (*Missing self hypothesis*) (44). Hence, downregulation or absence of MHC molecules that bind inhibitory receptors such as killer immunoglobulin-like receptors (KIRs) or CD94/NKG2A on NK cells, leads to lysis of tumor cells by NK cells. Similarly, signals provided by interaction of stress-induced ligands on tumor cells with activating receptors such as NKG2A or FcγRIII expressed on NK cells contributes to the recognition and elimination of tumor cells by NK cells (45, 46).

Identification of the molecular basis for NK target-cell recognition has allowed study of the ability of NK-mediated cytotoxicity to eradicate malignancy after MHC mismatched allogeneic stem cell transplantation. Ruggeri and colleagues found that a KIR-HLA mismatch was associated with reduced frequency of GVHD, a lower relapse rate and improved overall outcome in patients with AML who received a haploidentical stem cell transplant (30). Since that first admirably clear demonstration, confusion has reigned, with conflicting results obtained by a multiplicity of groups. Clearly, our understanding of activating and suppressive ligands for NK-cell receptors and the ways in which these interact is far from complete. Until this information is available, accurate prediction of outcome will remain difficult (47–49). Additional methodological obstacles also need to be resolved to optimize the clinical use of allogeneic NK-cell preparations, and these include the development of isolation techniques for removing NK cells from leukapheresis product without contamination with alloreactive T cells and a standardization of the absolute numbers and functional status of NK cells to achieve comparability within and between studies (50).

2.2.2.2. Adoptive Immunotherapy with Virus-Specific Cytotoxic T Lymphocytes

Viral infections are one of the commonest causes of morbidity and mortality after stem cell transplant, and are more prevalent as the degree of antigen mismatching between donor and recipient is increased. Cord blood transplantation in particular is associated with often intractable virus infections and is becoming recognized as a major limitation of the approach. The commonest problematic viral infections after stem cell transplantation are reactivated herpes viruses, including cytomegalovirus (CMV), which typically causes pneumonitis and hepatitis and the gamma herpes virus Epstein-Barr Virus (EBV), which may cause a rapidly fatal lymphoproliferative disease (LPD). In children and recipients of cord blood transplants, adenoviral disease is also common. Adoptive transfer of virus-specific T cells appears to effectively prevent and treat these infections after transplant. Infusion of even small numbers of specific cells (10^6 or less) may be sufficient for benefit, since the lymphodepletion of the immediate post-transplant period is associated with the release of homeostatic cytokines such as IL7 and IL15, which augment the expansion of virus-specific T cells when they encounter their antigen.

2.2.2.2.1. Autologous Virus-Specific T Cells

Riddell and colleagues pioneered the use of cytomegalovirus (CMV)-specific CD8+ T-cell clones to prevent CMV reactivation in allogeneic HSCT recipients (51). They activated and expanded donor-derived CTLs by coculturing with CMV-infected autologous fibroblasts. Neither viremia nor disease activation were detected in any of the treated patients. However, CMV-specific CTL clones did not persist. Subsequent studies showed that presence of endogenous CD4+ T cells are necessary for the maintenance of anti-viral activity in vivo (52–54).

We reported the use of donor-derived polyclonal but EBV-specific CTL lines to treat and prevent EBV-associated lymphoproliferative disease (LPD) after allogeneic HSCT (55–57). Since 1993, over 110 stem cell recipients have received donor-derived EBV-specific CTL lines. None of the patients in our prophylaxis group developed PTLD, in contrast to an incidence of 11.5% in 44 patients in the control group. Elevated EBV-DNA levels declined within 1–3 weeks of first T-cell infusion and EBV-specific CTLs have also been found effective in 10 of 12 patients with bulky EBV lymphoma (58). Other groups have confirmed that adoptive immunotherapy with EBV-specific CTLs effectively prevents and treats EBV-LPD after hemopoietic stem cell or solid organ transplantation (59–62).

Improvements in methodology to simplify and accelerate manufacture of these viral-specific CTLs have followed. We have developed a culture method to generate, in a single culture, CTL lines that have anti-viral activity for EBV, CMV, and Adv, and mini-bioreactors in which to prepare these cells in a closed system. We can now use plasmid mediated transduction of antigen-presenting cells to force expression of CMV, Adv and EBV-associated antigens without the need to manufacture EBV-transformed lymphoblastoid cell lines. In combination, these techniques allow us to make sufficient CTLs for patient treatment in <10 days instead of >10 weeks. Other groups have developed even faster techniques, in which T cells activated by viral antigens are selected by columns specific for activation markers such as CD25 or gamma-interferon. Early results with this approach are promising but it may be of limited value when the frequency of antigen responding cells is low, for example, for adenoviruses generally, or for all viruses in cord blood samples.

2.2.2.2.2. Allogeneic Virus-Specific T Cells

Ideally, virus-specific CTLs should be immediately available from a cryopreserved line. The cost of doing this for each patient at risk is prohibitive, but Crawford and colleagues generated a bank of polyclonal EBV-CTL lines expressing common HLA antigens and gave the best matched cells to subjects who developed EBV lymphoproliferation after solid organ transplantation (63). More recently they reported results of a phase-II multicenter trial in which they treated 33 patients with EBV-LPD with an overall response rate of 64% at 5 weeks and 52% at 6 months (64). These impressive results have led us to develop a similar multicenter study to evaluate whether our trivirus-specific CTL lines may have similar activity against EBV,CMV and adenovirus in partially HLA matched allogeneic patients.

2.2.3. Adoptive Immunotherapy for Treatment of Tumors

2.2.3.1. Virus-Related Malignancy

The encouraging results of adoptive immunotherapy with EBV-specific CTLs in the immunocompromised host led us to extend this strategy to EBV-associated tumors (lymphoma and nasopharyngeal cancer) that develop in the immunocompetent subject. Unlike EBV-LPD, which expresses the highly immunogenic viral latency antigens EBNA1, EBNA2, and EBNA3, these other EBV tumors express a limited number of poorly processed (EBNA1) or weakly stimulatory (LMP1 and LMP2) EBV derived antigens. We have therefore used CTLs specific for these EBV antigens, beginning with the cells directed to LMP2. The CTLs were generated from patients with Hodgkin's disease by using mDC that are engineered to overexpress LMP2. The infusion of polyclonal LMP2-specific T cells containing both CD4$^+$ and CD8$^+$ T cells increases LMP2-specific T-cell responses, and lead to complete tumor regression in 8 of 12 patients with EBV+ lymphoma (65).

Similar results have been obtained in EBV+ Nasopharyngeal carcinoma (NPC), a tumor which originates from the epithelial cells of the nasopharynx (66). Like EBV+ lymphomas, NPCs express the same restricted set of weakly immunogenic viral antigens including EBNA1, LMP1, and LMP2. Treatment of EBV-positive NPC with polyclonal EBV-specific CTLs has produced complete clinical responses in patients with limited tumor burden (67, 68). One of the main limitations of treatment of NPC with EBV-specific CTL is the failure of in vivo expansion of adoptively transferred cells. To overcome this deficiency, we conducted another clinical study in which patients with recurrent NPC received a lymphodepleting anti-CD45 monoclonal antibody before EBV-specific CTL infusion. Such lymphodepletion increased the expansion of adoptively transferred EBV-specific CTL, but unfortunately with little discernible improvement to the anti-tumor activity (69).

2.2.3.2. Cytotoxic T Cells to Non-viral Antigens

Many different types of tumor-associated or tumor-specific antigens have been described and are reviewed in (6, 70). Among the most widely studied are the tumor testes antigens, which are expressed by a range of tumors, including melanoma. For example, CTL clones specific for MART (melanoma Ag recognized by T cells) have been successfully used to treat patients with metastatic melanoma (71). Although infused CTLs localized to tumor sites and induce clinical responses, tumor antigen-loss variants were observed in three patients who subsequently relapsed, highlighting the risk of escape mutants when targeting a single epitope by a clone of CTLs.

3. Genetic Modification of T Cells

There is considerable interest in genetically modifying T cells so that they may be used for cancer therapy. Most tumor-associated antigens are self-proteins to which the immune system has limited responsiveness, due to the development of tolerance by clonal deletion or anergy (72). Hence, tumor antigen-specific T cells isolated from patients with cancer may have low affinity TCRs, limiting their cytotoxic activity against tumor cells (73). Investigators have overcome this limitation by expressing transgenic T-cell receptor α and β chains of high affinity, or by expressing a synthetic chimeric antigen receptor (CAR), which has the binding domains of, for example, a monoclonal antibody, and the endodomains of the T-cell receptor to ensure signaling and T-cell activation once the CAR has been engaged. Interest in genetic modification of T cells has also arisen as a means of incorporating countermeasures to the multiplicity of immune evasion strategies used by potentially immunogenic tumor cells.

3.1. Artificial αβ T-Cell Receptors

The cDNAs for the α and β chains of the TCR are cloned from class I HLA-restricted TCRs of tumor-reactive cytotoxic T cells and transferred to fresh T cells by an integrating vector, potentially giving the recipient cells the same antigen specificity as the donor T cells (74). This approach allows rapid production of large numbers of tumor antigen-specific T cells. Preclinical studies have shown that infusion of αβ TCR transgenic T cells can eradicate tumors in vivo (75, 76). Recently, Morgan and colleagues treated melanoma patients with T cells genetically modified with MART-1 specific TCRs and reported regression of metastatic lesions in two patients together with prolonged persistence of CTLs (77). The same procedure has also been applied to generate T cells specific for the minor histocompatibility antigens HA-1- or HA-2- to treat leukemic relapse after HLA-mismatched HSCT (78, 79) and to common oncoproteins such as MDM2 and WT-1 (76, 80). To date, however, success has been less than desired, and a major constraint is the development of hybrid TCR which contain a mixture of donor and recipient T-cell receptors. These are usually functionless, but may produce autoreactivity.

3.2. Chimeric Antigen Receptors (CARs)

Chimeric TCRs are usually generated by joining the light and heavy chain variable regions of a monoclonal antibody expressed as a single-chain Fv (scFv) molecule to the transmembrane and cytoplasmic signaling domains derived from CD3 δ chain or Fc receptor γ chain through a flexible spacer (81, 82). Thus they combine the antigen specificity of an antibody and the cytotoxic properties of a T cell in a single fusion molecule. Since CARs bind to target antigens in an HLA-unrestricted manner, they are resistant to many of the tumor immune evasion mechanisms, such as downregulation of HLA class I molecules or failure to process or present proteins, used by tumor cells to escape immune attack. First-generation CARs, incorporated the cytoplasmic region (endodomains) from the CD3 δ or the Fc receptor γ chains as their signaling domain. But although these receptors successfully redirected T-cell cytotoxicity, they failed to stimulate T-cell proliferation and survival in vivo, likely because of the lack of appropriate costimulatory signals to T cells following engagement of the CAR. Hence the efficacy of these first generation CAR-T cells has been modest in phase I clinical trials in patients with lymphoma, ovarian or renal cancer (83–85). Second generation CARs were constructed by incorporating signaling domains from costimulatory molecules such as CD28, OX40, and 4-1BB within the endodomain, and improved antigen-specific T-cell activation and expansion (86, 87). An alternative approach is to express CARs in antigen-specific T cells, which will then also be activated and expanded through engagement of their native αβ TCR by antigen on professional antigen-presenting cells, with attendant co-stimulation. We have shown that EBV-specific CTLs engineered with a CAR specific for the disialoganglioside antigen GD2a on neuroblastoma cells had better in vivo persistence compared with unselected T cells engineered with the identical CAR, and could be associated with tumor responses including complete remission (88).

3.3. Engineering T cells to Overcome Immune Evasion Strategies

One of the main challenges to effective adoptive T-cell therapy is the lack of in vivo expansion and maintenance of ex vivo manipulated, adoptively transferred T cells because of various tumor-induced immune evasion mechanisms. Gene transfer technologies allow us to modify T cells and restore their functionality in a hostile environment. For example, many tumor cells or their associated stroma produce TGF-β, which favors the development of immune tolerance and T-cell anergy (89), inducing T effector cell growth arrest with induction of Tregs. Zhang and colleagues demonstrated that dnTGF-β RII transfection improved the persistence of T cells and that infusion of modified cells eliminated tumor in a mouse prostate cancer model (90). Subsequently, our group showed that antigen-specific T cells expressing dnTGF-β RII were resistant to the anti-proliferative effects of TGF-β and retained their effector function in vivo (91). T cells may also be modified to express cytokine or cytokine receptor genes that mimic the milieu found during lymphoid regeneration and restoration of homeostasis, such as IL-2, IL-7, or IL-15 (92–94). As yet we do not know how safe or effective these transgenic cytokines and their receptors will be (95, 96).

4. Future Applications and Implementation of Cell Therapies for Cancer

With the recent approval of the first cell therapeutic for cancer (Dendreon), and the publication of increasing numbers of reports of complete tumor responses after cellular immunotherapy, there is increasing hope that this methodology will finally take its place among other more conventional cancer therapeutics. Much remains to be done to ensure the effectiveness and safety of these cell therapies and to develop economic models to support their development to licensure, but we are confident that well within the next decade this approach will cease being almost entirely experimental and will be considered a significant component of standard cancer therapy.

References

1. Kim, E. S., Vokes, E. E., and Kies, M. S. (2004) Cetuximab in cancers of the lung and head & neck. *Semin Oncol 31*, 61–67.
2. Mendelsohn, J. (1997) Epidermal growth factor receptor inhibition by a monoclonal antibody as anticancer therapy. *Clin Cancer Res 3*, 2703–2707.
3. Piccart-Gebhart, M. J., Procter, M., Leyland-Jones, B., Goldhirsch, A., Untch, M., Smith, I., Gianni, L., Baselga, J., Bell, R., Jackisch, C., Cameron, D., Dowsett, M., Barrios, C. H., Steger, G., Huang, C. S., Andersson, M., Inbar, M., Lichinitser, M., Lang, I., Nitz, U., Iwata, H., Thomssen, C., Lohrisch, C., Suter, T. M., Ruschoff, J., Suto, T., Greatorex, V., Ward, C., Straehle, C., McFadden, E., Dolci, M. S., and Gelber, R. D. (2005) Trastuzumab after adjuvant chemotherapy in HER2-positive breast cancer. *N Engl J Med 353*, 1659–1672.
4. Weiner, G. J., and Link, B. K. (2004) Monoclonal antibody therapy of B cell lymphoma. *Expert Opin Biol Ther 4*, 375–385.
5. Giaccone, G. (2005) Epidermal growth factor receptor inhibitors in the treatment of non-small-cell lung cancer. *J Clin Oncol 23*, 3235–3242.
6. Graziano, D. F., and Finn, O. J. (2005) Tumor antigens and tumor antigen discovery. *Cancer Treat Res 123*, 89–111.
7. Renkvist, N., Castelli, C., Robbins, P. F., and Parmiani, G. (2001) A listing of human tumor antigens recognized by T cells. *Cancer Immunol Immunother 50*, 3–15.
8. Van Der Bruggen, P., Zhang, Y., Chaux, P., Stroobant, V., Panichelli, C., Schultz, E. S., Chapiro, J., Van Den Eynde, B. J., Brasseur, F., and Boon, T. (2002) Tumor-specific shared antigenic peptides recognized by human T cells. *Immunol Rev 188*, 51–64.

9. Drake, C. G., Jaffee, E., and Pardoll, D. M. (2006) Mechanisms of immune evasion by tumors. *Adv Immunol 90*, 51–81.

10. Smyth, M. J., Godfrey, D. I., and Trapani, J. A. (2001) A fresh look at tumor immunosurveillance and immunotherapy. *Nat Immunol 2*, 293–299.

11. Cho, H. J., Takabayashi, K., Cheng, P. M., Nguyen, M. D., Corr, M., Tuck, S., and Raz, E. (2000) Immunostimulatory DNA-based vaccines induce cytotoxic lymphocyte activity by a T-helper cell-independent mechanism. *Nat Biotechnol 18*, 509–514.

12. Stevenson, F. K., Ottensmeier, C. H., Johnson, P., Zhu, D., Buchan, S. L., McCann, K. J., Roddick, J. S., King, A. T., McNicholl, F., Savelyeva, N., and Rice, J. (2004) DNA vaccines to attack cancer, *Proc Natl Acad Sci U S A 101*(2), 14646–14652.

13. Stevenson, F. K., Rice, J., Ottensmeier, C. H., Thirdborough, S. M., and Zhu, D. (2004) DNA fusion gene vaccines against cancer: from the laboratory to the clinic. *Immunol Rev 199*, 156–180.

14. McConkey, S. J., Reece, W. H., Moorthy, V. S., Webster, D., Dunachie, S., Butcher, G., Vuola, J. M., Blanchard, T. J., Gothard, P., Watkins, K., Hannan, C. M., Everaere, S., Brown, K., Kester, K. E., Cummings, J., Williams, J., Heppner, D. G., Pathan, A., Flanagan, K., Arulanantham, N., Roberts, M. T., Roy, M., Smith, G. L., Schneider, J., Peto, T., Sinden, R. E., Gilbert, S. C., and Hill, A. V. (2003) Enhanced T-cell immunogenicity of plasmid DNA vaccines boosted by recombinant modified vaccinia virus Ankara in humans. *Nat Med 9*, 729–735.

15. Woodland, D. L. (2004) Jump-starting the immune system: prime-boosting comes of age. *Trends Immunol 25*, 98–104.

16. Boczkowski, D., Nair, S. K., Snyder, D., and Gilboa, E. (1996) Dendritic cells pulsed with RNA are potent antigen-presenting cells in vitro and in vivo. *J Exp Med 184*, 465–472.

17. Gottschalk, S., Edwards, O. L., Sili, U., Huls, M. H., Goltsova, T., Davis, A. R., Heslop, H. E., and Rooney, C. M. (2003) Generating CTLs against the subdominant Epstein-Barr virus LMP1 antigen for the adoptive immunotherapy of EBV-associated malignancies. *Blood 101*, 1905–1912.

18. Holmes, L. M., Li, J., Sticca, R. P., Wagner, T. E., and Wei, Y. (2001) A Rapid, Novel Strategy to Induce Tumor Cell-Specific Cytotoxic T Lymphocyte Responses Using Instant Dendritomas. *J Immunother (1991) 24*, 122–129.

19. Mackensen, A., Herbst, B., Chen, J. L., Kohler, G., Noppen, C., Herr, W., Spagnoli, G. C., Cerundolo, V., and Lindemann, A. (2000) Phase I study in melanoma patients of a vaccine with peptide-pulsed dendritic cells generated in vitro from CD34(+) hematopoietic progenitor cells. *Int J Cancer 86*, 385–392.

20. Radford, K. J., Jackson, A. M., Wang, J. H., Vassaux, G., and Lemoine, N. R. (2003) Recombinant E. coli efficiently delivers antigen and maturation signals to human dendritic cells: presentation of MART1 to CD8+ T cells. *Int J Cancer 105*, 811–819.

21. Kikuchi, T., Akasaki, Y., Irie, M., Homma, S., Abe, T., and Ohno, T. (2001) Results of a phase I clinical trial of vaccination of glioma patients with fusions of dendritic and glioma cells. *Cancer Immunol Immunother 50*, 337–344.

22. Lin, A. M., Hershberg, R. M., and Small, E. J. (2006) Immunotherapy for prostate cancer using prostatic acid phosphatase loaded antigen presenting cells. *Urol Oncol 24*, 434–441.

23. Small, E. J., Schellhammer, P. F., Higano, C. S., Redfern, C. H., Nemunaitis, J. J., Valone, F. H., Verjee, S. S., Jones, L. A., and Hershberg, R. M. (2006) Placebo-controlled phase III trial of immunologic therapy with sipuleucel-T (APC8015) in patients with metastatic, asymptomatic hormone refractory prostate cancer. *J Clin Oncol 24*, 3089–3094.

24. Moretta, L., Ferlazzo, G., Bottino, C., Vitale, M., Pende, D., Mingari, M. C., and Moretta, A. (2006) Effector and regulatory events during natural killer-dendritic cell interactions. *Immunol Rev 214*, 219–228.

25. Degli-Esposti, M. A., and Smyth, M. J. (2005) Close encounters of different kinds: dendritic cells and NK cells take centre stage. *Nat Rev Immunol 5*, 112–124.

26. Raulet, D. H. (2004) Interplay of natural killer cells and their receptors with the adaptive immune response. *Nat Immunol 5*, 996–1002.

27. Becknell, B., and Caligiuri, M. A. (2005) Interleukin-2, interleukin-15, and their roles in human natural killer cells. *Adv Immunol 86*, 209–239.

28. Rosenberg, S. A., Lotze, M. T., Muul, L. M., Leitman, S., Chang, A. E., Ettinghausen, S. E., Matory, Y. L., Skibber, J. M., Shiloni, E., Vetto, J. T., and et al. (1985) Observations on the systemic administration of autologous lymphokine-activated killer cells and recombinant interleukin-2 to patients

with metastatic cancer. *N Engl J Med 313*, 1485–1492.

29. Atkins, M. B., Lotze, M. T., Dutcher, J. P., Fisher, R. I., Weiss, G., Margolin, K., Abrams, J., Sznol, M., Parkinson, D., Hawkins, M., Paradise, C., Kunkel, L., and Rosenberg, S. A. (1999) High-dose recombinant interleukin 2 therapy for patients with metastatic melanoma: analysis of 270 patients treated between 1985 and 1993. *J Clin Oncol 17*, 2105–2116.

30. Ruggeri, L., Capanni, M., Urbani, E., Perruccio, K., Shlomchik, W. D., Tosti, A., Posati, S., Rogaia, D., Frassoni, F., Aversa, F., Martelli, M. F., and Velardi, A. (2002) Effectiveness of donor natural killer cell alloreactivity in mismatched hematopoietic transplants. *Science 295*, 2097–2100.

31. Bishop, M. R., Fowler, D. H., Marchigiani, D., Castro, K., Kasten-Sportes, C., Steinberg, S. M., Gea-Banacloche, J. C., Dean, R., Chow, C. K., Carter, C., Read, E. J., Leitman, S., and Gress, R. (2004) Allogeneic lymphocytes induce tumor regression of advanced metastatic breast cancer. *J Clin Oncol 22*, 3886–3892.

32. Horowitz, M. M., Gale, R. P., Sondel, P. M., Goldman, J. M., Kersey, J., Kolb, H. J., Rimm, A. A., Ringden, O., Rozman, C., Speck, B., and et al. (1990) Graft-versus-leukemia reactions after bone marrow transplantation. *Blood 75*, 555–562.

33. Kolb, H. J., Mittermuller, J., Clemm, C., Holler, E., Ledderose, G., Brehm, G., Heim, M., and Wilmanns, W. (1990) Donor leukocyte transfusions for treatment of recurrent chronic myelogenous leukemia in marrow transplant patients. *Blood 76*, 2462–2465.

34. Gilleece, M. H., and Dazzi, F. (2003) Donor lymphocyte infusions for patients who relapse after allogeneic stem cell transplantation for chronic myeloid leukaemia. *Leuk Lymphoma 44*, 23–28.

35. Kolb, H. J., Schattenberg, A., Goldman, J. M., Hertenstein, B., Jacobsen, N., Arcese, W., Ljungman, P., Ferrant, A., Verdonck, L., Niederwieser, D., van Rhee, F., Mittermueller, J., de Witte, T., Holler, E., and Ansari, H. (1995) Graft-versus-leukemia effect of donor lymphocyte transfusions in marrow grafted patients. *Blood 86*, 2041–2050.

36. Mackinnon, S., Papadopoulos, E. B., Carabasi, M. H., Reich, L., Collins, N. H., Boulad, F., Castro-Malaspina, H., Childs, B. H., Gillio, A. P., Kernan, N. A., and et al. (1995) Adoptive immunotherapy evaluating escalating doses of donor leukocytes for relapse of chronic myeloid leukemia after

bone marrow transplantation: separation of graft-versus-leukemia responses from graft-versus-host disease. *Blood 86*, 1261–1268.

37. Amrolia, P. J., Muccioli-Casadei, G., Yvon, E., Huls, H., Sili, U., Wieder, E. D., Bollard, C., Michalek, J., Ghetie, V., Heslop, H. E., Molldrem, J. J., Rooney, C. M., Schlinder, J., Vitetta, E., and Brenner, M. K. (2003) Selective depletion of donor alloreactive T cells without loss of antiviral or antileukemic responses. *Blood 102*, 2292–2299.

38. Solomon, S. R., Mielke, S., Savani, B. N., Montero, A., Wisch, L., Childs, R., Hensel, N., Schindler, J., Ghetie, V., Leitman, S. F., Mai, T., Carter, C. S., Kurlander, R., Read, E. J., Vitetta, E. S., and Barrett, A. J. (2005) Selective depletion of alloreactive donor lymphocytes: a novel method to reduce the severity of graft-versus-host disease in older patients undergoing matched sibling donor stem cell transplantation. *Blood 106*, 1123–1129.

39. Bonini, C., Ferrari, G., Verzeletti, S., Servida, P., Zappone, E., Ruggieri, L., Ponzoni, M., Rossini, S., Mavilio, F., Traversari, C., and Bordignon, C. (1997) HSV-TK gene transfer into donor lymphocytes for control of allogeneic graft-versus-leukemia. *Science 276*, 1719–1724.

40. Shariat, S. F., Desai, S., Song, W., Khan, T., Zhao, J., Nguyen, C., Foster, B. A., Greenberg, N., Spencer, D. M., and Slawin, K. M. (2001) Adenovirus-mediated transfer of inducible caspases: a novel "death switch" gene therapeutic approach to prostate cancer. *Cancer Res 61*, 2562–2571.

41. Straathof, K. C., Spencer, D. M., Sutton, R. E., and Rooney, C. M. (2003) Suicide genes as safety switches in T lymphocytes. *Cytotherapy 5*, 227–230.

42. Thomis, D. C., Marktel, S., Bonini, C., Traversari, C., Gilman, M., Bordignon, C., and Clackson, T. (2001) A Fas-based suicide switch in human T cells for the treatment of graft-versus-host disease. *Blood 97*, 1249–1257.

43. Tiberghien, P., Ferrand, C., Lioure, B., Milpied, N., Angonin, R., Deconinck, E., Certoux, J. M., Robinet, E., Saas, P., Petracca, B., Juttner, C., Reynolds, C. W., Longo, D. L., Herve, P., and Cahn, J. Y. (2001) Administration of herpes simplex-thymidine kinase-expressing donor T cells with a T-cell-depleted allogeneic marrow graft. *Blood 97*, 63–72.

44. Ljunggren, H. G., and Karre, K. (1990) In search of the 'missing self': MHC molecules and NK cell recognition. *Immunol Today 11*, 237–244.

45. Lanier, L. L. (1998) NK cell receptors. *Annu Rev Immunol 16*, 359–393.

46. Parham, P. (2005) MHC class I molecules and KIRs in human history, health and survival. *Nat Rev Immunol 5*, 201–214.

47. Farag, S. S., Bacigalupo, A., Eapen, M., Hurley, C., Dupont, B., Caligiuri, M. A., Boudreau, C., Nelson, G., Oudshoorn, M., van Rood, J., Velardi, A., Maiers, M., Setterholm, M., Confer, D., Posch, P. E., Anasetti, C., Kamani, N., Miller, J. S., Weisdorf, D., and Davies, S. M. (2006) The effect of KIR ligand incompatibility on the outcome of unrelated donor transplantation: a report from the center for international blood and marrow transplant research, the European blood and marrow transplant registry, and the Dutch registry. *Biol Blood Marrow Transplant 12*, 876–884.

48. Passweg, J. R., Koehl, U., Uharek, L., Meyer-Monard, S., and Tichelli, A. (2006) Natural-killer-cell-based treatment in haematopoietic stem-cell transplantation. *Best Pract Res Clin Haematol 19*, 811–824.

49. Ruggeri, L., Mancusi, A., Capanni, M., Urbani, E., Carotti, A., Aloisi, T., Stern, M., Pende, D., Perruccio, K., Burchielli, E., Topini, F., Bianchi, E., Aversa, F., Martelli, M. F., and Velardi, A. (2007) Donor natural killer cell allorecognition of missing self in haploidentical hematopoietic transplantation for acute myeloid leukemia: challenging its predictive value. *Blood 110*, 433–440.

50. Ljunggren, H. G., and Malmberg, K. J. (2007) Prospects for the use of NK cells in immunotherapy of human cancer. *Nat Rev Immunol 7*, 329–339.

51. Riddell, S. R., Watanabe, K. S., Goodrich, J. M., Li, C. R., Agha, M. E., and Greenberg, P. D. (1992) Restoration of viral immunity in immunodeficient humans by the adoptive transfer of T cell clones. *Science 257*, 238–241.

52. Einsele, H., Rauser, G., Grigoleit, U., Hebart, H., Sinzger, C., Riegler, S., and Jahn, G. (2002) Induction of CMV-specific T-cell lines using Ag-presenting cells pulsed with CMV protein or peptide. *Cytotherapy 4*, 49–54.

53. Einsele, H., Roosnek, E., Rufer, N., Sinzger, C., Riegler, S., Loffler, J., Grigoleit, U., Moris, A., Rammensee, H. G., Kanz, L., Kleihauer, A., Frank, F., Jahn, G., and Hebart, H. (2002) Infusion of cytomegalovirus (CMV)-specific T cells for the treatment of CMV infection not responding to antiviral chemotherapy. *Blood 99*, 3916–3922.

54. Walter, E. A., Greenberg, P. D., Gilbert, M. J., Finch, R. J., Watanabe, K. S., Thomas, E. D., and Riddell, S. R. (1995) Reconstitution of cellular immunity against cytomegalovirus in recipients of allogeneic bone marrow by transfer of T-cell clones from the donor. *N Engl J Med 333*, 1038–1044.

55. Heslop, H. E., Ng, C. Y., Li, C., Smith, C. A., Loftin, S. K., Krance, R. A., Brenner, M. K., and Rooney, C. M. (1996) Long-term restoration of immunity against Epstein-Barr virus infection by adoptive transfer of gene-modified virus-specific T lymphocytes. *Nat Med 2*, 551–555.

56. Leen, A. M., and Heslop, H. E. (2008) Cytotoxic T lymphocytes as immune-therapy in haematological practice. *Br J Haematol 143*, 169–179.

57. Rooney, C. M., Smith, C. A., Ng, C. Y., Loftin, S., Li, C., Krance, R. A., Brenner, M. K., and Heslop, H. E. (1995) Use of gene-modified virus-specific T lymphocytes to control Epstein-Barr-virus-related lymphoproliferation. *Lancet 345*, 9–13.

58. Gottschalk, S., Ng, C. Y., Perez, M., Smith, C. A., Sample, C., Brenner, M. K., Heslop, H. E., and Rooney, C. M. (2001) An Epstein-Barr virus deletion mutant associated with fatal lymphoproliferative disease unresponsive to therapy with virus-specific CTLs. *Blood 97*, 835–843.

59. Comoli, P., Basso, S., Zecca, M., Pagliara, D., Baldanti, F., Bernardo, M. E., Barberi, W., Moretta, A., Labirio, M., Paulli, M., Furione, M., Maccario, R., and Locatelli, F. (2007) Preemptive therapy of EBV-related lymphoproliferative disease after pediatric haploidentical stem cell transplantation. *Am J Transplant 7*, 1648–1655.

60. Gustafsson, A., Levitsky, V., Zou, J. Z., Frisan, T., Dalianis, T., Ljungman, P., Ringden, O., Winiarski, J., Ernberg, I., and Masucci, M. G. (2000) Epstein-Barr virus (EBV) load in bone marrow transplant recipients at risk to develop posttransplant lymphoproliferative disease: prophylactic infusion of EBV-specific cytotoxic T cells. *Blood 95*, 807–814.

61. Imashuku, S., Goto, T., Matsumura, T., Naya, M., Yamori, M., Hojo, M., Hibi, S., and Todo, S. (1997) Unsuccessful CTL transfusion in a case of post-BMT Epstein-Barr virus-associated lymphoproliferative disorder (EBV-LPD). *Bone Marrow Transplant 20*, 337–340.

62. O'Reilly, R. J., Doubrovina, E., Trivedi, D., Hasan, A., Kollen, W., and Koehne, G. (2007) Adoptive transfer of antigen-specific T-cells of donor type for immunotherapy of

viral infections following allogeneic hemato-poietic cell transplants. *Immunol Res 38*, 237–250.

63. Haque, T., Wilkie, G. M., Taylor, C., Amlot, P. L., Murad, P., Iley, A., Dombagoda, D., Britton, K. M., Swerdlow, A. J., and Crawford, D. H. (2002) Treatment of Epstein-Barr-virus-positive post-transplantation lymphoproliferative disease with partly HLA-matched allogeneic cytotoxic T cells. *Lancet 360*, 436–442.

64. Haque, T., Wilkie, G. M., Jones, M. M., Higgins, C. D., Urquhart, G., Wingate, P., Burns, D., McAulay, K., Turner, M., Bellamy, C., Amlot, P. L., Kelly, D., MacGilchrist, A., Gandhi, M. K., Swerdlow, A. J., and Crawford, D. H. (2007) Allogeneic cytotoxic T-cell therapy for EBV-positive posttransplantation lymphoproliferative disease: results of a phase 2 multicenter clinical trial. *Blood 110*, 1123–1131.

65. Bollard, C. M., Gottschalk, S., Leen, A. M., Weiss, H., Straathof, K. C., Carrum, G., Khalil, M., Wu, M. F., Huls, M. H., Chang, C. C., Gresik, M. V., Gee, A. P., Brenner, M. K., Rooney, C. M., and Heslop, H. E. (2007) Complete responses of relapsed lymphoma following genetic modification of tumor-antigen presenting cells and T-lymphocyte transfer. *Blood 110*, 2838–2845.

66. Niedobitek, G. (2000) Epstein-Barr virus infection in the pathogenesis of nasopharyngeal carcinoma. *Mol Pathol 53*, 248–254.

67. Chua, D., Huang, J., Zheng, B., Lau, S. Y., Luk, W., Kwong, D. L., Sham, J. S., Moss, D., Yuen, K. Y., Im, S. W., and Ng, M. H. (2001) Adoptive transfer of autologous Epstein-Barr virus-specific cytotoxic T cells for nasopharyngeal carcinoma. *Int J Cancer 94*, 73–80.

68. Straathof, K. C., Bollard, C. M., Popat, U., Huls, M. H., Lopez, T., Morriss, M. C., Gresik, M. V., Gee, A. P., Russell, H. V., Brenner, M. K., Rooney, C. M., and Heslop, H. E. (2005) Treatment of nasopharyngeal carcinoma with Epstein-Barr virus--specific T lymphocytes. *Blood 105*, 1898–1904.

69. Louis, C. U., Straathof, K., Bollard, C. M., Gerken, C., Huls, M. H., Gresik, M. V., Wu, M. F., Weiss, H. L., Gee, A. P., Brenner, M. K., Rooney, C. M., Heslop, H. E., and Gottschalk, S. (2009) Enhancing the in vivo expansion of adoptively transferred EBV-specific CTL with lymphodepleting CD45 monoclonal antibodies in NPC patients. *Blood 113*, 2442–2450.

70. Stevenson, F. K., Rice, J., and Zhu, D. (2004) Tumor vaccines. *Adv Immunol 82*, 49–103.

71. Yee, C., Thompson, J. A., Byrd, D., Riddell, S. R., Roche, P., Celis, E., and Greenberg, P. D. (2002) Adoptive T cell therapy using antigen-specific CD8+ T cell clones for the treatment of patients with metastatic melanoma: in vivo persistence, migration, and antitumor effect of transferred T cells. *Proc Natl Acad Sci U S A 99*, 16168–16173.

72. Ochsenbein, A. F., Klenerman, P., Karrer, U., Ludewig, B., Pericin, M., Hengartner, H., and Zinkernagel, R. M. (1999) Immune surveillance against a solid tumor fails because of immunological ignorance. *Proc Natl Acad Sci U S A 96*, 2233–2238.

73. Teague, R. M., Sather, B. D., Sacks, J. A., Huang, M. Z., Dossett, M. L., Morimoto, J., Tan, X., Sutton, S. E., Cooke, M. P., Ohlen, C., and Greenberg, P. D. (2006) Interleukin-15 rescues tolerant CD8+ T cells for use in adoptive immunotherapy of established tumors. *Nat Med 12*, 335–341.

74. Dembic, Z., Haas, W., Weiss, S., McCubrey, J., Kiefer, H., von Boehmer, H., and Steinmetz, M. (1986) Transfer of specificity by murine alpha and beta T-cell receptor genes. *Nature 320*, 232–238.

75. Kessels, H. W., Wolkers, M. C., van den Boom, M. D., van der Valk, M. A., and Schumacher, T. N. (2001) Immunotherapy through TCR gene transfer. *Nat Immunol 2*, 957–961.

76. Xue, S. A., Gao, L., Hart, D., Gillmore, R., Qasim, W., Thrasher, A., Apperley, J., Engels, B., Uckert, W., Morris, E., and Stauss, H. (2005) Elimination of human leukemia cells in NOD/SCID mice by WT1-TCR gene-transduced human T cells. *Blood 106*, 3062–3067.

77. Morgan, R. A., Dudley, M. E., Wunderlich, J. R., Hughes, M. S., Yang, J. C., Sherry, R. M., Royal, R. E., Topalian, S. L., Kammula, U. S., Restifo, N. P., Zheng, Z., Nahvi, A., de Vries, C. R., Rogers-Freezer, L. J., Mavroukakis, S. A., and Rosenberg, S. A. (2006) Cancer regression in patients after transfer of genetically engineered lymphocytes. *Science 314*, 126–129.

78. Heemskerk, M. H., Hoogeboom, M., de Paus, R. A., Kester, M. G., van der Hoorn, M. A., Goulmy, E., Willemze, R., and Falkenburg, J. H. (2003) Redirection of antileukemic reactivity of peripheral T lymphocytes using gene transfer of minor histocompatibility antigen HA-2-specific T-cell receptor complexes expressing a conserved alpha joining region. *Blood 102*, 3530–3540.

79. Mutis, T., Blokland, E., Kester, M., Schrama, E., and Goulmy, E. (2002) Generation of minor histocompatibility antigen HA-1-specific cytotoxic T cells restricted by nonself HLA molecules: a potential strategy to treat relapsed leukemia after HLA-mismatched stem cell transplantation. *Blood 100*, 547–552.

80. Stanislawski, T., Voss, R. H., Lotz, C., Sadovnikova, E., Willemsen, R. A., Kuball, J., Ruppert, T., Bolhuis, R. L., Melief, C. J., Huber, C., Stauss, H. J., and Theobald, M. (2001) Circumventing tolerance to a human MDM2-derived tumor antigen by TCR gene transfer. *Nat Immunol 2*, 962–970.

81. Gross, G., Waks, T., and Eshhar, Z. (1989) Expression of immunoglobulin-T-cell receptor chimeric molecules as functional receptors with antibody-type specificity. *Proc Natl Acad Sci U S A 86*, 10024–10028.

82. Kershaw, M. H., Darcy, P. K., Trapani, J. A., and Smyth, M. J. (1996) The use of chimeric human Fc(epsilon) receptor I to redirect cytotoxic T lymphocytes to tumors. *J Leukoc Biol 60*, 721–728.

83. Kershaw, M. H., Westwood, J. A., Parker, L. L., Wang, G., Eshhar, Z., Mavroukakis, S. A., White, D. E., Wunderlich, J. R., Canevari, S., Rogers-Freezer, L., Chen, C. C., Yang, J. C., Rosenberg, S. A., and Hwu, P. (2006) A phase I study on adoptive immunotherapy using gene-modified T cells for ovarian cancer. *Clin Cancer Res 12*, 6106–6115.

84. Lamers, C. H., Sleijfer, S., Vulto, A. G., Kruit, W. H., Kliffen, M., Debets, R., Gratama, J. W., Stoter, G., and Oosterwijk, E. (2006) Treatment of metastatic renal cell carcinoma with autologous T-lymphocytes genetically retargeted against carbonic anhydrase IX: first clinical experience. *J Clin Oncol 24*, e20–22.

85. Till, B. G., Jensen, M. C., Wang, J., Chen, E. Y., Wood, B. L., Greisman, H. A., Qian, X., James, S. E., Raubitschek, A., Forman, S. J., Gopal, A. K., Pagel, J. M., Lindgren, C. G., Greenberg, P. D., Riddell, S. R., and Press, O. W. (2008) Adoptive immunotherapy for indolent non-Hodgkin lymphoma and mantle cell lymphoma using genetically modified autologous CD20-specific T cells. *Blood 112*, 2261–2271.

86. Finney, H. M., Akbar, A. N., and Lawson, A. D. (2004) Activation of resting human primary T cells with chimeric receptors: costimulation from CD28, inducible costimulator, CD134, and CD137 in series with signals from the TCR zeta chain. *J Immunol 172*, 104–113.

87. Maher, J., Brentjens, R. J., Gunset, G., Riviere, I., and Sadelain, M. (2002) Human T-lymphocyte cytotoxicity and proliferation directed by a single chimeric TCRzeta/CD28 receptor. *Nat Biotechnol 20*, 70–75.

88. Pule, M. A., Savoldo, B., Myers, G. D., Rossig, C., Russell, H. V., Dotti, G., Huls, M. H., Liu, E., Gee, A. P., Mei, Z., Yvon, E., Weiss, H. L., Liu, H., Rooney, C. M., Heslop, H. E., and Brenner, M. K. (2008) Virus-specific T cells engineered to coexpress tumor-specific receptors: persistence and antitumor activity in individuals with neuroblastoma. *Nat Med 14*, 1264–1270.

89. Siegel, P. M., and Massague, J. (2003) Cytostatic and apoptotic actions of TGF-beta in homeostasis and cancer. *Nat Rev Cancer 3*, 807–821.

90. Zhang, Q., Yang, X., Pins, M., Javonovic, B., Kuzel, T., Kim, S. J., Parijs, L. V., Greenberg, N. M., Liu, V., Guo, Y., and Lee, C. (2005) Adoptive transfer of tumor-reactive transforming growth factor-beta-insensitive CD8+ T cells: eradication of autologous mouse prostate cancer. *Cancer Res 65*, 1761–1769.

91. Bollard, C. M., Rossig, C., Calonge, M. J., Huls, M. H., Wagner, H. J., Massague, J., Brenner, M. K., Heslop, H. E., and Rooney, C. M. (2002) Adapting a transforming growth factor beta-related tumor protection strategy to enhance antitumor immunity. *Blood 99*, 3179–3187.

92. Hsu, C., Hughes, M. S., Zheng, Z., Bray, R. B., Rosenberg, S. A., and Morgan, R. A. (2005) Primary human T lymphocytes engineered with a codon-optimized IL-15 gene resist cytokine withdrawal-induced apoptosis and persist long-term in the absence of exogenous cytokine. *J Immunol 175*, 7226–7234.

93. Heemskerk, B., Liu, K., Dudley, M. E., Johnson, L. A., Kaiser, A., Downey, S., Zheng, Z., Shelton, T. E., Matsuda, K., Robbins, P. F., Morgan, R. A., and Rosenberg, S. A. (2008) Adoptive cell therapy for patients with melanoma, using tumor-infiltrating lymphocytes genetically engineered to secrete interleukin-2. *Hum Gene Ther 19*, 496–510.

94. Vera, J. F., Hoyos, V., Savoldo, B., Quintarelli, C., Giordano Attianese, G. M., Leen, A. M., Liu, H., Foster, A. E., Heslop, H. E., Rooney, C. M., Brenner, M. K., and Dotti, G. (2009) Genetic Manipulation of Tumor-specific Cytotoxic T Lymphocytes to Restore Responsiveness to IL-7. *Mol Ther.*

95. Gattinoni, L., Powell, D. J., Jr., Rosenberg, S. A., and Restifo, N. P. (2006) Adoptive

immunotherapy for cancer: building on success. *Nat Rev Immunol 6*, 383–393.

96. Wagner, H. J., Bollard, C. M., Vigouroux, S., Huls, M. H., Anderson, R., Prentice, H. G., Brenner, M. K., Heslop, H. E., and Rooney, C. M. (2004) A strategy for treatment of Epstein-Barr virus-positive Hodgkin's disease by targeting interleukin 12 to the tumor environment using tumor antigen-specific T cells. *Cancer Gene Ther 11*, 81–91.

97. Cuenca, A., Cheng, F., Wang, H., Brayer, J., Horna, P., Gu, L., Bien, H., Borrello, I. M., Levitsky, H. I., and Sotomayor, E. M. (2003) Extra-lymphatic solid tumor growth is not immunologically ignored and results in early induction of antigen-specific T-cell anergy: dominant role of cross-tolerance to tumor antigens. *Cancer Res 63*, 9007–9015.

98. Staveley-O'Carroll, K., Sotomayor, E., Montgomery, J., Borrello, I., Hwang, L., Fein, S., Pardoll, D., and Levitsky, H. (1998) Induction of antigen-specific T cell anergy: An early event in the course of tumor progression. *Proc Natl Acad Sci USA 95*, 1178–1183.

99. Horna, P., Cuenca, A., Cheng, F., Brayer, J., Wang, H. W., Borrello, I., Levitsky, H., and Sotomayor, E. M. (2006) In vivo disruption of tolerogenic cross-presentation mechanisms uncovers an effective T-cell activation by B-cell lymphomas leading to antitumor immunity. *Blood 107*, 2871–2878.

100. Sotomayor, E. M., Borrello, I., Rattis, F. M., Cuenca, A. G., Abrams, J., Staveley-O'Carroll, K., and Levitsky, H. I. (2001) Cross-presentation of tumor antigens by bone marrow-derived antigen-presenting cells is the dominant mechanism in the induction of T-cell tolerance during B-cell lymphoma progression. *Blood 98*, 1070–1077.

101. Koneru, M., Schaer, D., Monu, N., Ayala, A., and Frey, A. B. (2005) Defective proximal TCR signaling inhibits CD8+ tumor-infiltrating lymphocyte lytic function. *J Immunol 174*, 1830–1840.

102. Mizoguchi, H., O'Shea, J. J., Longo, D. L., Loeffler, C. M., McVicar, D. W., and Ochoa, A. C. (1992) Alterations in signal transduction molecules in T lymphocytes from tumor-bearing mice. *Science 258*, 1795–1798.

103. Whiteside, T. L. (2006) Immune suppression in cancer: effects on immune cells, mechanisms and future therapeutic intervention. *Semin Cancer Biol 16*, 3–15.

104. Marincola, F. M., Jaffee, E. M., Hicklin, D. J., and Ferrone, S. (2000) Escape of human solid tumors from T-cell recognition: molecular mechanisms and functional significance. *Adv Immunol 74*, 181–273.

105. Rivoltini, L., Carrabba, M., Huber, V., Castelli, C., Novellino, L., Dalerba, P., Mortarini, R., Arancia, G., Anichini, A., Fais, S., and Parmiani, G. (2002) Immunity to cancer: attack and escape in T lymphocyte-tumor cell interaction. *Immunol Rev 188*, 97–113.

106. Blank, C., Gajewski, T. F., and Mackensen, A. (2005) Interaction of PD-L1 on tumor cells with PD-1 on tumor-specific T cells as a mechanism of immune evasion: implications for tumor immunotherapy. *Cancer Immunol Immunother 54*, 307–314.

107. Kryczek, I., Zou, L., Rodriguez, P., Zhu, G., Wei, S., Mottram, P., Brumlik, M., Cheng, P., Curiel, T., Myers, L., Lackner, A., Alvarez, X., Ochoa, A., Chen, L., and Zou, W. (2006) B7-H4 expression identifies a novel suppressive macrophage population in human ovarian carcinoma. *J Exp Med 203*, 871–881.

108. Leach, D. R., Krummel, M. F., and Allison, J. P. (1996) Enhancement of antitumor immunity by CTLA-4 blockade. *Science 271*, 1734–1736.

109. Watanabe, N., Gavrieli, M., Sedy, J. R., Yang, J., Fallarino, F., Loftin, S. K., Hurchla, M. A., Zimmerman, N., Sim, J., Zang, X., Murphy, T. L., Russell, J. H., Allison, J. P., and Murphy, K. M. (2003) BTLA is a lymphocyte inhibitory receptor with similarities to CTLA-4 and PD-1. *Nat Immunol 4*, 670–679.

110. Akasaki, Y., Liu, G., Chung, N. H., Ehtesham, M., Black, K. L., and Yu, J. S. (2004) Induction of a CD4+ T regulatory type 1 response by cyclooxygenase-2-overexpressing glioma. *J Immunol 173*, 4352–4359.

111. Gabrilovich, D. I., Chen, H. L., Girgis, K. R., Cunningham, H. T., Meny, G. M., Nadaf, S., Kavanaugh, D., and Carbone, D. P. (1996) Production of vascular endothelial growth factor by human tumors inhibits the functional maturation of dendritic cells. *Nat Med 2*, 1096–1103.

112. Gerlini, G., Tun-Kyi, A., Dudli, C., Burg, G., Pimpinelli, N., and Nestle, F. O. (2004) Metastatic melanoma secreted IL-10 down-regulates CD1 molecules on dendritic cells in metastatic tumor lesions. *Am J Pathol 165*, 1853–1863.

113. Li, M. O., Wan, Y. Y., Sanjabi, S., Robertson, A. K., and Flavell, R. A. (2006) Transforming growth factor-beta regulation of immune responses. *Annu Rev Immunol 24*, 99–146.

114. Waldmann, T. A. (2006) Effective cancer therapy through immunomodulation. *Annu Rev Med 57*, 65–81.

115. Andreola, G., Rivoltini, L., Castelli, C., Huber, V., Perego, P., Deho, P., Squarcina,

P., Accornero, P., Lozupone, F., Lugini, L., Stringaro, A., Molinari, A., Arancia, G., Gentile, M., Parmiani, G., and Fais, S. (2002) Induction of lymphocyte apoptosis by tumor cell secretion of FasL-bearing microvesicles. *J Exp Med 195*, 1303–1316.

116. Giovarelli, M., Musiani, P., Garotta, G., Ebner, R., Di Carlo, E., Kim, Y., Cappello, P., Rigamonti, L., Bernabei, P., Novelli, F., Modesti, A., Coletti, A., Ferrie, A. K., Lollini, P. L., Ruben, S., Salcedo, T., and Forni, G. (1999) A "stealth effect": adenocarcinoma cells engineered to express TRAIL elude tumor-specific and allogeneic T cell reactions. *J Immunol 163*, 4886–4893.

117. Hahne, M., Rimoldi, D., Schroter, M., Romero, P., Schreier, M., French, L. E., Schneider, P., Bornand, T., Fontana, A., Lienard, D., Cerottini, J., and Tschopp, J. (1996) Melanoma cell expression of Fas(Apo-1/CD95) ligand: implications for tumor immune escape. *Science 274*, 1363–1366.

118. O'Connell, J., Houston, A., Bennett, M. W., O'Sullivan, G. C., and Shanahan, F. (2001) Immune privilege or inflammation? Insights into the Fas ligand enigma. *Nat Med 7*, 271–274.

119. Perillo, N. L., Pace, K. E., Seilhamer, J. J., and Baum, L. G. (1995) Apoptosis of T cells mediated by galectin-1. *Nature 378*, 736–739.

120. Uyttenhove, C., Pilotte, L., Theate, I., Stroobant, V., Colau, D., Parmentier, N., Boon, T., and Van den Eynde, B. J. (2003) Evidence for a tumoral immune resistance mechanism based on tryptophan degradation by indoleamine 2,3-dioxygenase. *Nat Med 9*, 1269–1274.

121. Almand, B., Resser, J. R., Lindman, B., Nadaf, S., Clark, J. I., Kwon, E. D., Carbone, D. P., and Gabrilovich, D. I. (2000) Clinical significance of defective dendritic cell differentiation in cancer. *Clin Cancer Res 6*, 1755–1766.

122. Colonna, M., Trinchieri, G., and Liu, Y. J. (2004) Plasmacytoid dendritic cells in immunity. *Nat Immunol 5*, 1219–1226.

123. Gabrilovich, D. I., Velders, M. P., Sotomayor, E. M., and Kast, W. M. (2001) Mechanism of immune dysfunction in cancer mediated by immature Gr-1+ myeloid cells. *J Immunol 166*, 5398–5406.

124. Kusmartsev, S., Nagaraj, S., and Gabrilovich, D. I. (2005) Tumor-associated CD8+ T cell tolerance induced by bone marrow-derived immature myeloid cells. *J Immunol 175*, 4583–4592.

125. Li, Q., Pan, P. Y., Gu, P., Xu, D., and Chen, S. H. (2004) Role of immature myeloid Gr-1+ cells in the development of antitumor immunity. *Cancer Res 64*, 1130–1139.

126. Munn, D. H., Sharma, M. D., Hou, D., Baban, B., Lee, J. R., Antonia, S. J., Messina, J. L., Chandler, P., Koni, P. A., and Mellor, A. L. (2004) Expression of indoleamine 2,3-dioxygenase by plasmacytoid dendritic cells in tumor-draining lymph nodes. *J Clin Invest 114*, 280–290.

127. Munn, D. H., Sharma, M. D., Lee, J. R., Jhaver, K. G., Johnson, T. S., Keskin, D. B., Marshall, B., Chandler, P., Antonia, S. J., Burgess, R., Slingluff, C. L., Jr., and Mellor, A. L. (2002) Potential regulatory function of human dendritic cells expressing indoleamine 2,3-dioxygenase. *Science 297*, 1867–1870.

128. Pinzon-Charry, A., Ho, C. S., Laherty, R., Maxwell, T., Walker, D., Gardiner, R. A., O'Connor, L., Pyke, C., Schmidt, C., Furnival, C., and Lopez, J. A. (2005) A population of HLA-DR+ immature cells accumulates in the blood dendritic cell compartment of patients with different types of cancer. *Neoplasia 7*, 1112–1122.

129. Pinzon-Charry, A., Maxwell, T., Prato, S., Furnival, C., Schmidt, C., and Lopez, J. A. (2005) HLA-DR+ immature cells exhibit reduced antigen-presenting cell function but respond to CD40 stimulation. *Neoplasia 7*, 1123–1132.

130. Sakaguchi, S. (2004) Naturally arising CD4+ regulatory t cells for immunologic self-tolerance and negative control of immune responses. *Annu Rev Immunol 22*, 531–562.

131. Zou, W. (2005) Immunosuppressive networks in the tumour environment and their therapeutic relevance. *Nat Rev Cancer 5*, 263–274.

132. Angulo, I., de las Heras, F. G., Garcia-Bustos, J. F., Gargallo, D., Munoz-Fernandez, M. A., and Fresno, M. (2000) Nitric oxide-producing CD11b(+)Ly-6G(Gr-1)(+)CD31(ER-MP12)(+) cells in the spleen of cyclophosphamide-treated mice: implications for T-cell responses in immunosuppressed mice. *Blood 95*, 212–220.

133. Mackall, C. L., Fleisher, T. A., Brown, M. R., Magrath, I. T., Shad, A. T., Horowitz, M. E., Wexler, L. H., Adde, M. A., McClure, L. L., and Gress, R. E. (1994) Lymphocyte depletion during treatment with intensive chemotherapy for cancer. *Blood 84*, 2221–2228.

134. Mohty, M., Gaugler, B., Faucher, C., Sainty, D., Lafage-Pochitaloff, M., Vey, N., Bouabdallah, R., Arnoulet, C., Gastaut, J. A., Viret, F., Wolfers, J., Maraninchi, D.,

Blaise, D., and Olive, D. (2002) Recovery of lymphocyte and dendritic cell subsets following reduced intensity allogeneic bone marrow transplantation. *Hematology 7*, 157–164.

135. Santosuosso, M., Divangahi, M., Zganiacz, A., and Xing, Z. (2002) Reduced tissue macrophage population in the lung by anticancer agent cyclophosphamide: restoration by local granulocyte macrophage-colony-stimulating factor gene transfer. *Blood 99*, 1246–1252.

136. Hakim, F. T., Cepeda, R., Kaimei, S., Mackall, C. L., McAtee, N., Zujewski, J., Cowan, K., and Gress, R. E. (1997) Constraints on CD4 recovery postchemotherapy in adults: thymic insufficiency and apoptotic decline of expanded peripheral CD4 cells. *Blood 90*, 3789–3798.

137. Mackall, C. L., Fleisher, T. A., Brown, M. R., Andrich, M. P., Chen, C. C., Feuerstein, I. M., Horowitz, M. E., Magrath, I. T., Shad, A. T., Steinberg, S. M., and et al. (1995) Age, thymopoiesis, and CD4+ T-lymphocyte regeneration after intensive chemotherapy. *N Engl J Med 332*, 143–149.

138. Mackall, C. L., Fleisher, T. A., Brown, M. R., Andrich, M. P., Chen, C. C., Feuerstein, I. M., Magrath, I. T., Wexler, L. H., Dimitrov, D. S., and Gress, R. E. (1997) Distinctions between CD8+ and CD4+ T-cell regenerative pathways result in prolonged T-cell subset imbalance after intensive chemotherapy. *Blood 89*, 3700–3707.

139. Kirkwood, J. M., Ibrahim, J., Lawson, D. H., Atkins, M. B., Agarwala, S. S., Collins, K., Mascari, R., Morrissey, D. M., and Chapman, P. B. (2001) High-dose interferon alfa-2b does not diminish antibody response to GM2 vaccination in patients with resected melanoma: results of the Multicenter Eastern Cooperative Oncology Group Phase II Trial E2696. *J Clin Oncol 19*, 1430–1436.

140. Miles, D., and Papazisis, K. (2003) Rationale for the clinical development of STn-KLH (Theratope) and anti-MUC-1 vaccines in breast cancer. *Clin Breast Cancer. Suppl 4*, S134–138.

141. Ibrahim, N. (2004) Humoral immune responses to naturally occuring STn in metastatic breast cancer patients (MBC pts) treated with STn-KLH vaccine (abstract). *Prom Am Soc Clin Oncol 23*.

142. Mayordoma, J. (2004) Long term follow up of patients concomitantly treated with hormone therapy in prospective controlled randomized multicenter clinical study comparing STn-KLH avccine with KLH control in stage IV breast cancer following first line chemotherapy (abstract). *Prom Am Soc Clin Oncol 23*.

143. De Marco, F., Hallez, S., Brulet, J. M., Gesche, F., Marzano, P., Flamini, S., Marcante, M. L., and Venuti, A. (2003) DNA vaccines against HPV-16 E7-expressing tumour cells. *Anticancer Res 23*, 1449–1454.

144. Kim, D., Hoory, T., Wu, T. C., and Hung, C. F. (2007) Enhancing DNA vaccine potency by combining a strategy to prolong dendritic cell life and intracellular targeting strategies with a strategy to boost CD4+ T cell. *Hum Gene Ther 18*, 1129–1139.

145. Yu, M., and Finn, O. J. (2006) DNA vaccines for cancer too. *Cancer Immunol Immunother 55*, 119–130.

146. Baskar, S., Nabavi, N., Glimcher, L. H., and Ostrand-Rosenberg, S. (1993) Tumor cells expressing major histocompatibility complex class II and B7 activation molecules stimulate potent tumor-specific immunity. *J Immunother Emphasis Tumor Immunol 14*, 209–215.

147. Berd, D., Maguire, H. C., Jr., McCue, P., and Mastrangelo, M. J. (1990) Treatment of metastatic melanoma with an autologous tumor-cell vaccine: clinical and immunologic results in 64 patients. *J Clin Oncol 8*, 1858–1867.

148. Dols, A., Smith, J. W., 2nd, Meijer, S. L., Fox, B. A., Hu, H. M., Walker, E., Rosenheim, S., Moudgil, T., Doran, T., Wood, W., Seligman, M., Alvord, W. G., Schoof, D., and Urba, W. J. (2003) Vaccination of women with metastatic breast cancer, using a costimulatory gene (CD80)-modified, HLA-A2-matched, allogeneic, breast cancer cell line: clinical and immunological results. *Hum Gene Ther 14*, 1117–1123.

149. Michael, A., Ball, G., Quatan, N., Wushishi, F., Russell, N., Whelan, J., Chakraborty, P., Leader, D., Whelan, M., and Pandha, H. (2005) Delayed disease progression after allogeneic cell vaccination in hormone-resistant prostate cancer and correlation with immunologic variables. *Clin Cancer Res 11*, 4469–4478.

150. Mitchell, M. S., Kan-Mitchell, J., Kempf, R. A., Harel, W., Shau, H. Y., and Lind, S. (1988) Active specific immunotherapy for melanoma: phase I trial of allogeneic lysates and a novel adjuvant. *Cancer Res 48*, 5883–5893.

151. Raez, L. E., Cassileth, P. A., Schlesselman, J. J., Sridhar, K., Padmanabhan, S., Fisher, E. Z., Baldie, P. A., and Podack, E. R. (2004) Allogeneic vaccination with a B7.1 HLA-A gene-modified adenocarcinoma cell line in

patients with advanced non-small-cell lung cancer. *J Clin Oncol 22*, 2800–2807.

152. Townsend, S. E., and Allison, J. P. (1993) Tumor rejection after direct costimulation of CD8+ T cells by B7-transfected melanoma cells. *Science 259*, 368–370.

153. Vermorken, J. B., Claessen, A. M., van Tinteren, H., Gall, H. E., Ezinga, R., Meijer, S., Scheper, R. J., Meijer, C. J., Bloemena, E., Ransom, J. H., Hanna, M. G., Jr., and Pinedo, H. M. (1999) Active specific immunotherapy for stage II and stage III human colon cancer: a randomised trial. *Lancet 353*, 345–350.

154. Boczkowski, D., Nair, S. K., Nam, J. H., Lyerly, H. K., and Gilboa, E. (2000) Induction of tumor immunity and cytotoxic T lymphocyte responses using dendritic cells transfected with messenger RNA amplified from tumor cells. *Cancer Res 60*, 1028–1034.

155. Chen, Z., Moyana, T., Saxena, A., Warrington, R., Jia, Z., and Xiang, J. (2001) Efficient antitumor immunity derived from maturation of dendritic cells that had phagocytosed apoptotic/necrotic tumor cells. *Int J Cancer 93*, 539–548.

156. Di Nicola, M., Carlo-Stella, C., Milanesi, M., Magni, M., Longoni, P., Mortarini, R., Anichini, A., Tomanin, R., Scarpa, M., and Gianni, A. M. (2000) Large-scale feasibility of gene transduction into human CD34+ cell-derived dendritic cells by adenoviral/polycation complex. *Br J Haematol 111*, 344–350.

157. Galea-Lauri, J., Wells, J. W., Darling, D., Harrison, P., and Farzaneh, F. (2004) Strategies for antigen choice and priming of dendritic cells influence the polarization and efficacy of antitumor T-cell responses in dendritic cell-based cancer vaccination. *Cancer Immunol Immunother 53*, 963–977.

158. Gong, J., Nikrui, N., Chen, D., Koido, S., Wu, Z., Tanaka, Y., Cannistra, S., Avigan, D., and Kufe, D. (2000) Fusions of human ovarian carcinoma cells with autologous or allogeneic dendritic cells induce antitumor immunity. *J Immunol 165*, 1705–1711.

159. He, Y., Zhang, J., Mi, Z., Robbins, P., and Falo, L. D., Jr. (2005) Immunization with lentiviral vector-transduced dendritic cells induces strong and long-lasting T cell responses and therapeutic immunity. *J Immunol 174*, 3808–3817.

160. Koido, S., Ohana, M., Liu, C., Nikrui, N., Durfee, J., Lerner, A., and Gong, J. (2004) Dendritic cells fused with human cancer cells: morphology, antigen expression, and T cell stimulation. *Clin Immunol 113*, 261–269.

161. Li, Y., Bendandi, M., Deng, Y., Dunbar, C., Munshi, N., Jagannath, S., Kwak, L. W., and Lyerly, H. K. (2000) Tumor-specific recognition of human myeloma cells by idiotype-induced CD8(+) T cells. *Blood 96*, 2828–2833.

162. Muller, M. R., Grunebach, F., Nencioni, A., and Brossart, P. (2003) Transfection of dendritic cells with RNA induces CD4- and CD8-mediated T cell immunity against breast carcinomas and reveals the immunodominance of presented T cell epitopes. *J Immunol 170*, 5892–5896.

163. Strobel, I., Berchtold, S., Gotze, A., Schulze, U., Schuler, G., and Steinkasserer, A. (2000) Human dendritic cells transfected with either RNA or DNA encoding influenza matrix protein M1 differ in their ability to stimulate cytotoxic T lymphocytes. *Gene Ther 7*, 2028–2035.

164. Timmerman, J. M., Czerwinski, D. K., Davis, T. A., Hsu, F. J., Benike, C., Hao, Z. M., Taidi, B., Rajapaksa, R., Caspar, C. B., Okada, C. Y., van Beckhoven, A., Liles, T. M., Engleman, E. G., and Levy, R. (2002) Idiotype-pulsed dendritic cell vaccination for B-cell lymphoma: clinical and immune responses in 35 patients. *Blood 99*, 1517–1526.

165. Titzer, S., Christensen, O., Manzke, O., Tesch, H., Wolf, J., Emmerich, B., Carsten, C., Diehl, V., and Bohlen, H. (2000) Vaccination of multiple myeloma patients with idiotype-pulsed dendritic cells: immunological and clinical aspects. *Br J Haematol 108*, 805–816.

166. Biagi, E., Rousseau, R., Yvon, E., Schwartz, M., Dotti, G., Foster, A., Havlik-Cooper, D., Grilley, B., Gee, A., Baker, K., Carrum, G., Rice, L., Andreeff, M., Popat, U., and Brenner, M. (2005) Responses to human CD40 ligand/human interleukin-2 autologous cell vaccine in patients with B-cell chronic lymphocytic leukemia. *Clin Cancer Res 11*, 6916–6923.

167. Eguchi, J., Kuwashima, N., Hatano, M., Nishimura, F., Dusak, J. E., Storkus, W. J., and Okada, H. (2005) IL-4-transfected tumor cell vaccines activate tumor-infiltrating dendritic cells and promote type-1 immunity. *J Immunol 174*, 7194–7201.

168. Kusumoto, M., Umeda, S., Ikubo, A., Aoki, Y., Tawfik, O., Oben, R., Williamson, S., Jewell, W., and Suzuki, T. (2001) Phase 1 clinical trial of irradiated autologous melanoma cells adenovirally transduced with human GM-CSF gene. *Cancer Immunol Immunother 50*, 373–381.

169. Pandha, H., Eaton, J., Greenhalgh, R., Soars, D., and Dalgleish, A. (2005) Immunotherapy of murine prostate cancer using whole tumor cells killed ex vivo by herpes simplex viral thymidine kinase/ganciclovir suicide gene therapy. *Cancer Gene Ther 12*, 572–578.

170. Pericle, F., Giovarelli, M., Colombo, M. P., Ferrari, G., Musiani, P., Modesti, A., Cavallo, F., Di Pierro, F., Novelli, F., and Forni, G. (1994) An efficient Th2-type memory follows CD8+ lymphocyte-driven and eosinophil-mediated rejection of a spontaneous mouse mammary adenocarcinoma engineered to release IL-4. *J Immunol 153*, 5659–5673.

171. Rousseau, R. F., Biagi, E., Dutour, A., Yvon, E. S., Brown, M. P., Lin, T., Mei, Z., Grilley, B., Popek, E., Heslop, H. E., Gee, A. P., Krance, R. A., Popat, U., Carrum, G., Margolin, J. F., and Brenner, M. K. (2006) Immunotherapy of high-risk acute leukemia with a recipient (autologous) vaccine expressing transgenic human CD40L and IL-2 after chemotherapy and allogeneic stem cell transplantation. *Blood 107*, 1332–1341.

172. Schirrmacher, V. (2005) Clinical trials of antitumor vaccination with an autologous tumor cell vaccine modified by virus infection: improvement of patient survival based on improved antitumor immune memory. *Cancer Immunol Immunother 54*, 587–598.

173. Brenner, M. K., Heslop, H., Krance, R., Horowitz, M., Strother, D., Nuchtern, J., Grilley, B., Martingano, E., and Cooper, K. (2000) Phase I study of chemokine and cytokine gene-modified autologous neuroblastoma cells for treatment of relapsed/refractory neuroblastoma using an adenoviral vector. *Hum Gene Ther 11*, 1477–1488.

174. Dilloo, D., Bacon, K., Holden, W., Zhong, W., Burdach, S., Zlotnik, A., and Brenner, M. (1996) Combined chemokine and cytokine gene transfer enhances antitumor immunity. *Nat Med 2*, 1090–1095.

175. Abdel-Wahab, Z., Dar, M., Osanto, S., Fong, T., Vervaert, C. E., Hester, D., Jolly, D., and Seigler, H. F. (1997) Eradication of melanoma pulmonary metastases by immunotherapy with tumor cells engineered to secrete interleukin-2 or gamma interferon. *Cancer Gene Ther 4*, 33–41.

176. Fearon, E. R., Pardoll, D. M., Itaya, T., Golumbek, P., Levitsky, H. I., Simons, J. W., Karasuyama, H., Vogelstein, B., and Frost, P. (1990) Interleukin-2 production by tumor cells bypasses T helper function in the generation of an antitumor response. *Cell 60*, 397–403.

177. Maass, G., Schmidt, W., Berger, M., Schilcher, F., Koszik, F., Schneeberger, A., Stingl, G., Birnstiel, M. L., and Schweighoffer, T. (1995) Priming of tumor-specific T cells in the draining lymph nodes after immunization with interleukin 2-secreting tumor cells: three consecutive stages may be required for successful tumor vaccination. *Proc Natl Acad Sci U S A 92*, 5540–5544.

178. Moller, P., Sun, Y., Dorbic, T., Alijagic, S., Makki, A., Jurgovsky, K., Schroff, M., Henz, B. M., Wittig, B., and Schadendorf, D. (1998) Vaccination with IL-7 gene-modified autologous melanoma cells can enhance the anti-melanoma lytic activity in peripheral blood of patients with a good clinical performance status: a clinical phase I study. *Br J Cancer 77*, 1907–1916.

179. Sun, Y., Jurgovsky, K., Moller, P., Alijagic, S., Dorbic, T., Georgieva, J., Wittig, B., and Schadendorf, D. (1998) Vaccination with IL-12 gene-modified autologous melanoma cells: preclinical results and a first clinical phase I study. *Gene Ther 5*, 481–490.

180. Czerniecki, B. J., Cohen, P. A., Faries, M., Xu, S., Roros, J. G., and Bedrosian, I. (2001) Diverse functional activity of CD83+ monocyte-derived dendritic cells and the implications for cancer vaccines. *Crit Rev Immunol 21*, 157–178.

181. De Vries, I. J., Krooshoop, D. J., Scharenborg, N. M., Lesterhuis, W. J., Diepstra, J. H., Van Muijen, G. N., Strijk, S. P., Ruers, T. J., Boerman, O. C., Oyen, W. J., Adema, G. J., Punt, C. J., and Figdor, C. G. (2003) Effective migration of antigen-pulsed dendritic cells to lymph nodes in melanoma patients is determined by their maturation state. *Cancer Res 63*, 12–17.

182. Jonuleit, H., Kuhn, U., Muller, G., Steinbrink, K., Paragnik, L., Schmitt, E., Knop, J., and Enk, A. H. (1997) Pro-inflammatory cytokines and prostaglandins induce maturation of potent immunostimulatory dendritic cells under fetal calf serum-free conditions. *Eur J Immunol 27*, 3135–3142.

183. Schuler-Thurner, B., Schultz, E. S., Berger, T. G., Weinlich, G., Ebner, S., Woerl, P., Bender, A., Feuerstein, B., Fritsch, P. O., Romani, N., and Schuler, G. (2002) Rapid induction of tumor-specific type 1 T helper cells in metastatic melanoma patients by vaccination with mature, cryopreserved, peptide-loaded monocyte-derived dendritic cells. *J Exp Med 195*, 1279–1288.

184. Lapenta, C., Santini, S. M., Spada, M., Donati, S., Urbani, F., Accapezzato, D.,

Franceschini, D., Andreotti, M., Barnaba, V., and Belardelli, F. (2006) IFN-alpha-conditioned dendritic cells are highly efficient in inducing cross-priming CD8(+) T cells against exogenous viral antigens. *Eur J Immunol 36*, 2046–2060.

185. Mosca, P. J., Hobeika, A. C., Clay, T. M., Nair, S. K., Thomas, E. K., Morse, M. A., and Lyerly, H. K. (2000) A subset of human monocyte-derived dendritic cells expresses high levels of interleukin-12 in response to combined CD40 ligand and interferon-gamma treatment. *Blood 96*, 3499–3504.

186. Czerniecki, B. J., Koski, G. K., Koldovsky, U., Xu, S., Cohen, P. A., Mick, R., Nisenbaum, H., Pasha, T., Xu, M., Fox, K. R., Weinstein, S., Orel, S. G., Vonderheide, R., Coukos, G., DeMichele, A., Araujo, L., Spitz, F. R., Rosen, M., Levine, B. L., June, C., and Zhang, P. J. (2007) Targeting HER-2/neu in early breast cancer development using dendritic cells with staged interleukin-12 burst secretion. *Cancer Res 67*, 1842–1852.

187. Mailliard, R. B., Wankowicz-Kalinska, A., Cai, Q., Wesa, A., Hilkens, C. M., Kapsenberg, M. L., Kirkwood, J. M., Storkus, W. J., and Kalinski, P. (2004) alpha-type-1 polarized dendritic cells: a novel immunization tool with optimized CTL-inducing activity. *Cancer Res 64*, 5934–5937.

188. Nair, S., McLaughlin, C., Weizer, A., Su, Z., Boczkowski, D., Dannull, J., Vieweg, J., and Gilboa, E. (2003) Injection of immature dendritic cells into adjuvant-treated skin obviates the need for ex vivo maturation. *J Immunol 171*, 6275–6282.

189. MartIn-Fontecha, A., Sebastiani, S., Hopken, U. E., Uguccioni, M., Lipp, M., Lanzavecchia, A., and Sallusto, F. (2003) Regulation of dendritic cell migration to the draining lymph node: impact on T lymphocyte traffic and priming. *J Exp Med 198*, 615–621.

SUBJECT INDEX

Note: The letters 'f', 't' and 'n' following locators refer to figures, tables and note numbers respectively.

P. Yotnda (ed.), Immunotherapy of Cancer, Methods in Molecular Biology 651,
DOI 10.1007/978-1-60761-786-0, © Springer Science+Business Media, LLC 2010

Breinigsville, PA USA
13 October 2010
247248BV00007B/3/P